MOLECULAR BIOLOGY
INTELLIGENCE
UNIT

The Biogenesis
of Cellular Organelles

Chris Mullins, Ph.D.
Division of Kidney, Urologic and Hematologic Diseases
National Institute of Diabetes and Digestive
and Kidney Diseases
National Institutes of Health
Bethesda, Maryland, U.S.A.

LANDES BIOSCIENCE / EUREKAH.COM
GEORGETOWN, TEXAS
U.S.A.

KLUWER ACADEMIC / PLENUM PUBLISHERS
NEW YORK, NEW YORK
U.S.A.

THE BIOGENESIS OF CELLULAR ORGANELLES

Molecular Biology Intelligence Unit

Landes Bioscience / Eurekah.com
Kluwer Academic / Plenum Publishers

Copyright ©2005 Eurekah.com and Kluwer Academic / Plenum Publishers

Kluwer Academic / Plenum Publishers, 233 Spring Street, New York, New York, U.S.A. 10013
http://www.wkap.nl/

Please address all inquiries to the Publishers:
Eurekah.com / Landes Bioscience, 810 South Church Street, Georgetown, Texas, U.S.A. 78626
Phone: 512/ 863 7762; FAX: 512/ 863 0081
http://www.eurekah.com
http://www.landesbioscience.com

ISBN: 0-306-47990-7

The Biogenesis of Cellular Organelles, edited by Chris Mullins, Landes / Kluwer dual imprint / Landes series: Molecular Biology Intelligence Unit

While the authors, editors and publisher believe that drug selection and dosage and the specifications and usage of equipment and devices, as set forth in this book, are in accord with current recommendations and practice at the time of publication, they make no warranty, expressed or implied, with respect to material described in this book. In view of the ongoing research, equipment development, changes in governmental regulations and the rapid accumulation of information relating to the biomedical sciences, the reader is urged to carefully review and evaluate the information provided herein.

Library of Congress Cataloging-in-Publication Data

The biogenesis of cellular organelles / [edited by] Chris Mullins.
     p. ; cm. -- (Molecular biology intelligence unit)
   Includes index.
   ISBN 0-306-47990-7
   1. Cell organelles--Formation. I. Mullins, Chris. II. Series: Molecular biology intelligence unit (Unnumbered)
   [DNLM: 1. Evolution, Molecular. 2. Organelles. QH 591 B615 2004]
   QH581.2.B55 2004
   571.6'5--dc22
                              2004019014

CONTENTS

EDITOR

Chris Mullins, Ph.D.
Division of Kidney, Urologic, and Hematologic Diseases
National Institute of Diabetes and Digestive
and Kidney Diseases
National Institutes of Health
Bethesda, Maryland, U.S.A.
Chapter 2

CONTRIBUTORS

Nihal Altan-Bonnet, Ph.D.
Cell Biology and Metabolism Branch
National Institute of Child Health
  and Human Development
National Institutes of Health
Bethesda, Maryland, U.S.A.
Chapter 5

Sean P. Curran, Ph.D.
Department of Chemistry
  and Biochemistry
University of California, Los Angeles
Los Angeles, California, U.S.A.
Chapter 8

Sui Huang, Ph.D.
Department of Cell and Molecular
  Biology
Northwestern University Medical School
Chicago, Illinois, U.S.A.
Chapter 7

Jerry Kaplan, Ph.D.
Department of Pathology
University of Utah School of Medicine
Salt Lake City, Utah, U.S.A.
Chapter 6

Carla M. Koehler, Ph.D.
Department of Chemistry
  and Biochemistry
University of California, Los Angeles
Los Angeles, California, U.S.A.
Chapter 8

Danielle Leuenberger, Ph.D.
Department of Chemistry
  and Biochemistry
University of California, Los Angeles
Los Angeles, California, U.S.A.
Chapter 8

Jennifer Lippincott-Schwartz, Ph.D.
Cell Biology and Metabolism Branch
National Institute of Child Health
  and Human Development
National Institutes of Health
Bethesda, Maryland, U.S.A.
Chapter 5

J. Paul Luzio, Ph.D.
Department of Clinical Biochemistry
Cambridge Institute
  for Medical Research
University of Cambridge
Addenbrooke's Hospital
Cambridge, United Kingdom
Chapter 1

Thomas F. J. Martin, Ph.D.
Department of Biochemistry
University of Wisconsin
Madison, Wisconsin, U.S.A.
Chapter 3

Diane McVey Ward, Ph.D.
Department of Pathology
University of Utah School of Medicine
Salt Lake City, Utah, U.S.A.
Chapter 6

Barbara M. Mullock, Ph.D.
Department of Clinical Biochemistry
Cambridge Institute
  for Medical Research
University of Cambridge
Addenbrooke's Hospital
Cambridge, United Kingdom
Chapter 1

Shelly L. Shiflett
Department of Pathology
University of Utah School of Medicine
Salt Lake City, Utah, U.S.A.
Chapter 6

Erik Snapp, Ph.D.
Cell Biology and Metabolism Branch
National Institute of Child Health
  and Human Development
National Institutes of Health
Bethesda, Maryland, U.S.A.
Chapter 4

Stanley R. Terlecky, Ph.D.
Department of Pharmacology
Wayne State University School
  of Medicine
Detroit, Michigan, U.S.A.
Chapter 9

Paul A. Walton, Ph.D.
Department of Anatomy and Cell
  Biology
University of Western Ontario
London, Ontario, Canada
Chapter 9

PREFACE

The evolution of modern cell biology tools, such as confocal imaging techniques and advanced electron microscopy methodologies, has allowed for ever improving structural and functional characterizations of the cell. Such methods complement classical genetics and biochemistry in the ongoing effort to define cellular science. This is especially apparent in the area of organelle biology. Studies dating back over 100 years to the present have revealed the elaborate collection of distinctive membrane-bound cytoplasmic subcompartments, termed organelles, within the eukaryotic cell and defined their roles in mediating numerous specialized functions in cellular physiology. Organelles play an essential role in the cell in large part through ensuring a tight regulatory and functional separation of distinct chemical reactions, such as cellular respiration, and molecular processes, such as protein degradation and DNA replication. Many organelles are common to virtually all cell types (e.g., the nucleus) while others reside only in certain differentiated cells (e.g., the lysosome-related lytic granules and melanosomes found in cytotoxic T lymphocytes and melanocytes, respectively). The unique characteristics of such heterogeneous cellular organelles are dictated by their particular biochemical composition and complement of biomolecules.

The Biogenesis of Cellular Organelles seeks to describe the cellular and molecular mechanisms mediating the biogenesis, maintenance, and function of key eukaryotic organelles. This work consists of an initial discussion of the evolution of organelle biogenesis theory from early studies through recent findings, overviews of the prominent cellular machineries involved in the biogenesis and maintenance of cellular organelles, and reviews of the function and biogenesis of a number of key organelles common to nearly all eukaryotic cells, including the endoplasmic reticulum, the Golgi apparatus, the lysosome, the nucleus, the mitochondria, and the peroxisome. All chapters strive to highlight recent findings and topical issues relating to organelle biology. The primary interests of this work are the biogenesis and functional events operating in mammalian cells and in some cases the analogous events in key lower eukaryotes, such as yeast and Drosophila. The reader should note that a wealth of organelles besides those covered here have also been described, such as the all important chloroplast present in plants and other photosynthetic organisms. The general themes of each chapter are as follows:

Chapter one offers a historical perspective of organelle biogenesis. This chapter recounts early discoveries that formed the foundation for the modern study of organelle biology, including the role of protein sorting in organelle maintenance and methods of organelle inheritance during cell division. In this chapter the progression from early findings to more recent discoveries in developing our current views of organelle function and biogenesis are highlighted.

Chapter two presents an in depth discussion of protein coats, which in concert with additional components of the cellular machinery operate to selectively sort proteins within intracellular and endocytic trafficking pathways. In this function protein coats serve as key mediators of organelle biogenesis and maintenance. The protein coat constituents described include the adaptor protein (AP) complexes and clathrin, which operate in the late-secretory and endocytic pathways, and the COP complexes, which operate in the early secretory pathway. The recently defined adaptor-related coat proteins, the GGAs and Stoned B family members, are also reviewed.

Chapter three describes the cooperative role played by lipids and proteins in maintaining organelle identity and function in the face of continuous biomolecular flux between compartments and to and from the plasma membrane. The key players mediating compartment identity described include the ARF and Rab GTPases, the inositol phospholipids, and members of the SNARE protein family.

Chapter four provides an extensive description of the organization, function, and maintenance of the endoplasmic reticulum. The remarkably dynamic nature and morphological variability of the endoplasmic reticulum are detailed along with its numerous cellular roles, including serving as the primary site for membrane protein synthesis and entry into the secretory pathway. The contribution of proliferation and differentiation of existing membranes to the generation of endoplasmic reticulum networks are also reviewed.

Chapter five reviews classical and recent findings relating to the Golgi apparatus, which functions as a site for post-translational modifications of glycoproteins and glycolipids and for the selective sorting of secretory proteins to the plasma membranes or target sites within the cell. The complex morphology of the Golgi, which allows compartmentalization of distinct Golgi functions, and the dynamics of its disassembly and reassembly during the cell cycle are highlighted.

Chapter six discusses the function and biogenesis of the lysosome. The role of the lysosome, and the analogous yeast vacuole, as the primary degradative compartment in the cell and current models for the biogenesis of lysosomes and related compartments are discussed. The participation of the protein sorting machinery in lysosomal maintenance and function are described. Also, the importance of the lysosome to cellular function is illustrated through discussions of a number of mutant phenotypes resulting from perturbation of lysosomal protein sorting.

Chapter seven offers a review of nuclear biogenesis, or nucleogenesis. This chapter focuses on the dynamic disassembly and reassembly of the nuclear envelope during mitotic division and the cellular machinery mediating these processes. The biogenesis of nucleoli, the nuclear structures that serve as sites for ribosome biosynthesis, is also detailed.

Chapter eight reviews the function, intricate structure, and biogenesis of the mitochondria, which serves as the site of cellular respiration. The unique nature of this organelle, which has prokaryotic origins and still retains it own small genome, is described, as is its essential nature in the physiology of the cell. The mode of mitochondrial biogenesis through growth and division of pre-existing mitochondria is detailed. The pathways for mitochondrial protein import and export and ion trafficking are also reviewed.

Chapter nine presents an overview of peroxisome biogenesis and function. Potential modes of formation of the peroxisome, which represent an organelle rich in metabolic enzymes and activities, are discussed along with cellular factors that contribute to its biogenesis and function. This work also details the numerous peroxisomal disorders in humans, which highlights the need to address the many unanswered questions regarding the biology of this important organelle.

While the discoveries described in *The Biogenesis of Cellular Organelles* and elsewhere illustrate our growing understanding of the fundamental processes mediating organelle biogenesis and function, they also remind us of how much remains to be discovered. The pursuit of knowledge regarding organelle biology is essential to understanding the basic science of the cell as well as human physiology. This is clearly evident from the growing observations that associate defects in organelle function to human disease. With the continued dedication of basic and clinical scientists to addressing these important questions ensured, the future of cellular biology is sure to be one of remarkable discovery.

Chris Mullins, Ph.D.
National Institutes of Health

I would like to acknowledge Dr. Josephine Briggs, Dr. Juan S. Bonifacino, and Dr. Leroy M. Nyberg, Jr. for their continuing encouragement and support and the National Research Council of the National Academies of Science for their sponsorship during the early stages of this project. Special thanks are extended to Dr. Rosa Puertollano for her kind and generous advice and assistance during the completion of this book. Most of all I thank the many contributors for their valuable time, exhaustive effort, and patience in the development of this project. This work is dedicated to them and all the basic and clinical researchers who strive to understand the biology of the eukaryotic cell.

CHAPTER 1

Theory of Organelle Biogenesis:

A Historical Perspective

Barbara M. Mullock and J. Paul Luzio

Abstract

O rganelles, defined as intracellular membrane-bound structures in eukaryotic cells, were described from the early days of light microscopy and the development of cell theory in the 19th century. During the 20th century, electron microscopy and subcellular fractionation enabled the discovery of additional organelles and, together with radiolabelling, allowed the first modern experiments on their biogenesis. Over the past 30 years, the development of cell-free systems and the use of yeast genetics have together established the major pathways of delivery of newly synthesised proteins to organelles and the vesicular traffic system used to transfer cargo between organelles in the secretory and endocytic pathways. Mechanisms of protein sorting, retrieval and retention have been described and give each organelle its characteristic composition. Insights have been gained into the mechanisms by which complex organelle morphology can be established. Organelle biogenesis includes the process of organelle inheritance by which organelles are divided between daughter cells during mitosis. Two inheritance strategies have been described, stochastic and ordered, which are not mutually exclusive. Among the major challenges of the future are the need to understand the role of self-organization in ensuring structural stability and the mechanisms by which a cell senses the status of its organelles and regulates their biogenesis.

Introduction

Today, cell biologists are almost overwhelmed by molecular detail about organelle composition, structure, function and biogenesis. Nevertheless during the molecular era, which has encompassed the past half century, a conceptual framework has developed to explain processes such as protein sorting, membrane traffic and organelle biogenesis. In this chapter we review this development, together with earlier work that established the existence of organelles and traffic to them. Necessarily, we cannot include specific detail about all organelles and we have concentrated, for the most part, on those found on the secretory and endocytic pathways.[1] We begin with some definitions.

Definitions

Organelles are defined as intracellular membrane-bound structures in eukaryotic cells, usually specialized for a particular function.[2] While many organelles are morphologically similar and perform essentially the same function in all eukaryotic cells, some are specialized and

The Biogenesis of Cellular Organelles, edited by Chris Mullins. ©2005 Eurekah.com and Kluwer Academic/Plenum Publishers.

occur only in particular cell types. Among the former are the nucleus, mitochondria and organelles in the secretory and endocytic pathways including the endoplasmic reticulum, Golgi complex, endosomes and lysosomes (vacuoles in yeast), whereas the latter include chloroplasts restricted to the plant kingdom. In mammalian cells there has been much study of cell type-specific specialist organelles and their relationship to common organelles. Many, if not all, of these are specialized structures in the secretory and endocytic pathways and include, for example, regulated secretory granules in neuroendocrine cells[3] and melanosomes,[4] which are clearly lysosome-like, in skin melanocytes.

Organelle biogenesis is the process by which new organelles are made. In a few cases, notably mitochondria and chloroplasts, some organelle proteins are encoded by the organelle's own genome. However, the amount of DNA in such organelles can encode only a very small number of the many proteins required.[5] In practice, the study of organelle biogenesis includes the mechanisms by which proteins and lipids, newly synthesized elsewhere in the cell, are delivered to organelles and the process by which organelles are divided between daughter cells during mitosis. In general it is thought that new organelles are derived by proliferation of preexisting organelles.[6] However, for some organelles on the secretory and endocytic pathways, e.g., the Golgi complex (see below), the extent to which they can be made de novo by a cell without a preexisting organelle or template remains a subject of controversy.[7]

The History of Organelle Recognition

Light Microscopy and Cell Theory

Recognition of organelles is only as feasible as the available techniques for observation. The light microscope was the essential first tool; once this existed "cells" could be and were observed, initially in plant material where substances such as cellulose made observation easier or in unicellular organisms. In 1833, Brown observed and described the nucleus, the first organelle.[8] In 1838, the many and various observations were converted into a cell theory by Schleiden, who proposed that all plant tissues were composed of nucleated cells.[9] The following year Schwann applied this cell theory to animal tissues.[10] Schleiden and Schwann assumed that cells were formed by some kind of crystallization of intracellular substance, in spite of observations on the binary fission of nucleus and cell in plants.[11] However, by 1855 Virchow proclaimed "Omnis cellula e cellula" (all cells from cells)[12,13] and in 1874 Flemming began to publish detailed and correct descriptions of mitosis, culminating in a comprehensive book in 1882.[14] The importance of the recognition of organelles to the development of cell theory is clear, since as Richmond[15] has described, "German cell theory primarily looked to cellular structures, such as the nucleus, rather than to processes as the focal points for vital organization".

Coincident with the emergence of Schleiden and Schwann's cell theory was the recognition that a membrane structure bounded cells (reviewed in ref. 16). The osmotic properties of plant cells led to Nageli defining the "plasmamembran" as a surface layer of protoplasm, denser and more viscous than the protoplasm as a whole. By the early 20th century, the osmotic properties of red blood cells had extended the concept of the plasma membrane to mammalian cells, but it was not until the classic experiment of Gorter and Grendel published in 1925[17] that the basic structure of the plasma membrane was shown to consist of a bilayer of phospholipid. In this experiment, the surface area of a compressed film of total lipid extracted from a known number of red blood cells was measured and found to be twice the total cell area. The phospholipid bilayer was incorporated as a central feature in many subsequent models of the structure of both the plasma membrane and intracellular membranes, culminating in the fluid mosaic model of Singer and Nicholson in which integral membrane proteins were distributed within the bilayer.[18]

The structure of the interphase nucleus was also extensively studied during the late 19th century. Brown[8] had suggested the possibility of a nuclear membrane and in 1882 Flemming[14] summarised the evidence for its reality. Following experiments using basic stains such as haematoxylin he also defined chromatin as "the substance in the cell nucleus which takes up color during nuclear staining" (although a stain specific for DNA was not described until 1924 by Feulgen and Rossenbeck[19]). The nucleolus had been observed as a feature of some nuclei many times; over 700 articles on the subject had appeared before the classic paper by Montgomery in 1898.[20,21]

Meanwhile, mitochondria had been seen with varying degrees of conviction by a number of scientists from Henle in 1841 onwards.[22] Altmann in 1890,[23] however, was the first to recognize the ubiquitous occurrence of mitochondria and to suggest that they carried out vital functions. The increasing use of chemicals, which preferentially stained some parts of the cell, led to more accurate descriptions of cell structure, although concerns over artefacts had to be addressed. In 1898, Golgi[24] demonstrated the existence of the Golgi complex by staining with heavy metals such as silver nitrate or osmium tetroxide. The reality of this organelle, however, continued to be doubted until the mid 1950s when electron micrographs became available.[25]

Electron Microscopy and Subcellular Fractionation

Mitochondria and the Golgi complex are at the limit of resolution by the light microscope; the visualization of smaller organelles had to wait for the development of electron microscopes. However, a parallel interest in taking cells apart and studying the nature of the separated components also yielded invaluable information; the existence of lysosomes was established before they were seen. Information as to the chemical nature and function of organelles was sought as early as 1934 by Bensley and Hoerr,[26] who made a crude preparation of mitochondria. Claude in 1940-1946 used similar procedures with a crucial difference.[27,28] He insisted on quantitative criteria, examining the total recovery of an enzyme or chemical constituent and its relative concentrations in the fractions he prepared by differential centrifugation, rather than preparing a single fraction. He also examined the size, shape and fine structure of the particulates in the separated fractions and used an isotonic medium for homogenisation. In 1948 Hogeboom, Schneider and Palade[29] improved his methodology by using a Potter-Elvehjem homogeniser to achieve quantitative gentle breakage of liver cells and sucrose in place of saline. They were then able to show that most of Claude's "large granules" had the elongated shape of mitochondria and stained with Janus Green, a specific stain for this organelle.

Enzymes such as cytochrome oxidase, which appeared mostly in the large granule fraction, were clearly mitochondrial. There were also enzymes such as glucose 6-phosphatase, which appeared primarily in the smaller "microsomal" fraction. However, the work of de Duve from 1949 onwards demonstrated the existence of a group of enzymes, which were sedimented in the large granule fraction only if relatively high speeds were used in its preparation. The large granule fraction could be separated into a heavy and a light fraction. The former contained the respiratory activity characteristic of mitochondria but the light fraction contained variegated hydrolases. These were only measurable when the preparation had been subjected to hypotonic media, detergents or other insults to membrane integrity. From these results, de Duve hypothesised the existence of organelles containing primarily hydrolases and named them lysosomes.[30]

Electron microscopy had meanwhile progressed to a generally available method of investigation. This necessitated the development of adequate fixing, staining, embedding and sectioning techniques as well as the development of the instruments themselves.[31] In 1952, Palade published high resolution pictures of mitochondria.[32] In 1954, Dalton and Felix (among others) published pictures of the Golgi complex,[33] which showed that it contained cisternae and

vesicles and stained with osmium tetroxide, as had the disputed structure seen by light microscopy. However, the electron microscope also revealed structures which the light microscope
was completely unable to resolve. The varying forms but almost ubiquitous existence of the
endoplasmic reticulum could be seen and shown to contribute largely to Claude's microsomal
fraction. By a lucky chance, Porter, Claude and Fullam first saw the endoplasmic reticulum in
whole tissue cells as a "lace-like" structure in 1945.[34] As sectioning techniques improved over
the next ten years, the endoplasmic reticulum had to be recognized in slices which were much
smaller than the mesh size of the reticulum. The continuous nature of the meshes could only be
demonstrated by tedious serial sectioning, although much more detailed structure could be
observed and many different tissues examined to show the ubiquity of the organelle.[35]

Lysosomes were identified with the pericanalicular dense bodies described by Rouiller in
1954 by examination of partially purified preparations and by the development of a method
for acid phosphatase localisation at both light and electron microscopic levels.[36] Peroxisomes
were reported by electron microscopy as microbodies in liver and kidney at about the same
time, although their identity with the bodies carrying non-latent uricase and other enzymes
involved with hydrogen peroxide was only established in the early sixties.[37]

Radiolabelling and the Dynamic Nature of Organelles

In addition to the clearly recognizable organelles, the electron microscope showed that
cells contained a multiplicity of vesicles; the components of the secretory and endocytic pathways. The dynamic nature of such vesicles and of most other organelles began to be revealed
when, in 1967, Jamieson and Palade used radioactive tracers and electron microscopic autora-
diography.[38] They showed that newly synthesized secretory proteins during, or shortly after,
synthesis, crossed the rough (ribosome-studded) endoplasmic reticulum and then moved from
the endoplasmic reticulum to the Golgi region and thence to secretory granules. By 1975,
Palade, if not every worker in the field, believed that movement of material through these
organelles depended on vesicular traffic.[39]

Appreciation of the endocytic system was more diffuse. Phagocytosis was observed as
early as 1887, but the fact that endocytosis was of widespread occurrence in animal cells was
recognized only in the mid 1950s by electron microscopy.[35] Coated pits and vesicles were
observed in oocytes as early as 1964,[40] but the ability of coated pits to concentrate endocytic
receptors before pinching off to form coated vesicles was only recognised in 1976.[41] In 1973
Heuser and Reece[42] suggested that plasma membrane components inserted during exocytosis
in synapses might be recycled. Quantitative electron microscopic investigations in 1976 by
Steinman, Brodie and Cohn[43] showed that tissue culture cells internalized plasma membrane
at a rate which greatly exceeded their biosynthetic capacity. Therefore, a mechanism had to
exist whereby endocytosed membrane could be recycled to the plasma membrane. Only by the
1980's was it widely accepted that endocytosed vesicles fused with an intracellular organelle
called the endosome from which recycling to the plasma membrane could occur and also delivery to lysosomes and the trans-Golgi network.[44] By this stage there was also widespread recognition of the various vesicle traffic pathways involved in exocytosis, endocytosis, transcytosis
and biogenesis of organelles.

Protein Synthesis and Targeting

Although Palade had established that newly synthesised secretory proteins crossed into
the lumen of the endoplasmic reticulum, it required the experiments of Blobel and his colleagues to establish that this sorting and targeting event was mediated by a sequence motif
within the primary sequence of the secretory protein, which was named the signal sequence.[45]
To test the predictions of the signal hypothesis, first announced in 1971, Blobel developed a
cell-free system in which protein translation and protein translocation across microsomal

membrane vesicles could be measured. This cell-free system was a powerful forerunner of many others established elsewhere which faithfully recapitulated individual steps in organelle biogenesis pathways. The signal hypothesis also led directly to the concept that specific sequences within a protein could direct its targeting to a particular organelle. Thus, different consensus sequences have since been recognized as targeting motifs for import into mitochondria,[46] chloroplasts,[47] peroxisomes,[48] nuclei[49] and for the targeting of membrane proteins on secretory and endocytic pathways. Subsequent to the discovery of consensus sequences targeting proteins to particular organelles, there has been much work over the past 20 years identifying the protein machinery required for transport into such organelles, leading to an extensive understanding of transport to the mitochondrial matrix,[46] inner membrane,[50] outer membrane,[51] into chloroplasts,[52] into peroxisomes[53] and through nuclear pores.[54] In addition to amino acid sequence motifs, secondary modifications have also been recognized as targeting motifs, for example mannose 6-phosphate to target acid hydrolases from the Golgi complex to lysosomes[55] and both glycosylation and glycosylphosphatidylinositol membrane anchors to target proteins to the apical surface of polarized epithelial cells.[56]

A further bequest of the signal hypothesis was that testing it provided support for the idea that in evolution the eukaryotic endoplasmic reticulum arose by invagination of the prokaryotic plasma membrane since signal sequences addressed to the eukaryotic endoplasmic reticulum function in translocation across the prokaryotic plasma membrane and signal sequences for bacterial secretory proteins function in translocation across the eukaryotic endoplasmic reticulum.[57] In contrast, it had earlier been suggested that uptake of a prokaryotic progenitor cell(s) was the evolutionary origin of mitochondria and chloroplasts,[58] a hypothesis largely supported by the results of subsequent genome analysis which were consistent with the origin of the mitochondrion being an endosymbiotic α-proteobacterium.[59]

Cell-Free Systems and Yeast Genetics

Vesicular traffic is now accepted as the central mechanism by which proteins are transported between donor and acceptor compartments on the secretory and endocytic pathways[60] (Fig. 1). The discovery of clathrin by Pearse in the 1970s[61] provided the first coat component of vesicles involved in membrane traffic. However, it was during the 1980s that elucidation of the molecular machinery of vesicular traffic started in earnest with the reconstitution of individual traffic steps in cell-free systems from animal cells[62] and the isolation of secretory mutants in yeast.[63] Probably the most informative of these early cell-free systems was one in which vesicular traffic between Golgi cisternae was reconstituted by incubating Golgi membranes with cytosol and ATP.[64] In this system a population of Golgi membranes derived from cells lacking N-acetylglucosamine transferase but containing the G protein of vesicular stomatitis virus (VSV) was incubated with an population of Golgi membranes from wild type cells. Vesicular traffic resulted in addition of radioactive N-acetylglucosamine to the VSV-G as a result of the activity of the transferase in the wild type Golgi membranes. This assay led directly to the discovery of COPI (coat protein I) coated vesicles[65] and the discovery of components of the general cytosolic fusion machinery required for vesicle fusion with acceptor membranes throughout the secretory and endocytic pathways.[66] Subsequently, using the same principles of incubating organelle membrane fractions with cytosol and ATP, many membrane traffic steps were reconstituted in cell-free systems. Similarly, cell-free assays were established to look at the breakdown and reformation of organelles during cell division.

The isolation of secretion (*sec*) mutants in the budding yeast *Saccharomyces cerevisiae*[63] provided a powerful approach to identify proteins required for traffic through the secretory pathway and to study their function. Throughout the 1980s and 1990s many proteins necessary for membrane traffic on the secretory pathway were identified almost at the same time, either by fractionating mammalian cytosol or through characterization of yeast mutants. These

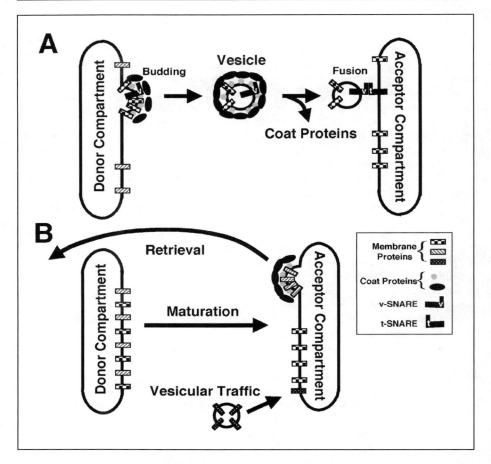

Figure 1. Mechanisms for organelle biogenesis in the secretory and endocytic pathways. A) Vesicular traffic. A coated vesicle buds from a donor organelle, loses its coat and fuses with an acceptor organelle. The coat made up of cytosolic proteins (denoted by black ovals and gray circles - refer to legend for designations of individual factors) both deforms the donor membrane to form the vesicle and sorts into the vesicle only those proteins (checked boxes) selected for delivery. Vesicle fusion with the acceptor membrane requires formation of a SNARE complex. Thus, the vesicle must contain a v-SNARE which forms a complex with a cognate t-SNARE in the acceptor membrane. B) Maturation. An organelle is formed from the preceding organelle in a pathway by retrieval of those proteins (hatched boxes) which should not be in the final organelle, using retrograde vesicular traffic to deliver them to an earlier stage in the pathway. Additional proteins (stippled boxes) may be delivered to the organelle by vesicular traffic from other sources (e.g., to endocytic compartments from the biosynthetic/secretory pathway). It should be noted that an organelle may be formed and/or maintain its composition by a mixture of the two mechanisms. Thus, when organelles are formed by anterograde vesicular traffic, retrieval may still be used to ensure that mis-sorted proteins are returned to their correct residence.

studies established the similarities of membrane traffic pathways at the molecular level in all eukaryotes.[60] The genetic screens in yeast which allowed isolation of the original temperaturesensitive and other *sec* mutants were followed by many others, for example those identifying genes affected in vacuolar protein sorting (*vps*) mutants[67,68] and those identifying genes involved in autophagy.[69] These latter screens led directly to our current understanding of the molecular mechanisms of biogenesis of the vacuole, of its mammalian equivalent the lysosome[70] and of autophagosomes in both yeast and mammalian cells.[69,70] In recent years, the development of cell-free systems to study homotypic yeast vacuole fusion, together with yeast genetics,[71] have led to a massive expansion in our understanding of what is effectively a multi-protein machine required to achieve vacuole membrane fusion, a process essential to vacuole biogenesis in the daughter bud of a dividing yeast.

Vesicle Budding and Delivery

When clathrin was purified and shown to be the major protein component of purified coated vesicles,[61] it was not clear whether it was simply the scaffold that makes the coat, involved in vesicle budding and/or also involved in sorting cargo into the vesicles. Very soon it was realized that there were at least two classes of clathrin coated vesicles in cells, one predominantly Golgi-associated, subsequently shown to be involved in budding from the trans-Golgi network and the other at the plasma membrane responsible for a major endocytic uptake route. The two classes of clathrin-coated vesicles were distinguished by the presence of two different heterotetrameric adaptor protein complexes, AP-1 at the trans-Golgi network and AP-2 at the plasma membrane. Electron microscopy, protein-protein interaction studies and most recently structural biology[72] have strongly suggested that adaptor complexes have similar structures, resembling Mickey Mouse, with a core or "head" consisting of medium (μ) and small subunits and the amino-terminal domains of two large subunits (α/γ and β), flanked by flexibly-hinged "ears" consisting of the carboxyterminal domains of the two large subunits. Work in several laboratories showed that the adaptors were involved in cargo sorting as well as recruitment of clathrin to the membrane.[73] Later, further family members were discovered including heterotetrameric AP-3 and AP-4 complexes that are not associated with clathrin and the more distantly related monomeric GGAs (Golgi-localised, γ-ear-containing, ARF-binding proteins).[74] All of these coat proteins function in post-Golgi membrane traffic pathways. In mammalian cells GGAs are important in trafficking mannose 6-phosphate receptors and associated newly synthesised mannose 6-phosphate–tagged acid hydrolases to the endosomes for delivery to lysosomes. AP-1 is most likely involved in traffic back to the trans-Golgi network of the empty mannose 6-phosphate receptors. AP-3 is required for efficient delivery of newly synthesised membrane proteins to lysosomes and lysosome-related organelles. Mutations in AP-3 occur naturally in animals including fruit flies (i.e., *Drosophila melanogaster*) and humans, leading to alterations of eye colour in the former and a rare genetic disease in the latter as a result of defects in delivery of proteins to lysosome-related organelles such as *Drosophila* eye pigment granules and platelet dense core granules, respectively. AP-4 may be involved in delivery to lysosomes and/or polarized sorting in epithelial cells. The formation of clathrin coated vesicles at either the plasma membrane or at intracellular sites is now recognised to require a host of accessory and regulatory proteins, many of which interact primarily with the carboxyterminal "ear" domains of the large subunits of the heterotetrameric AP complexes. Once mechanical invagination of the donor membrane to form the vesicle is complete, pinching off occurs, mediated at least in part by the action of the GTPase dynamin.[75]

While clathrin and AP complexes provide the major coat components for vesicle traffic in post-Golgi pathways, different coats are required for traffic between the endoplasmic reticulum and the Golgi complex. The first coat to be identified for vesicular traffic in this part of the secretory pathway was COPI using the cell-free assays described above. In such assays it was found that non-hydrolyzable analogues of GTP, such as GTP-γS can block traffic and this was accompanied by the accumulation of 70nm coated vesicles. The COPI coat on these vesicles contains eight polypeptides, one being the small GTPase ARF (ADP-ribosylation factor) responsible for coat recruitment to the membrane and the remainder being associated in an equimolar coat protomer (coatomer) complex.[60] Weak sequence similarities and information about coatomer interactions have led to the suggestion that the molecular architecture of the COPI coat is similar to that of the AP/clathrin coats.[76] It is now thought that the major traffic pathway mediated by COPI coated vesicles is the retrograde pathway from the Golgi complex to the endoplasmic reticulum necessary for the retrieval of escaped resident endoplasmic reticulum proteins and for the recycling of membrane proteins required for vesicle traffic and membrane fusion.[77] Whereas COPI coated vesicles were first discovered through cell-free assays (although it was rapidly realised that the mammalian coatomer γ-COP is homologous to yeast Sec21p), the COPII coat, required for vesicles to bud from the endoplasmic reticulum for traffic to the Golgi complex, was identified by analysis of yeast *sec* mutants. The COPII coat consists of the small GTPase Sar1p, responsible for coat recruitment to the endoplasmic reticulum membrane, and the heterodimeric protein complexes Sec23/24p and Sec13/31p. These five proteins are necessary and sufficient to produce COPII vesicles from endoplasmic reticulum microsomes or from chemically defined liposomes.[78] COPII coated vesicles were the first vesicles to be reconstituted solely from purified components. Indeed they might be regarded as the first organelles to be reconstituted solely from purified components since they fulfill the essential criteria to be called organelles in being intracellular membrane-bound structures in eukaryotic cells.

Vesicular traffic between donor and acceptor organelles in the secretory and endocytic pathways requires not only vesicle formation, but subsequent loss of the vesicle coat and fusion with the acceptor organelle. In addition, it often requires interactions of the vesicle with the cytoskeleton: with microtubules via kinesin or dynein motor proteins for long distance movement and/or via unconventional myosins for efficient short distance movement through actin rich regions of the cell. Once the vesicle reaches its target acceptor organelle, membrane fusion can occur, utilizing a common cytosolic fusion machinery and cognate interacting membrane proteins specific to the particular vesicle and organelle. Discovery of the common cytosolic fusion machinery derived from the observation that low concentrations of the alkylating agent N-ethylmaleimide (NEM) inhibited many membrane traffic steps reconstituted in cell-free systems. Using essentially brute force biochemistry, Rothman's group purified the soluble cytosolic NEM sensitive protein required to reconstitute membrane fusion in their cell-free Golgi assay, calling it NSF (NEM-sensitive factor).[66] This protein had ATPase activity and its sequence showed similarity to that of yeast Sec18p. The discovery of NSF led rapidly to the finding of proteins, called SNAPs (soluble NSF atachment proteins) which bind it to membranes. The next stage was discovery of SNAP receptors, or SNAREs, which are integral membrane proteins that confer specificity on individual fusion reactions.[60,79] The first of these were identified in mammalian brain, a tissue highly specialized for the membrane fusion required for neurotransmission at synapses. These studies led to the proposal of the SNARE hypothesis in which each transport vesicle bears a unique address marker or v-SNARE and each target membrane a unique t-SNARE, thus allowing targeting specificity to be achieved by the v-SNARES binding to matching t-SNAREs.[60,79,80] Importantly in yeast, whereas mutations in *SEC18* and *SEC17* (the gene encoding the yeast homologue of α-SNAP) had effects throughout the secretory and endocytic pathways, when SNARE mutants were isolated it was found that individual alleles often affected only trafficking steps related to the organelles with which a particular SNARE was associated.[81] In the few cases where a SNARE complex required for membrane fusion has been fully characterized it consists of four interacting α-helices aligned in parallel. A classification of SNAREs based on sequence alignments of the helical domains and structural features observed in the crystal structure of the synaptic SNARE fusion complex[82] has been proposed. This separates SNAREs into Q-SNAREs and R-SNAREs, with four-helix SNARE complex bundles being composed of three Q-SNAREs and one R-SNARE.[83,84] Q and R represent the glutamine and arginine residues observed in the central hydrophilic layer of the helical bundle.

Although cognate SNARE proteins can be reconstituted into liposomes and themselves act as phospholipid bilayer fusion catalysts,[80,85,86] membrane fusion within the cell requires the functional involvement of other proteins. Most current models of fusion suggest three steps, tethering of the vesicle to the target organelle, SNARE complex formation and phospholipid bilayer fusion. A class of small GTPases known as rab proteins was identified as generally important when it was shown that different rabs localize to different organelles on the secretory and endocytic pathways.[87] Rab proteins have been proposed to play a variety of roles in membrane fusion, and current evidence suggests a major function in the recruitment of tethering and docking proteins at an early stage in membrane interaction.[88] Tethering has been defined as involving links that extend over distances > 25 nm from a given membrane surface, and docking as holding membranes within a bilayer's distance, < 5-10 nm of one another.[88] Following tether recruitment and oligomeric assembly of the tethers, SNARE complex formation occurs. Fusion may also require downstream events after SNARE complex formation. In yeast vacuole fusion, a process which has been reconstituted in cell-free assays, Ca^{2+} release from the vacuole lumen is required in a post-docking phase of fusion[89] and there is increasing evidence that Ca^{2+} may have a function late in the fusion process in other membrane fusion events.[90] Once fusion has taken place the SNARE complex will reside in the target organelle membrane, necessitating separation of the complex, mediated by the ATPase activity of NSF followed by retrieval of the v-SNARE for further rounds of fusion.

Sorting, Retrieval and Retention

Vesicular traffic between organelles on the secretory pathway is the mechanism by which proteins and lipids are delivered and removed. To allow the organelles to retain their integrity as well as to ensure efficient traffic of cargo by vesicles requires mechanisms for sorting proteins into vesicles, to retrieve proteins that have been inappropriately delivered to another organelle and to retain proteins in an organelle (Fig. 1). Efficient sorting of cell surface membrane receptors into clathrin coated pits was recognized at an early stage in their biochemical characterization. By the late 1970s it was recognised that while some receptors are concentrated into clathrin-coated pits, other plasma membrane proteins are effectively excluded such that the pits act as molecular filters.[91,92] An important clue about the molecular basis of such sorting came from analysis of the sequence of the low density lipoprotein receptor in a patient with familial hypocholesterolemia, patient J.D.[93] In fibroblasts from this patient, receptor numbers on the cell surface were normal but they were not concentrated into coated pits. The mutation leading to this phenotype was an amino acid substitution in the cytoplasmic domain resulting in a cysteine replacing a tyrosine. Subsequent work showed that cytoplasmic tail motifs of the form NPXY(where X is any amino acid) as in the low density lipoprotein receptor, YXXØ (where Ø is a bulky hydrophobic amino acid), or dileucine motifs could act as efficient endocytosis signals as a result of their interaction with the clathrin adaptor AP-2.[94] Membrane proteins without such motifs cannot be efficiently internalized. Cytoplasmic tail sequence motifs containing tyrosine and dileucine are now recognized as being important not only for internalization from the cell surface but also for targeting to organelles within the secretory and endocytic pathways. Different coated vesicle adaptor proteins show subtle differences in specificity for such sequences. The structural basis for such differences is unclear. However, the way in which a YXXØ motif binds to the μ subunit of AP-2 has been determined by X-ray crystallography.[95] The recent solving of the complete structure of the core of AP-2 has shown that the μ binding site for YXXØ is blocked, implying a large structural change in the molecule to allow AP-2 to recruit receptors into clathrin-coated pits.[72]

Not only is there sorting into vesicles for anterograde traffic in the secretory and endocytic pathways, but also sorting into vesicles for retrieval. The concept of retrieval derived initially from studies of lumenal proteins in the endoplasmic reticulum. Munro and Pelham[96] showed that a number of lumenal proteins in mammalian endoplasmic reticulum have the sequence KDEL at their carboxy-terminus (HDEL in *S. cerevisiae*) and that if this is deleted the proteins escape and are secreted. Subsequently, Pelham's laboratory identified the recycling receptor, Erd2p that is responsible for the retrieval of such proteins from the Golgi complex.[97,98] In this retrieval pathway, membrane proteins with di-lysine motifs in their cytoplasmic tails bind to COPI.[77] The structural basis for this interaction is not yet understood.

The identity of an organelle is not maintained solely by retrieval but also by retention. Perhaps the clearest example of this is in the cisternae of the Golgi complex where a variety of glycosyl transferases must be retained to carry out their function in the biosynthesis of glyco-proteins. These enzymes are type II membrane proteins with trans-membrane domains that are, on average, five amino acids shorter than the trans-membrane domains of plasma mem-brane proteins.[99] During the 1990s it was recognised that the length of the trans-membrane domain rather than its amino acid composition is important to localization, since in the case of sialyl transferase, replacement of the trans-membrane domain by 17 leucines provides efficient retention whereas a longer stretch of leucines does not.[99] However, in the case of N-acetylglucosaminyltransferase I, part of the lumenal stalk domain appeared to be sufficient and necessary for retention.[100] Two hypotheses have been proposed to explain retention of glycosyl transferases in the Golgi complex, one based on phospholipid bilayer thickness,[99] which differs between the Golgi complex and the plasma membrane, and the other entitled "kin recognition" based on the formation of glycosyltransferase hetero-oligomers.[101] For an individual membrane protein, it is feasible that both length of trans-membrane domain and interaction with other membrane proteins may contribute to retention. In the trans-Golgi network, the localization of the protein TGN38 depends on both retention provided by the trans-membrane domain and retrieval provided by a YXXØ motif in the cytoplasmic tail.[102]

Organization into Complex Structures

Organelle biogenesis is not simply a question of delivering newly synthesized proteins and lipids to a specific intracellular site but may also require the establishment of a complex archi-tecture. A dramatic example of this is seen in the case of the Golgi complex where it is clear that the observed morphology in part reflects the interaction of the structure with the cytoskeleton via appropriate motor proteins[103] and in part the function of matrix proteins in the organiza-tion of the cisternae.[104,105] A further complication, particularly for organelles on the secretory and endocytic pathways, is the requirement to maintain morphological form and associated functional integrity despite the large volume of through traffic of both proteins and lipids. In the case of the Golgi complex, there has long been a debate about how secreted proteins pass through it.[106] The work of Rothman and colleagues described above on reconstituting traffic through the Golgi complex in a cell-free system suggested anterograde vesicular traffic between the Golgi cisternae. However, electron microscopy studies of large macromolecules, including algal scales and collagen aggregates favoured a maturation model with new cisternae forming on the cis-side and mature ones fragmenting from the trans-side. The cisternal maturation model has been refined to encompass data on retrograde vesicular traffic in COPI coated vesicles such that the present consensus is that most, if not all, anterograde movement through the Golgi complex is the result of cisternal progression with retrograde vesicular traffic ensuring that the polarized distribution of Golgi enzymes in the cisternal stack is maintained (Fig. 1).[107] A recent three dimensional reconstruction of the Golgi complex from data obtained by high voltage electron microscopy has suggested that tubular and vesicular structures can bud at every level of the Golgi stack.[108] Structurally, using conventional electron microscopy tech-niques, and functionally, the trans-Golgi network can be distinguished from the cisternal stack and is defined as the site for sorting to different post-Golgi destinations.[109] Both clathrin-coated vesicles and noncoated tubular structures appear to bud from the trans-Golgi network.

Experiments in which secreted proteins tagged with green fluorescent protein have been imaged as they leave the Golgi complex in living cells have shown that large tubular carriers are particularly important for constitutive traffic to the cell surface.[110] In many neuroendocrine cell types, regulated secretory granules are also formed at the trans-Golgi network. Despite the biogenesis of such organelles being amongst the first to be studied by radiolabelling pulse-chase techniques (see above), the mechanisms by which proteins are sorted into these granules remain unclear, with "sorting for entry" and "sorting by retention" models still the subject of much debate.[3]

In the endocytic pathway, the biogenesis of individual organelles has been less well studied with the exception of lysosomes and the yeast vacuole.[111-113] This has partly been due to the pleiomorphic morphology of endosomes, partly to the difficulty of identifying marker proteins that, at steady state, are mainly localized in endosomes and partly because the molecular mechanisms of membrane traffic through the pathway have only started to be understood in the last few years. As in the secretory pathway, vesicular traffic between individual organelles does not explain all steps in the pathway. Clathrin-coated vesicles budding from the plasma membrane comprise a very important, but not sole, mechanism of delivery from the plasma membrane to early endosomes (defined historically as the first endosomal compartment to be entered by endocytosed ligands). Traffic from early to late endosomes, found deeper within the cell, has been studied extensively and is mediated by large endocytic carrier vesicles which some regard as matured early endosomes.[114,115] Delivery from late endosomes to lysosomes involves "kiss and run" and direct fusion between the two organelles. Such fusion is SNARE-mediated and results in a hybrid organelle from which lysosomes are reformed. In addition to heterotypic fusion between late endosomes and lysosomes, the endocytic pathway is characterized by the occurrence of homotypic fusions between early endosomes and between late endosomes. These homotypic fusion events are also SNARE-mediated[116,117] and allow continuous remodelling of these organelles. Organelles in the late endocytic pathway are characterised by the presence of numerous internal vesicles, leading to the alternative description of late endosomes as multivesicular bodies. Some cell surface receptors are sorted into such vesicles after internalization from the plasma membrane and prior to degradation. Recently, insights have been gained into the molecular mechanisms by which proteins are sorted into these vesicles, which have a different lipid composition from the limiting membrane of the organelle. Such mechanisms include partitioning into lipid microdomains, dependent on the composition of trans-membrane domains, and ubiquitination of cytoplamic tail domains followed by recognition of the ubiquinated domain by protein complexes involved in inward vesiculation.[118,119]

Organelle Inheritance

Organelle biogenesis is closely linked to organelle inheritance in cell division. During the cell cycle, each organelle must double in size, divide and be delivered appropriately to the daughter cells. Historically, the inheritance of organelles was recognised as occurring over the same period of the late 19th and early 20th centuries as the basic mechanics of mitosis were being described.[13,120-122] In summarizing a large amount of earlier work, Warren and Wickner[120] categorized two organelle inheritance strategies that have been described. The first is stochastic, relying on the presence of multiple copies of an organelle randomly distributed throughout the cytoplasm and the second is ordered, often, but not always, using the mitotic spindle as a means of partitioning (Fig. 2). The morphology of many organelles may differ in different cell types, which itself may be related to the use of one or other of these strategies to a greater or lesser extent. Mitochondria, for example are, in many cells, multiple copies of small bean shaped structures, but in the budding yeast *S. cerevisiae* form an extensive tubular reticulum beneath the plasma membrane which partitions in an ordered way into the bud. The steady-state morphology of mitochondria which continuously grow, divide and fuse throughout the cell cycle is

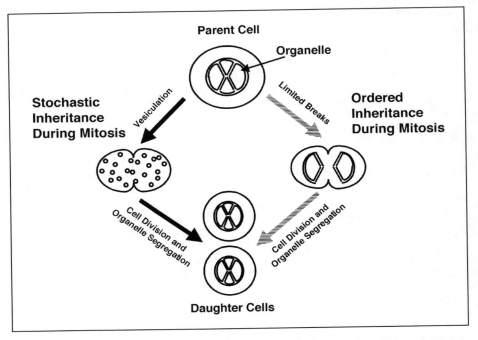

Figure 2. Mechanisms for organelle inheritance during mitosis. In the "stochastic inheritance" model (solid arrows), an organelle, shown here as an anastomosed, reticular network with all the membrane having a common composition, vesiculates to form many vesicles. These are apportioned by chance to the daughter cells where the organelle is reassembled. It has been estimated that the Golgi complex of a fibroblastic cell would, if completely vesiculated, generate ~80,000 vesicles of 0.1µm diam.[137] In the "ordered inheritance" model (hatched arrows), specific and limited breaks in the organelle occur such that, once the fragments are correctly aligned in the dividing cell, each daughter receives half.

itself largely determined by the frequency of fission events and fusion.[123] It should be noted that growth and division of mitochondria also requires coordination of these processes for the inner and outer membranes. In contrast to mitochondria, the endoplasmic reticulum is always a single copy organelle, albeit a dynamic reticulum. This breaks down into tubular vesicular elements during cell division to a variable extent. It often fragments little, thus segregation of equal amounts into daughter cells during mitosis may rely mainly on the uniform and extensive distribution of the endoplasmic reticulum network throughout the cytoplasm of the mother cell. In *S. cerevisiae* the endoplasmic reticulum becomes anchored at the bud tip pulling the network into the bud as it enlarges.[124] Whereas the bulk of the endoplasmic reticulum often does not fragment during mitosis, inheritance of the nuclear envelope, the outer membrane of which is continuous with the endoplasmic reticulum, is more complex since it has to break down during mitosis of animal cells to allow separation of the chromatids. At the end of mitosis the nuclear envelope rapidly reassembles around daughter chromosomes. During the 1980s, nuclear envelope breakdown in animal cells was shown to involve depolymerisation of the lamina underlying the membrane, fragmentation of the membrane and disassembly of nuclear pore complexes.[125] This was accompanied by reversible phosphorylation of many nuclear envelope proteins thought to lead to the formation of a discrete population of vesicles which could fuse at the end of mitosis to reform the envelope. Using *Xenopus* oocytes, which contain many nuclear components stored for use in early development, it was observed that injection of bacteriophage lambda DNA or its addition to cell-free extracts was sufficient to trigger nuclear assembly.[126] The availability of this cell-free system enabled study, at the molecular level, of the pathway of nuclear assembly, including nuclear envelope vesicle fusion.[127] Recently, it has been suggested that the nuclear envelope does not have to vesiculate completely during mitosis, but that phosphorylation may allow redistribution of nuclear envelope membrane proteins back into the endoplasmic reticulum.[128] The lack of requirement for membrane vesiculation has raised the question of how the nuclear envelope ruptures, resolved by recent evidence that it is literally torn apart by motor protein attachment and movement along microtubules.[128]

Perhaps the greatest recent controversy concerning organelle inheritance relates to how the Golgi complex is divided between daughter cells at mitosis.[7] Two models have been proposed to explain this. In the first, proposed by Warren, the Golgi complex breaks down into vesicle clusters and shed vesicles which are distributed stochastically between the daughter cells where they reassemble in telophase.[129] Cell-free assays have led to the identification of some of the molecular machinery for disassembly and reassembly.[130] In the second model, proposed by Lippincott-Schwartz, endoplasmic reticulum is the partioning unit, with the Golgi complex merging with the endoplasmic reticulum during prometaphase and emerging from it during telophase.[131] A key observation in developing this second model was that inhibition of traffic from the endoplasmic reticulum to the Golgi complex results in disintegration of the latter. Some of the discrepancies between the two models may be resolved by data from Warren's group who have shown that whilst Golgi membrane enzymes may, to a greater or lesser extent, redistribute to the endoplasmic reticulum during mitosis, matrix proteins do not, thus allowing the disassembled matrix to become the partitioning units on which the Golgi complex is reassembled after mitosis.[132,133] A further twist has come from the study of the protozoan *Toxoplasma gondii* which has a single Golgi that divides as a result of lateral cisternal growth followed by medial fission.[134] Even in mammalian cells, Golgi fragmentation-dispersion may not be obligatory for equal partitioning. Kondo and colleagues recently found that prevention of Golgi dissassembly, by microinjection of a nonphosphorylated mutant form of a soluble protein required for this process, had no effect on equal partitioning of the Golgi to daughter cells.[135]

Challenges

It is now clear that intracellular organelles are very dynamic structures, yet at steady state they exhibit characteristic morphology and architecture that are easily observed by microscopy. Recently Misteli[133] has suggested that the generation of an overall stable configuration in such dynamic structures is consistent with organelle morphology being determined by self-organization. This is defined as "the capacity of a macromolecular complex or organelle to determine its own structure based on the functional interaction of its components". Self-organization will ensure structural stability without loss of plasticity. Self-organization is an interesting concept, but how organelles self-organize is unclear. What is certain is that future investigations will lead us to a better understanding of the molecular machinery of organelle biogenesis and inheritance. Such investigations are likely to address a number of questions to which we have few answers at present. These include the role of lipids, in particular lipid-protein interactions in microdomains, in determining morphology and the regulation of the size, shape and number of organelles in cells.

Acknowledgements

We thank the Medical Research Council and the Wellcome Trust for supporting our experimental work on lysosome biogenesis and post-Golgi membrane traffic pathways.

References

1. Mellman I, Warren G. The road taken: Past and future foundations of membrane traffic. Cell 2000; 100:99-112.
2. In: Kendrew J, ed. The Encyclopedia of Molecular Biology. Oxford: Blackwell Science, 1994.
3. Tooze SA. Biogenesis of secretory granules in the trans-Golgi network of neuroendocrine and endocrine cells. Biochim Biophys. Acta 1998; 1404:231-244.
4. Raposo G, Marks MS. The dark side of lysosome-related organelles: Specialization of the endocytic pathway for melanosome biogenesis. Traffic 2002; 3:237-248.
5. Schatz G. What mitochondria have told me. Mol Biol Cell 2001; 12:777-778.
6. Nunnari J, Walter P. Regulation of organelle biogenesis. Cell 1996; 84:389-394.
7. Check E. Will the real Golgi please stand up. Nature 2002; 416:780-781.
8. Brown R. Observations on the organs and mode of fecundation in Orchidae and Asclepiadeae. Trans Linn Soc (Lond) 1833; 16:685-743.
9. Schleiden MJ. Beiträge zur Phytogenesis. Müller's Arch Anat Physiol Wiss Med 1838; 136-176.
10. Schwann T. Mikroskopische untersuchungen über die uberstimmung in der Struktur und dem Wachsthum der Thiere und Pflanzen. Berlin: Verlag der Sander'schen Buchhandlung, 1839.
11. Von Mohl H. Über die vermehrung der pflanzenzellen durch theilung (Inaugural dissertation, Tübingen). 1835.
12. Virchow R. Cellular-Pathologie. Arch für Path Anat 1855; VIII:3-39.
13. Wilson EB. The cell in development and heredity. 3rd ed. NY: MacMillan Co., 1925.
14. Flemming W. Zellsubstanz, Kern und Zelltheilung. Leipzig: FCW Vogel, 1882.
15. Richmond M. Thomas Henry Huxley's developmental view of the cell. Nature Rev Mol Cell Biol 2002; 3:61-65.
16. Robertson JD. Membrane structure. J Cell Biol 1981; 91:189s-204s.
17. Gorter E, Grendel R. On biomolecular layers of lipids on the chromocytes of the blood. J Exp Med 1925; 41 439-443.
18. Singer SJ, Nicolson GL. The fluid mosaic model of the structure of cell membranes. Science 1972; 175:720-731.
19. Feulgen RJ, Rossenbeck H. Mikroscopisch-chemischer Nachweis einer Nucleinsäure vom Typus der Thymonucleinsäure und die darauf beruhende elective Färbung von Zellkernen in mikroscopischen Präparaten. Hoppe-Seyler's Zeit physiol Chem 1924; 135:203-248.
20. Montgomery TH. Comparative cytological studies with especial reference to the morphology of the nucleolus. J Morphology 1898; XV:204-265.
21. Miller Jr OL. The nucleolus, chromosomes and visualization of genetic activity. J Cell Biol 1981; 91:15s-27s.
22. Ernster L, Schatz G. Mitochondria: A historical review. J Cell Biol 1981; 91:227s-255s.
23. Altmann R. Die Elementarorganismen und ihre Beziehungen zu den Zellen. Leipzig, Veit: 1890.
24. Golgi C. Sur la structure des cellules nerveuses. Arch Ital Biol 1898; 30:60-71.
25. Farquhar MG, Palade GE. Golgi apparatus (complex) – (1954-1981) – from artifact to center stage. J Cell Biol 1981; 91:77s-103s.
26. Bensley RR, Hoerr N. Studies on cell structure by freeze-drying method; preparation and properties of mitochondria. Anat Rec 1934; 60:449-455.
27. Claude A. Fractionation of mammalian liver cells by differential centrifugation II. Experimental procedures and results. J Exp Med 1946; 84:61-89.
28. De Duve C, Beaufay H. A short history of tissue fractionation. J Cell Biol 1981; 91:293s-299s.
29. Hogeboom GH, Schneider WC, Palade GE. Cytochemical studies of mammalian tissues 1. Isolation of intact mitochondria from rat liver; some biochemical properties of mitochondria and submicroscopic particulate material. J Biol Chem 1948; 172:619-635.
30. De Duve C. Exploring cells with a centrifuge. Science 1975; 189:186-194.
31. Pease DC, Porter KR. Electron microscopy and ultramicrotomy. J Cell Biol 1981; 91:287s-292s.
32. Palade GE. Fine structure of mitochondria. Anat Rec 1952; 114:427-451.
33. Dalton AJ, Felix MD. Cytologic and cytochemical characteristics of the Golgi substance of epithelial cells of the epididymis – in situ, in homogenates and after homogenisation. Am J Anat 1954; 94:171-208.

34. Porter KR, Claude A, Fullam EF. A study of tissue culture cells by electron microscopy. J Exp Med 1945; 81:233-246.
35. Palade GE. The endoplasmic reticulum. J Biophys Biochem Cytol 1956; 2:85-97.
36. Bainton DF. The discovery of lysosomes. J Cell Biol 1981; 91:66s-76s.
37. De Duve C, Baudhuin P. Peroxisomes (microbodies and related particles). Physiol Rev 1966; 46:323-357.
38. Jamieson JD, Palade GE. Intracellular transport of secretory proteins in the pancreatic exocrine cell. I. Role of the peripheral elements of the Golgi complex. J Cell Biol 1967; 34:577-596.
39. Palade G. Intracellular aspects of the process of protein synthesis. Science1975; 189:347-358.
40. Roth TF, Porter KR. Yolk protein uptake in the oocyte of the mosquito Aedes aegypti. J Cell Biol 1964; 20:313-332.
41. Anderson RGW, Goldstein JL, Brown MS. Localisation of low density lipoprotein receptors on plasma membrane of normal human fibroblasts and their absence in cells from a familial hypercholesterolemia homozygote. Proc Natl Acad Sci USA 1976; 73:2434-2438.
42. Heuser JE, Reese TS. Evidence for recycling of synaptic vesicle membrane during neurotransmitter release at the frog neuromuscular junction. J Cell Biol 1973; 57:315-344.
43. Steinman RM, Brodie SE, Cohn ZA. Membrane flow during pinocytosis. A stereologic analysis. J Cell Biol 1976; 68:665-687.
44. Hopkins CR. The importance of the endosome in intracellular traffic. Nature 1983; 304:684-685.
45. Blobel G. Protein targeting (Nobel lecture). Chembiochem 2000; 1:86-102.
46. Rassow J, Pfanner N. The protein import machinery of the mitochondrial membranes. Traffic 2000; 1:457-464.
47. Cline K, Henry R. Import and routing of nucleus-encoded chloroplast proteins. Ann Rev Cell Dev Biol 1996; 12:1-26.
48. Subramani S, Protein import into peroxisomes and biogenesis of the organelle. Ann Rev Cell Devel Biol 1993; 9:445-478.
49. Görlich D, Kutay U. Transport between the cell nucleus and the cytoplasm. Ann Rev Cell Dev. Biol 1999; 15:607-660.
50. Tokatlidis K, Schatz G. Biogenesis of mitochondrial inner membrane proteins. J Biol Chem 1999; 274:35285-35288.
51. Mihara K. Targeting and insertion of nuclear-encoded preproteins into the mitochondrial outer membrane. BioEssays 2000; 22:364-371.
52. Schleiff E, Soll J. Travelling of proteins through membranes: Translocation into chloroplasts. Planta 2000; 211:449-456.
53. Purdue PE, Lazarow PB. Peroxisome biogenesis. Ann Rev Cell Dev Biol 2001; 17:701-752.
54. Bayliss R, Corbett AH, Stewart M. The molecular mechanism of transport of macromolecules through nuclear pore complexes. Traffic 2000; 1:448-456.
55. Kornfeld S, Mellman I. The biogenesis of lysosomes. Ann Rev Cell Dev Biol 1989; 5:483-525.
56. Benting JH, Rietveld AG, Simons K. N-Glycans mediate the apical sorting of a GPI-anchored, raft-associated protein in Madin-Darby canine kidney cells. J Cell Biol 1999; 146:313-320.
57. Blobel G. Intracellular protein topogenesis. Proc Natl Acad Sci USA 1980; 77:1496-1500.
58. Margulis L. Origin of eukaryotic cells. New Haven: Yale University Press, 1970.
59. Kurland CG, Andersson SGE. Origin and evolution of the mitochondrial proteome. Microbiol Mol Biol Rev 2000; 64:786-820.
60. Rothman J. Mechanisms of intracellular protein transport. Nature1994; 372:55-63.
61. Pearse BM. Clathrin: A unique protein associated with intracellular transfer of membrane by coated vesicles. Proc Natl Acad Sci USA 1976; 73:1255-1259.
62. Fries E, Rothman JE. Transport of vesicular stomatitis virus glycoprotein in a cell-free extract. Proc Natl Acad Sci USA 1980; 77:3870-3874.
63. Novick P, Field C, Schekman R. Identification of 23 complementation groups required for post-translational events in the yeast secretory pathway. Cell 1980; 21:205-215.
64. Balch WE, Dunphy WG, Braell WA et al. Reconstitution of the transport of protein between successive compartments of the Golgi measured by the coupled incorporation of N-acetylglucosamine. Cell 1984; 39:405-416.

65. Balch W, Glick BS, Rothman JE. Sequential intermediates in the pathway of intercompartmental transport in a cell-free system. Cell 1984; 39:525-536.
66. Block MR, Glick BS, Wilcox CA et al. Purification of an N-ethylmaleimide-sensitive protein catalyzing vesicular transport. Proc Natl Acad Sci USA 1988; 85:7852-7856.
67. Robinson JS, Klionsky DJ, Banta LM et al. Protein sorting in Saccharomyces cerevisiae: Isolation of mutants defective in the delivery and processing of multiple vacuolar hydrolases. Mol Cell Biol 1988; 8:4936-4948.
68. Raymond CK, Howald-Stevenson I, Vater CA et al. Morphological classification of the yeast vacuolar protein sorting mutants: Evidence for a prevacuolar compartment in Class E vps mutants. Mol Biol Cell 1992; 3:1389-1402.
69. Noda T, Suzuki K, Ohsumi Y. Yeast autophagosomes: De novo formation of a membrane structure. Trends Cell Biol 2002; 12:231-235.
70. Seaman MNJ, Luzio JP. Lysosomes and other late compartments of the endocytic pathway. In: Endocytosis: Frontiers in Molecular Biology. Oxford: Oxford University Press, 2001:111-148.
71. Seeley ES, Kato M, Margolis N et al. Genomic analysis of homotypic vacuole fusion. Mol Biol Cell 2002; 13:782-794.
72. Collins BM, McCoy AJ, Kent HM et al. Molecular architecture and fuctional model of endocytic AP-2 complex. Cell 2002; 109:523-535.
73. Pearse BM, Robinson MS. Clathrin, adaptors, and sorting. Ann Rev Cell Biol 1990; 6:151-171.
74. Robinson MS, Bonifacino JS. Adaptor-related proteins. Curr Opin Cell Biol 2001; 13:444-453.
75. Kelly RB. New twists for dynamin. Nature Cell Biol 1999; 1:E8-E9.
76. Eugster A, Frigerio G, Dale M et al. COP I domains required for coatomer integrity, and novel interactions with ARF and ARF-GAP. EMBO J 2000; 19:3905-3917.
77. Letourneur F, Gaynor EC, Hennecke S et al. Coatomer is essential for retrieval of dilysine-tagged proteins to the endoplasmic reticulum. Cell 1994; 79:1199-1207.
78. Matsuoka K, Orci L, Amherdt M et al. COPII-coated vesicle formation reconstituted with purified coat proteins and chemically defined liposomes. Cell 1998; 93:263-275.
79. Sollner T, Whiteheart SW, Brunner M et al. Protein SNAP receptors implicated in vesicle targeting and fusion. Nature 1993; 362:318-324.
80. McNew JA, Parlati F, Fukuda R et al. Compartmental specificity of cellular membrane fusion encoded in SNARE proteins. Nature 2000; 407:153-159.
81. Pelham HR. SNAREs and the secretory pathway-lessons from yeast. Exp Cell Res 1999; 247:1-8.
82. Sutton RB, Fasshauer D, Jahn R et al. Crystal structure of a SNARE complex involved in synaptic exocytosis at 2.4 A resolution. Nature1998; 395:347-353.
83. Fasshauer D, Sutton RB, Brunger AT et al. Conserved structural features of the synaptic fusion complex: SNARE proteins reclassified as Q- and R-SNAREs. Proc Natl Acad Sci USA 1998; 95:15781-15786.
84. Bock JB, Matern HT, Peden AA et al. A genomic perspective on membrane compartment organization. Nature 2001; 409:839-841.
85. Weber T, Zemelman BV, McNew JA et al. SNAREpins: Minimal machinery for membrane fusion. Cell 1998; 92:759-772.
86. Fukuda R, McNew JA, Weber T et al. Functional architecture of an intracellular membrane t-SNARE. Nature 2000; 407:198-202.
87. Chavrier P, Parton RG, Hauri HP. Localization of low molecular weight GTP binding proteins to exocytic and endocytic compartments. Cell 1990; 62:317-329.
88. Pfeffer SR. Transport-vesicle targeting: Tethers before SNAREs. Nature Cell Biol 1999 1:E17-E22.
89. Peters C, Mayer A. Ca2+/calmodulin signals the completion of docking and triggers a late step of vacuole fusion. Nature 1998; 396:575-580.
90. Pryor PR, Buss F, Luzio JP. (2000) Calcium, calmodulin and the endocytic pathway. ELSO Gaz. 2000; 2:(http://www.the-elso-gazette.org/magazines/issue2/reviews/reviews1_pr.asp).
91. Goldstein J, Anderson RG, Brown MS. Coated pits, coated vesicles, and receptor-mediated endocytosis. Nature 1979; 279:679-685.
92. Bretscher MS, Thomson JN, Pearse BM. Coated pits act as molecular filters. Proc Natl Acad Sci USA 1980; 77:4156-4159.

93. Davis CG, Lehrman MA, Russell DW et al. The J.D. mutation in familial hypercholesterolemia: Amino acid substitution in cytoplasmic domain impedes internalization of LDL receptors. Cell 1986; 45:15-24.

94. Bonifacino JS, Dell'Angelica EC. Molecular bases for the recognition of tyrosine-based sorting signals. J Cell Biol 1999; 145:923-926.

95. Owen DJ, Evans PR. A structural explanation for the recognition of tyrosine-based endocytotic signals. Science 1998; 282:1327-1332.

96. Munro S, Pelham HR. A C-terminal signal prevents secretion of luminal ER proteins. Cell 1987; 48:899-907.

97. Semenza JC, Hardwick KG, Dean N et al. ERD2, a yeast gene required for the receptor-mediated retrieval of luminal ER proteins from the secretory pathway. Cell 1990; 61:1349-1357.

98. Lewis MJ, Sweet DJ, Pelham HR. The ERD2 gene determines the specificity of the luminal ER protein retention system. Cell 1990; 61:1359-1363.

99. Bretscher MS, Munro S. Cholesterol and the Golgi apparatus. Science 1993; 261:1280-1281.

100. Nilsson T, Rabouille C, Hui N et al. The role of the membrane-spanning domain and stalk region of N-acetylglucosaminyltransferase I in retention, kin recognition and structural maintenance of the Golgi apparatus in HeLa cells. J Cell Sci 1996; 109:1975-1989.

101. Nilsson T, Slusarewicz P, Hoe MH et al. Kin recognition. A model for the retention of Golgi enzymes. FEBS Lett 1993; 330:1-4.

102. Reaves BJ, Banting G, Luzio JP. Lumenal and transmembrane domains play a role in sorting type I membrane proteins on endocytic pathways. Mol Biol Cell 1998; 9:1107-1122.

103. Burkhardt JK. The role of microtubule-based motor proteins in maintaining the structure and function of the Golgi complex. Biochim Biophys Acta 1998; 1404:113-126.

104. Pfeffer SR. Constructing a Golgi complex. J Cell Biol 2001; 155:873-876.

105. Barr FA. The Golgi apparatus: Going round in circles? Trends Cell Biol 2002; 12:101-104.

106. Pelham HR, Rothman JE. The debate about transport in the Golgi—two sides of the same coin? Cell 2000; 102:713-719.

107. Pelham HR. Traffic through the Golgi apparatus. J Cell Biol 2001; 155:1099-1101.

108. Marsh BJ, Mastronarde DN, Buttle KF et al. Organellar relationships in the Golgi region of the pancreatic beta cell line, HIT-T15, visualized by high resolution electron tomography. Proc Natl Acad Sci USA 2001; 98:2399-2406.

109. Griffiths G, Simons K. The trans Golgi network: Sorting at the exit site of the Golgi complex. Science 1986; 234:438-443.

110. Lippincott-Schwartz J, Roberts TH, Hirschberg K. Secretory protein trafficking and organelle dynamics in living cells. Ann Rev Cell Dev Biol 2000; 16:557-589.

111. Bryant NJ, Stevens TH. Vacuole biogenesis in Saccharomyces cerevisiae: Protein transport pathways to the yeast vacuole. Microbiol Mol Biol Rev 1998; 62:230-247.

112. Luzio JP, Rous BA, Bright NA et al. Lysosome-endosome fusion and lysosome biogenesis. J Cell Sci 2000; 113:1515-1524.

113. Mullins C, Bonifacino JS. The molecular machinery for lysosome biogenesis. Bioessays 2001; 23:333-343.

114. Gruenberg J, Maxfield FR. Membrane transport in the endocytic pathway. Curr Opin Cell Biol. 1995; 7:552-563.

115. Gu F, Gruenberg J. Biogenesis of transport intermediates in the endocytic pathway. FEBS Lett 1999; 452:61-66.

116. Antonin W, Holroyd C, Fasshauer D et al. A SNARE complex mediating fusion of late endosomes defines conserved properties of SNARE structure and function. EMBO J 2000; 19:6453-6464.

117. Antonin W, Fasshauer D, Becker S et al. Crystal structure of the endosomal SNARE complex reveals common structural principles of all SNAREs. Nat Struct Biol 2002; 9:107-111.

118. Piper RC, Luzio JP. Late endosomes: Sorting and partitioning in multivesicular bodies. Traffic 2001; 2:612-621.

119. Raiborg C, Bache KG, Gillooly DJ et al. Hrs sorts ubiquitinated proteins into clathrin-coated microdomains of early endosomes. Nat Cell Biol 2002; 4:394-398.

120. Warren G, Wickner W. Organelle inheritance. Cell 1996; 84:395-400.

121. Mitchison TJ, Salmon ED. Mitosis: A history of division. Nat Cell Biol 2001; 3:E17-21.

122. Paweletz N. Walther Flemming: Pioneer of mitosis research. Nature Reviews Molecular Cell Biology 2001; 2:72-75.
123. Shaw JM, Nunnari J. Mitochondrial dynamics and division in budding yeast. Trends Cell Biol 2002; 12:178-184.
124. Fehrenbacher KL, Davis D, Wu M et al. Endoplasmic reticulum dynamics, inheritance, and cytoskeletal interactions in budding yeast. Mol Biol Cell 2002; 13:854-865.
125. Gerace L, Burke B. Functional organization of the nuclear envelope. Ann Rev Cell Biol 1988; 4:335-374.
126. Newport J. Nuclear reconstitution in vitro: Stages of assembly around protein-free DNA. Cell 1987; 48:205-217.
127. Grant TM, Wilson KL. Nuclear Assembly. Ann Rev Cell Dev Biol 1997; 13:669-695.
128. Aitchison JD, Rout MP. A tense time for the nuclear envelope. Cell 2002; 108:301-304.
129. Shima DT, Haldar K, Pepperkok R et al. Partitioning of the Golgi apparatus during mitosis in living HeLa cells. J Cell Biol 1997; 137:1211-1228.
130. Rabouille C, Kondo H, Newman R et al. Syntaxin 5 is a common component of the NSF- and p97-mediated reassembly pathways of Golgi cisternae from mitotic Golgi fragments in vitro. Cell 1998; 92:603-610.
131. Zaal KJ, Smith CL, Polishchuk RS et al. Golgi membranes are absorbed into and reemerge from the ER during mitosis. Cell 1999; 99:589-601.
132. Seemann J, Pypaert M, Taguchi T et al. Partitioning of the matrix fraction of the Golgi apparatus during mitosis in animal cells. Science 2002; 295:848-851.
133. Horter J, Warren G. Golgi architecture and inheritance. Ann Rev Cell Dev Biol 2002; 18:379-420.
134. Pelletier L, Stern CA, Pypaert M et al. Golgi biogenesis in Toxoplasma gondii. Nature 2002; 418:548-552.
135. Uchiyama K, Jokitalo E, Lindman M et al. The localization and phosphorylation of p47 are important for Golgi disassembly-assembly during the cell cycle. J Cell Biol 2003; 161:1067-1079.
136. Misteli T. The concept of self-organization in cellular architecture. J Cell Biol 2001; 155:181-185.
137. Warren G. Membrane traffic and organelle division. Trends Biochem Sci 1985; 10:439-443.

CHAPTER 2

Protein Coats As Mediators of Intracellular Sorting and Organelle Biogenesis

Chris Mullins

Abstract

Protein sorting through the secretory and endocytic pathways is essential for many aspects of cell function, including the biogenesis and maintenance of numerous intracellular organelles. Efficient protein trafficking requires a complex machinery of regulatory and structural factors. Key components of this machinery include protein coats, which mediate selective recruitment of cargo and transport-vesicle formation and targeting. Through these functions, a diversity of protein coats, often with the aid of accessory factors, regulates protein type and number within secretory and endocytic organelles and at the cell surface. Recent studies both in model organisms and humans have provided new insights into the traditional view of protein coat structure and function. In addition, genetic and genome-based analyses have revealed novel coat components as well as the distinct sorting events in which they participate. The significance of these findings to secretory and endocytic sorting, and their relevance to the biogenesis of organelles comprising these pathways, are the subjects of the present review.

Introduction

Sorting of soluble and membrane proteins between intracellular compartments and the cell surface is a process fundamental to virtually all eukaryotic cells. Efficient and accurate trafficking of proteins, as well as accompanying biomolecules such as carbohydrates and lipids, is essential to a myriad of events requiring tight temporal and spatial control of protein composition and quantity. Examples include regulation of cell-surface receptors; uptake of nutrients and other molecules; secretion of hormones, neurotransmitters, and immune factors; quality-control/turnover of cellular and exogenous proteins; and establishment of cell polarity. Protein trafficking is also critical for the biogenesis and maintenance of cellular organelles and the plasma membrane through the selective delivery of resident structural and enzymatic factors. The importance of protein sorting to mammalian physiology, and particularly to organelle biology, is demonstrated by the variety of disorders resulting from its disruption.[1,2]

Protein sorting is typically described in terms of two general transport routes termed the "secretory" and "endocytic" sorting pathways (Fig. 1). Proteins enter the secretory pathway through translocation into the endoplasmic reticulum (ER) either cotranslationally (at distinct regions of the ER with associated ribosomes) or post-translationally. Here many nascent (i.e., immature) proteins are folded and receive post-translational modifications. From the ER, secretory proteins are

The Biogenesis of Cellular Organelles, edited by Chris Mullins. ©2005 Eurekah.com and Kluwer Academic/Plenum Publishers.

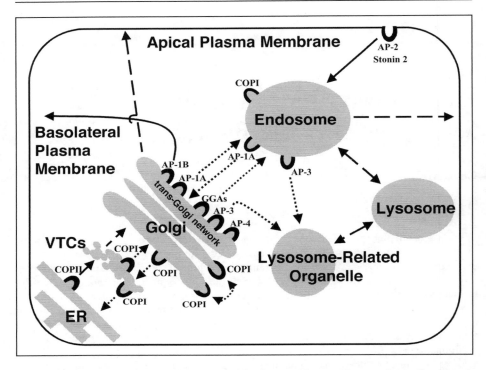

Figure 1. Schematic representation of the secretory and endocytic pathways and proposed sites of protein coat function. Key organelles and sorting steps comprising the secretory and endocytic sorting pathways and the localizations of protein coats and steps they have been demonstrated (solid lines), or strongly suggested (short-dash lines), to mediate are indicated. Some key, but less defined, sorting routes that may involve protein-coats are also shown (long-dash lines). Proposed endosomal structures (including early, late, and recycling) are summarized as one compartment for simplicity, though coats/pathways presented would generally involve an early endosome. Processes presented are primarily based on data from mammalian systems. However, many of these pathways, as well as additional, novel pathways, are more clearly defined in genetic models such as yeast and Drosophila (not indicated, see text for details). See text for abbreviations and relevant references.

sorted to the Golgi apparatus, where they are subjected to further modifications. A region of the Golgi referred to as the trans-Golgi network (TGN) acts as the secretory pathway's "Grand Central Station". From here proteins are selectively sorted to appropriate organelles, such as degradative lysosomes; the plasma membrane; or to secretory granules for exit out of the cell. The ER-to-Golgi segment is often referred to as the "early" secretory pathway, while post-Golgi sorting routes are commonly termed the "late" secretory pathway. The trafficking of newly synthesized proteins (as opposed to recycling proteins) along these routes to their ultimate destinations is commonly termed "biosynthetic sorting". Within the secretory pathway proteins may move in a "forward" (e.g., ER-to-Golgi) and, at certain steps, in a "backward" (e.g., Golgi-to-ER) direction, termed anterograde and retrograde transport, respectively. The endocytic pathway involves the endocytosis (i.e., internalization) of proteins from the plasma membrane and transport to the endosomal system, which consists of a number of putative, distinct compartments. Endocytosed proteins are initially sorted to early endosomes. From early endosomes proteins appear to be sorted to the Golgi, to recycling endosomes for transport back to the plasma membrane, or to late endosomes. Late endosomes serve as sites for sorting to degradative lysosomes and "lysosome-like organelles", cell-type specific compartments that share properties with conventional lysosomes, and/or mature into these compartments directly.[2,3]

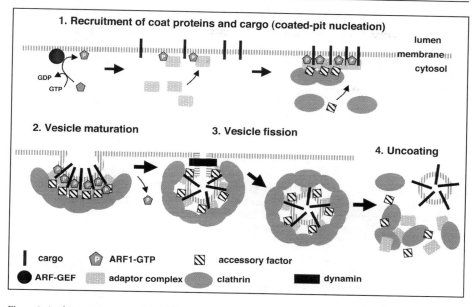

Figure 2. A schematic representation of the sequential stages of protein-coated transport vesicle formation. Here a clathrin-coated vesicle containing AP complexes serves as the model, though many of the basic processes are common to other types of coated vesicles. Initially, ARF1 is recruited to donor membrane sites by an ARF-GEF, which mediates GDP -> GTP exchange on ARF1 (step 1). Membrane-bound (i.e., activated) ARF1•GTPs then recruit AP complexes, though it is not clear if each ARF1•GTP recruits one or multiple complexes. AP complexes in turn recruit appropriate cargo; clathrin molecules, which form a lattice work required for structural integrity; and probably a variety of accessory factors (here collectively represented by one symbol) to the site of coated-pit nucleation. Forming clathrin-coated cargo vesicles mature (step 2) then undergo fission (also referred to as "pinching off") through the action of factors including the GTPase dynamin (step 3). Mature vesicles traffick to acceptor membrane sites, though they are generally believed to undergo coat dissociation before they arrive (step 4). This outline is highly simplified with numerous lipid and protein mediators omitted for the sake of simplicity (see references herein for additional detail).

Sorting from donor to acceptor membranes in the secretory and endocytic pathways is primarily conducted via vesicular and tubulovesicular transport intermediates.[4] While molecular events can vary widely, a basic model for vesicle formation at donor sites involves initial recruitment of a small GTPase, such as members of the ADP-ribosylation factor (ARF) family or Sar1p, to the membrane (Fig. 2, step 1).[5] For the ARFs this requires the ARF-guanine nucleotide exchange factor (GEF), which mediate GDP-to-GTP exchange on soluble ARF•GDP (i.e., inactive ARF) resulting in membrane-bound ARF•GTP (i.e., active ARF). Membrane-bound Sec12p performs this function for Sar1p. The activated GTPase then acts to recruit the three major classes of electron-dense, multi-component protein-coats important for cargo selection and vesicle formation/integrity: clathrin-containing, COPI, and COPII.[6] Clathrin-coats are comprised of the scaffolding protein clathrin and an "adaptor" component, such as an adaptor protein (AP) complex or monomeric "adaptor-related" protein, and localize to the late-secretory and endocytic pathways (Fig. 1). Adaptors typically function in recruiting membrane protein cargo, clathrin, and one or more "accessory-factor" (Fig. 2, step 1). The structurally and functionally distinct COPI and COPII coats also recruit select cargo and accessory factors, though they do not contain or associate with clathrin or adaptors. COPI and COPII are localized largely to the early-secretory pathway (Fig. 1). Polymerization of the coat and actions of additional protein and lipid mediators produce membrane deformations that lead to bud formation and eventually vesicle maturation (Fig. 2, step 2). For clathrin-coated vesicles (CCVs), ARF GTPase-activating proteins (GAPs) stimulate ARF hydrolysis of bound GTP, thus inactivating and releasing ARF•GDP from the membrane. Studies of CCV formation suggest a dynamic exchange of clathrin between the forming cage and the cytoplasm occurs at this point to promote coat rearrangements required for vesicle maturation.[7] Following maturation, the coated vesicle undergoes fission (or "pinching-off") from the donor membrane (Fig. 2, step 3). In the case of CCVs, this step involves the GTPase dynamin. Dynamin, in association with other accessory factors, forms a "collar" around the "neck" of the budding vesicle and facilitates fission through an undetermined mechanism requiring GTP hydrolysis. In the case of COP-coated vesicles, fission appears to result directly from completion of coat assembly. It is generally believed that following vesicle fission, but before arrival at the target membranes, protein coats are dissociated from transport vesicles in an uncoating reaction (Fig. 2, step 4). Removal of clathrin coats appears to involve the Hsc70 uncoating ATPase, auxilin, and probably other factors, while COP coats are disassociated through GAP-stimulated ATP hydrolysis by ARF or other associated ARF-like GTPases. The subsequent processes of vesicle targeting and docking and fusion with acceptor membranes are dependent on numerous additional factors. For example, the Rab family of small GTPases associate with membranes and appear to function in vesicle targeting, probably through interacting with cytoskeletal motors, and in vesicle docking/fusion events at target membranes, possibly through recruitment or activation of additional effectors.[8] The highly conserved, largely membrane-associated group of N-ethylmeimide-sensitive factor (NSF) attachment protein receptors, or SNARES, is also important for vesicle docking/fusion.[9] Selective interactions of cognate SNARES on vesicles (v-SNARES) with those at target sites (t-SNARES) facilitate mixing and fusion of vesicle and acceptor membranes, which results in cargo delivery. Finally, it is important to remember proteins sort through numerous means besides vesicular transport. Proteins are internalization via plasma membrane invaginations termed "caveolae", which represent a subset of the specialized lipid microdomains commonly referred to as "rafts", and through "bulk flow" processes like phagocytosis. Sorting can be mediated through homotypic (e.g., endosome-endosome) and heterotypic (e.g., secretory granule-plasma membrane) membrane fusions. Heterotypic fusions are common to cells that undergo "regulated secretion" of proteins housed in secretory granules or, in some cell types, secretory lysosomes. For reviews of these transport mechanisms see refs. 2,3,10-12.

Obviously even a simple description of the secretory and endocytic sorting machinery reveals a multitude of important factors. A complete survey of all players is well beyond the scope of this work. The present review will, therefore, focus primarily on the structure and function of the major classes of protein coats. First, two constituents of clathrin-containing coats, clathrin and the AP complexes, will be discussed followed by descriptions of COPI and COPII coats. Finally, the potential roles of two newly-described coats containing adaptor-related proteins will be addressed. Recent findings relating protein coat-function to the biogenesis of organelles comprising the endocytic and secretory pathways are also emphasized.

Clathrin: A Scaffold for Protein Coats

The clathrin protein acts at sorting sites of the late secretory pathway, including the TGN, endosomes, and plasma membrane, to drive the formation of cargo vesicles.[6,13] To perform this function, clathrin, which exists as a heterohexamer unit termed the triskelia, is recruited from the cytoplasm to the cytoplasmic face of donor membranes. Here clathrin triskelions assemble into a multimeric molecular scaffold to provide the mechanical force and structural integrity needed for membrane deformations leading to vesicle formation. Clathrin is ubiquitously expressed in all cell types and across all eukaryotic species examined from yeast to humans, indicating it performs an important and highly conserved function. Interestingly, recent studies suggest a newly-discovered second clathrin protein in humans may mediate muscle cell-specific TGN sorting steps through associations with the actin cytoskeleton.[14]

The structure of clathrin and assembled clathrin-coats on cargo vesicles has been studied in fine detail. Early studies using rotary-shadowing electron microscopy revealed the general "shape" of the clathrin triskelion and its composition of three heavy chain (190 kDa) - light chain (~25 kDa) pairs (Fig. 3A).[15] Following this initial description, the evolutionarily conserved heavy chain proved of particular interest for understanding the relationship between clathrin structure and function. This highly extended ~1675 amino acid subunit contains at its amino-terminus a "globular" domain and a short linker segment (together comprising residues ~1-500) that connects to the much larger "leg" region, itself consisting of distal and proximal (site of light chain association) domains, followed by the carboxy-terminus, which links to other heavy chains forming the vertex of the triskelion. Crystallographic studies reveal the "globular" domain folds into a seven-blade β-sheet propeller structure, which probably provides multiple sites for interactions with adaptor and accessory proteins, while the linker consists of repeating α-helical zig zags.[16] Clathrin triskelions in turn pack into highly complex 3-dimensional lattices, also referred to as "cages" or "baskets", up to 2000Å in diameter with the amino-terminal "globular" domain pointing inward (Fig. 3A and ref. 6).

Numerous factors, many of which were characterized in studies of neuronal synaptic vesicle (SV) formation, interact with clathrin to facilitate assembly and disassembly of clathrin lattices. Adaptors, adaptor-related proteins (see later sections), and the AP180 (neural form)/CALM (nonneural form) protein[17] all recruit clathrin to membrane sites of coated-vesicle formation. The β-arrestins (comprising two widely expressed homologues, β-arrestin 1 and β-arrestin 2/arrestin 3) also appear to recruit clathrin, and additional coat components, to sites of endocytosis for some G-protein-coupled receptors, including the β2-adrenergic receptor.[18-20] Importantly, a peptide corresponding to the clathrin-interacting sequence of β-arrestin 2 binds within grooves of the β-propellers at the clathrin heavy chain amino-terminus, suggesting a general mode by which clathrin interacts with other factors.[21] Amphiphysin (comprising the neural expressed amphiphysin I and the broadly expressed amphiphysin II)[22] and epsin (comprising two similar neural proteins, epsin I and II)[23,24] appear to recruit clathrin and additional coat components to the plasma membrane through interactions at multiple internal clathrin-binding sequences. In addition, amphiphysin, through its carboxy-terminal SH3 (Src-homology region 3) domain, interacts with dynamin and synaptojanin, a phosphatase involved in regulating levels of phosphoinostitides involved in endocytosis.[25] Auxilin, a member of the DnaJ family, binds clathrin with high affinity and, in cooperation with heat-shock protein hsp70c, participates in clathrin-uncoating prior to vesicle fusion with acceptor membrane sites.[26] These and other proteins that directly interact with clathrin contain one or more clathrin-binding motifs, or "clathrin-boxes", conforming to the five amino acid consensus sequence L (L,I) (D,E,N) (L,F) (D,E) and, in some cases, additional nonconsensus variants, such as PWDLW in the case of the human amphiphysins.[27] Finally, while these represent a select subset of proteins with described or presumed clathrin interactions, it should be remembered that numerous other factors are involved in clathrin-mediated sorting (for descriptions refer to refs. 13,28,29 and later sections).

As with many protein coat constituents, studies in genetic models have provided insight into clathrin function in coat formation and protein sorting in vivo. Cells of the budding yeast *Saccharomyces cerevisiae* lacking the clathrin heavy chain (Δ*chc1*) display slow growth; defective endocytosis; mislocalization of Golgi proteins; and, depending on the genetic background, inviability.[30-32] Similar phenotypes, as well as defective vesiculation, are observed in a light chain deletion mutant (Δ*clc1*), though this may be indirect due to heavy chain instability.[33] A temperature sensitive heavy chain mutant (*chc1-521*) displays the additional phenotype of defective biosynthetic sorting from the Golgi, though for unknown reasons sorting recovers over

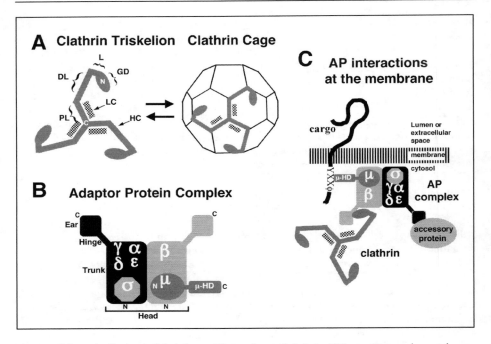

Figure 3. Schematic diagrams of clathrin, an AP complex, and clathrin-AP interactions at the membrane. A) The clathrin triskelion consists of three heavy chains (HC) and three light chains (LC). The HC is further subdivided into an amino-terminal globular domain (GD); linker (L); distal leg (DL); and a carboxy-terminal proximal leg (PL) domain, which joins with two other PL domains to form the vertex of three heavy chains. Triskelia assemble into a closed hexagonal lattice-work (here highly simplified), referred to as a clathrin cage or basket, which disassembles upon coat disassociation. The relative position of an individual triskelion in a clathrin cage is indicated. B) AP complexes consist of one β-adaptin; one γ, α, δ, or ε-adaptin, for AP-1-4, respectively; one μ-adaptin; and one σ-adaptin subunit. Relative positions of carboxyl-terminal "Ear", "Hinge", "Trunk", and regions comprising amino-terminal "Head" domains of large adaptins, as well as μ-homology domain (μ-HD) of μ-adaptin, are indicated. Subunits are drawn roughly to scale. C) At sites of transport-vesicle formation, AP complexes recruit cargo through interactions between the μ-HD of μ-adaptin and tyrosine-based (i.e., YXXΦ) sorting signals present on cytosolic domains of membrane proteins. For those AP complexes that recruit clathrin, the β-adaptin subunit interacts via one or more sites in its carboxyl-terminal "Hinge/Ear" region with the clathrin globular domain. Additional interactions between AP complex subunits and clathrin have also been reported (not pictured, see text for details). The "Ear" of the second large adaptin has been implicated in recruitment of accessory factors. See text for relevant references.

time.[34] Genetic screens using the *chc1-521* mutant identified dynamin-related Vps1p and synaptojanin-like Inp53p as players in clathrin-mediated sorting at the yeast Golgi.[35] In addition, the *chc1-521* mutation displays genetic interactions with deletion mutations of yeast adaptor AP-1,[36,37] as well as novel adaptor-related proteins (discussed in more detail below).[38] In contract to yeast, deletion of the clathrin heavy chain in *Drosophilia melanogaster* is lethal, suggesting a lack of factors capable of functional overlap with this coat protein and the importance of clathrin to viability.[39]

Adaptor Protein Complexes: Adaptors for Coats of the Late-Secretory and Endocytic Pathways

AP complexes serve as adaptors for clathrin-coats, and probably some nonclathrin-coats, operating among compartments of the late-secretory and endocytic pathways and the plasma membrane.[40,41] As protein coat adaptors, AP complexes perform key functions at the cytoplasmic surface of donor membranes, including: selective recruitment of protein cargo to sites of vesicle formation; recruitment of accessory factors involved in vesicle formation; and, at least for some AP complexes, linking clathrin to the forming vesicle.

To date, four AP complexes have been described in mammals: AP-1 through AP-4. Each AP complex is comprised of four protein subunits, or "adaptins": two large adaptins (β1-4 and one each of $\gamma/\alpha/\delta/\epsilon$ for AP-1-4, respectively, ~90-130 kDa), one medium adaptin (μ1-4, ~50 kDa), and one small adaptin (σ1-4, ~20 kDa) (Fig. 3B). In addition, a number of adaptin isoforms have been identified, suggesting alternative holo-complexes may perform specific sorting functions in some cell types. Electron microscopy studies have revealed the association of AP subunits yields a shape reminiscent of a "head" with one "ear" protruding from each of the two large adaptins and connected by a flexible "hinge" or "linker" region. Adaptin subunits bear a high degree of sequence homology across eukaryotic genera, suggesting an evolutionarily conserved function for AP complexes.[40]

Each of the four adaptin subunits comprising mammalian AP complexes has an ascribed function in coated-vesicle formation and selective sorting (Fig. 3C). Due to their ability to bind clathrin in vitro, the β-adaptins of AP-1 and AP-2 are believed to recruit clathrin to the forming vesicle in vivo.[42] Beta-3 also interacts with clathrin in vitro suggesting it performs a similar role in clathrin-coat assembly for AP-3,[43] though this is still a matter of debate. These in vitro β-adaptin-clathrin interactions are dependent on clathrin-binding motifs in the β1-3 hinge-domains.[42-44] The ear domain of β2, which does not contain a consensus clathrin-binding motif, is also implicated in clathrin-binding, as well as recruitment of accessory proteins.[45] Interestingly, β4 displays no apparent clathrin-binding.[46,47] The ear-domains of γ- and α-adaptin appear to target AP-1 and AP-2, respectively, to appropriate membranes.[48] In addition, the γ-adaptin ear recruits γ-synergin, a cytosolic protein of unknown function, to membranes. Gamma-synergin contains an EH (Eps15 homology) domain, known to mediate protein-protein interactions.[49] Though this EH motif is not required for AP-1 binding, it may recruit additional factors to the site of AP-1 function. Recent work by Doray and Kornfeld[50] demonstrates clathrin binds at multiple sites on γ-adaptin, including sites representing probable new variants of the clathrin-binding motif. Interactions between γ-adaptin of yeast AP-1 and clathrin have also been reported.[51] The α-adaptin ear, probably through a single binding-site, interacts with multiple ligands that participate in vesicle formation and sorting at the plasma membrane.[52] The μ-adaptins interact with distinct "sorting signals" in the cytosolic tails of membrane protein cargo. Cytosolic sorting signals, though somewhat heterogeneous, are often grouped into two main classes, tyrosine based, which includes NPXY and YXXØ signal types (where N is asparagine; P is proline; Y is tyrosine; X is any residue; and Ø is a bulky hydrophobic residue, such as phenylalanine (F), leucine (L), isoleucine (I), valine (V), or methionine (M)), and dileucine signals, which includes LL and LI signal types.[53-55] Interactions between the μ-adaptins and tyrosine-based signals serve to selectively recruit and concentrate cargo at sites of nascent transport-vesicle formation, thereby providing much of the specificity in sorting of the respective AP complexes. It has been suggested μ-adaptins[56] and/or the β-adaptins[57] interact with dileucine signals, though the significance of these interactions is controversial. The σ-adaptin subunit appears to function, at least in part, to strengthen interactions between the large adaptins.[58]

While similar in overall structure and respective subunit function, AP complexes display different distributions in the cell. This and other findings, largely from studies in model organisms, suggest unique functions for each AP complex in secretory and endocytic sorting. The characteristics of individual AP complexes are described in the following sections.

AP-1

The AP-1 complex primarily localizes to the TGN and to a lesser extent to endosomal compartments (Fig. 1). At the TGN, AP-1 is believed to mediate clathrin recruitment and selective sorting of CCVs containing cargo, including certain lysosomal and plasma membrane proteins, on to the endosomal system. AP-1 is itself recruited to membranes by membrane-bound ARF1•GTP.[59] Addition of brefeldin A (BFA), an inhibitor of ARF GTP- GDP exchange, results in redistribution of AP-1 to the cytosol.[60,61] Polarized cell-specific AP-1B has recently been identified as an alternative complex to the ubiquitous AP-1 (i.e., AP-1A) complex. AP-1B is similar to AP-1A but contains the epithelial-specific μ1B isoform.[62] This complex mediates targeting of select membrane proteins, such as the low density lipoprotein receptor (LDLR) and lysosomal-associated membrane protein 1 (Lamp1), from the TGN to basolateral membranes[63-65] and possibly post-endocytically.[66]

A number of early studies implicated AP-1 in sorting the cation-dependent (CD)- and cation-independent (CI)-mannose 6-phosphate receptors (MPRs), two major components of TGN-derived cargo vesicles.[67,68] The MPRs themselves mediate sorting of numerous soluble hydrolases to endosomes/lysosomes through recognition of mannose 6-phosphate moieties added to these proteins post-translationally. Protein cargos, such as the MPRs, do not appear to be required for efficient AP-1 recruitment and subsequent CCV formation at the TGN,[69] thought this is a matter of debate.[70] Selectivity in sorting is largely provided by μ1-adaptin, which recognizes distinct tyrosine-based sorting signals,[71,72] such as those present in the tails of the MPRs. New findings indicate AP-1 does not interact with di-leucine signals present in MPR cytosolic tail regions,[73,74] though these signals are known to be required for MPR sorting at the TGN.[67,73]

The importance of AP-1 to the development of higher eukaryotes is clear from genetic studies in mice that show disruption of the γ-adaptin gene is lethal (i.e., no homozygote mutant embryos developed past day 4.5 post-coitus).[75] In a separate study, disruption of μ1A also failed to yield homozygote mutants, though embryos developed sufficiently for the establishment of epithelial cell cultures.[76] Interestingly, these cells, which probably still form AP-1B, display inefficient endosome-TGN trafficking, which suggests a role for AP-1A in recycling.[64,76] In contrast to mammals, *S. cerevisiae* mutants containing genetic disruptions for all four AP-1 subunits individually or in combination display no growth or sorting phenotypes.[36,37] Individual AP-1 mutants do show synthetic defects in sorting from the yeast Golgi when combined with clathrin mutations.[36,37] Supporting the genetic interactions are findings that yeast AP-1 β and γ-adaptins interact with clathrin in vitro.[51]

Together, studies of AP-1 reveal that much remains to be learned concerning this adaptor's role in protein transport. It also appears likely that alternative sorting machineries participate, and potentially overlap, with AP-1 in selective sorting at the TGN and/or endosomes.

AP-2

AP-2 localizes to the plasma membrane where it recruits protein cargo and clathrin and mediates endocytosis and sorting of proteins in CCVs to early endosomes (Fig. 1). AP-2-mediated endocytosis at the cell surface is important for a number of processes including regulation of levels of cell-surface receptors, ion channels, and transporters; internalization of extracellular molecules; and formation and cycling of SVs in neural cells. The μ2-adaptin subunit weakly, but selectively, interacts with distinct sets of tyrosine-based sorting signals in vitro.[72,77,78] Such tyrosine signal–μ2-adaptin interactions are strengthened by the presence of clathrin and phospholipids.[79] In addition, phosphorylation of μ2 on a single threonine residue by a novel adaptor-related serine/threonine kinase increases AP-2 binding to membranes and sorting signals.[80-82] Recent descriptions of the AP-2 atomic structure reveal membrane-binding sites in α-adaptin and μ2 and suggest AP-2 may undergo conformational changes at the membrane to allow sorting-signal recognition/binding.[83,84] These and other findings suggest AP-2-mediated cargo recruitment at the plasma membrane is highly regulated.

Numerous accessory factors that interact with AP-2 to participate in endocytic vesicle formation and protein internalization have been identified from studies of clathrin-coated SV formation.[28,29] Amphiphysin concentrates at neuronal presynaptic termini and appears to recruit AP-2 through interactions with α-adaptin[52,85] and the clathrin heavy chain.[22] Beta-arrestin 2 binds β2-adaptin through a carboxyl-terminal sequence to facilitate agonist-induced internalization of some G-protein coupled receptors.[86] EPS15 (epidermal growth factor protein substrate 15) interacts with AP-2 ear-domains via carboxyl-terminal DPF (aspartic acid (D)-proline (P)-phenylalanine(F)) repeats. EPS15 also interacts with epsin and synaptojanin (which comprises two phosphoinositide phosphatase isoforms possibly involved in uncoating) via two amino-terminal EH (EPS15 homology) repeats.[28] Interactions between AP-2 and EPS15 appear to aid in recruiting growth factor receptors as endocytic cargo.[87] Epsin, the primary binding-partner for the EPS15 EH domains,[88] interacts with the α-adaptin ear of AP-2 via its central DPW (aspartic acid (D)-proline (P)-tryptophane (W)) domain and with clathrin via two cooperative clathrin-binding motifs.[23,24] Auxilin also interacts with AP-2 and clathrin probably as a function of its role in vesicle uncoating.[26,89] The neuronal-specific AP180 protein binds the β2-adaptin ear[45] and interacts with clathrin via multiple DLL (aspartate (D)-leucine (L)-leucine (L)) repeats.[17] This association of AP-2 and AP180 strengthens the affinity of both proteins for clathrin, suggesting these coat proteins cooperate in clathrin recruitment in neuronal cells.[90] AP-2 recruitment to the plasma membrane does not require ARF proteins,[91] and is thus not sensitive to BFA. Instead AP-2 recruitment appears to involve the membrane protein synaptotagmin.[92] Members of the synaptotagmin family contain two cytosolic C2-domains, C2A and the similar C2B domain, which bind AP-2 via a cluster of lysine residues.[93] Synaptotagmin, possibly in cooperation with phospholipids, strengthens AP-2-membrane associations and facilitates the formation of coated-pits (an early stage of coated-vesicle formation).[94] AP-2 function also appears to be regulated through interactions with phosphoinositides (PI) at the membrane. A recent study suggests binding of PIs by μ2 may regulate AP-2/clathrin-mediated endocytosis in neurons.[95] In addition to AP-2-containing clathrin-coats and the accessory factors named here, an array of additional players participate in regulated endocytosis (for a more complete survey see refs. 28, 29).

Analyses of AP-2 function have been performed in a number of genetic model organisms. Disruption of AP-2 subunit genes in *S. cerevisiae* does not produce an observable defect in viability or sorting,[37,96] even in combination with clathrin mutations.[95] Studies in *Caenorhabditis elegans* using RNA-mediated interference (RNAi) are inconclusive regarding the importance of AP-2 to endocytosis, but do reveal an essential requirement for development.[98,99] Mutations in Drosophila α-adaptin result in severe impairment of SV formation and development.[100] In addition, Drosophila α-adaptin interacts with the Numb protein, which influences cell fate during fly development.[101] Mutations in the α-adaptin ear domain abolish this interaction and lead to developmental defects similar to those seen in a *numb* mutant.[101] These roles for AP-2 detailed in genetic models are supported by studies in human cell lines that show interference with AP-2 function using a dominant-negative form of μ2 leads to severe defects in endocytosis in vivo.[102]

AP-3

The AP-3 complex appears to associate with the TGN and/or endosomes (Fig. 1), though its precise intracellular localization remains unclear. AP-3 is recruited from the cytosol to membranes by ARF1•GTP in a reaction blocked by BFA.[61] At the TGN, and possibly endosomes, AP-3 mediates selective sorting of membrane proteins to lysosomes as well as lysosome-related compartments such as melanosomes, platelet dense granules, visual pigment granules, and MHC class II compartments.[2] Other recent investigations suggest AP-3 is required for lysosomal delivery from the TGN via a route bypassing endosomal compartments.[103] An AP-3 complex containing neural-specific adaptin isoforms β3B (β-NAP) and μ3B has been implicated in SV formation from endosomal-like compartments in vitro.[104]

Extensive characterization of μ3-adaptin-sorting signal interactions show AP-3 prefers tyrosine-based signals resembling those in lysosomal membrane proteins such as Lamp 2 and Lamp 3/CD63.[72] Furthermore, ablating μ3-adaptin through anti-sense oligonucleotides inhibits TGN sorting of lysosomal membrane proteins Lamp 1 and Lamp 3/CD63, but not sorting of M6PRs, which involves AP-1.[105] Interestingly, μ3-adaptin interacts with a cytosolic segment of M6PR containing dileucine and tyrosine-based sorting signals,[106] though the significance of this interaction remains unclear.

AP-3 is proposed to recruit clathrin in a manner similar to AP-1 and AP-2 based on studies showing: AP-3 colocalizes with clathrin in vivo,[43] β3-adaptin interacts with clathrin via a consensus clathrin-binding motif in vitro,[21,43] and AP-3 can link clathrin to synthetic liposomes.[107] However, other reports revealed: little AP-3 on isolated CCV preparations,[108] the absence of clathrin on AP-3 vesicles budding from endosomes,[109] and β3-adaptin with its putative clathrin-binding domain mutated retains function in vivo.[110] In addition, deletion of the yeast clathrin heavy chain does not affect AP-3-dependent sorting of some vacuolar proteins.[34,111] One explanation for these findings is that this unique complex may participate in both clathrin- and nonclathrin coated vesicle sorting.

Genetic studies in model organisms and humans have probably yielded more insight into AP-3 function than for any of the other identified AP complexes. Disruption of the genes encoding yeast AP-3 subunits results in mis-sorting of the vacuolar hydrolase alkaline phosphatase (ALP) and the vacuolar t-SNARE Vam3p.[111-113] AP-3-mediated protein sorting via this "ALP-pathway" does not require clathrin, unlike sorting pathways mediated by yeast AP-1 and AP-2.[114] However, in some cases other proteins, such as Vps41p,[115] may substitute for clathrin in AP-3-coated vesicles. In Drosophila mutations in each of the four AP-3 subunits have been linked to eye color phenotypes resulting from defects in the biogenesis of visual pigment granules, a lysosome-like organelle.[116-119] In contrast to the proposed involvement of mammalian AP-3 in SV formation in vitro,[104,109,120] Drosophila AP-3 does not appear to be involved in SV formation in vivo.[118] The importance of AP-3 to lysosomes and related organelles is also seen in mouse coat-color mutants *mocha* and *pearl*, which contain defects in δ- and β3A-adaptins, respectively.[121,122] These mutants display various phenotypes associated with defective sorting to and biogenesis of melanosomes, platelet dense granules, and lysosomes. The importance of AP-3 for lysosomal sorting in humans has been elegantly demonstrated through studies of genetic disorders resulting from mutations in AP-3 genes. Patients with the Hermansky-Pudlak Syndrome (HPS) display hypopigmentation, clotting defects, and lysosomal abnormalities similar to those seen in AP-3 mutant mice. A form of HPS, termed HPS type 2, has been shown to result specifically from a mutation in the β3-adaptin gene, which in turn leads to defects in sorting to and biogenesis of melanosomes, platelet dense granules, and lysosomes.[123] Together these results clearly demonstrate the importance of AP-3 in biosynthetic sorting to and maintenance of lysosomes and lysosome-related organelles across all eukaryotic species examined.

AP-4

AP-4, the most recently identified member of the AP complex family, is localized to the cytoplasmic face of the TGN (Fig. 1), probably as a component of nonclathrin coats.[46,47] Like AP-1 and AP-3, AP-4 is recruited to membranes by ARF1•GTP in a reaction that can be inhibited by BFA.[124] AP-4 recruitment appears to require specific, and probably cooperative, interactions between ε- and μ4-adaptins with ARF I "switch regions" I and II,[124] which undergo conformational changes during GTP-GDP exchange[125,126] and act as binding sites for effector molecules.[127] Interestingly, AP-4 is not present in yeast, Drosophila, or *C. elegans*, though it is expressed in mammals as well as *Dictyostelium discoideum* and *Arabidopsis thaliana*.[40] This suggests that AP-4 is involved in cellular functions distinct to select eukaryotes. Like all μ-adaptins, μ4 displays a preference for a subset of tyrosine-based sorting signals.[128] The μ4-adaptin subunit also interacts in vitro with naturally occurring tyrosine-signals found in lysosomal membrane proteins including Lamp 2 and Lamp 3/CD63.[47,128] These interactions, as well as its cellular localization, argue for a role for AP-4 in biosynthetic sorting to the endosomal/lysosomal system. In addition, a recent report by Simmen et al[129] suggests a role for AP-4 in basolateral sorting in polarized epithelial cells. Additional work is needed to further elaborate the role of AP-4 in intracellular protein transport.

COP Complexes: Protein Coats of the Early Secretory Pathway

Bi-directional protein transport between organelles of the early-secretory pathway, specifically the ER and Golgi, is primarily mediated by the functionally and structurally distinct coat protein complexes, or COPs.[130,131] Two COPs have been described: COPI, also referred to as coatomer; and COPII. Like protein coats operating in the late-secretory and endocytic pathways, the COPs recruit cargo at membrane donor sites and facilitate the biogenesis and selective sorting of transport vesicles. In contrast to many other secretory pathway coats, COP coats do not contain clathrin or a separate adaptor component.

COPI and COPII appear to operate primarily in retrograde and anterograde sorting, respectively, at the highly dynamic and morphologically intricate interface between the ER and cis (early)-Golgi compartments (Fig. 1).[130] Following translation/translocation, secretory proteins sort from the ER at ribosome-free exit sites, or transitional elements (TEs), containing membrane-associated COPII. Following budding at TEs, COPII coats disassociate from cargo vesicles, which then fuse with a collection of membrane structures termed the vesicular tubular clusters (VTCs). These transient VTCs appear to move along microtubule tracks to cis-Golgi elements where they fuse resulting in the delivery of cargo.[132] COPI-coated vesicles form at cis-Golgi compartments and at VTCs. These COPI cargo vesicles traffic back to the ER, thus replenishing membranes and escaped resident and sorting machinery proteins. Some evidence suggests COPI vesicles also traffick from VTCs to the Golgi in an anterograde direction. The COPs thereby act in concert to ensure a tight coupling biosynthetic sorting and recycling in the early secretory pathway. Distinct characteristics and functions of these coats are discussed in the following sections.

COPI

The COPI coat was originally identified through in vitro assays of ER–Golgi transport.[133] Isolation of COPI-coated vesicles revealed the coat to be composed of a 600kDa protein complex, referred to as coatomer, and an ARF GTPase (Fig. 4).[134] Coatomer in turn is comprised of seven nonidentical subunits ranging from ~160kDa to ~20kDa: α-, β-, β'-, γ-, δ-, ε-, and ζ-COP.[135] Immunochemical studies revealed COPI coats primarily localize to VTC membranes and cis-Golgi membranes, but not to late-Golgi structures such as the TGN.[132,136]

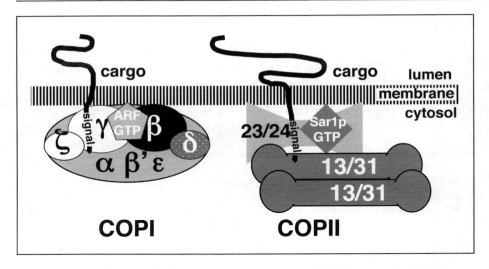

Figure 4. Schematic diagram of COP-coat proteins. Components of COPI (coatomer) and COPII coats and possible interactions at sites of transport vesicle formation are presented. Membrane proteins appear to be recruited through interactions with γ-COP and the Sec23/24 complex of COPI and COPII, respectively. Sorting signals in the cytosolic tails of cargo can vary widely (see text for details). COPI and COPII subunits appear to be recruited to membranes by membrane-bound ARF1•GTP and Sar1p•GTP, respectively. Individual COPI and COPII subunit arrangement and stoichiometry of COPII subcomplexes Sec23/24 and Sec13/31 remains unclear, though model presented represents most recent ideas. COPII model presented is derived largely from studies in yeast. COPI and COPII subunits are drawn roughly to scale. See text for relevant references.

COPI subunits are largely conserved from mammals to yeast and share sequence similarities with AP complex subunits.[6,40]

A role for COPI coats in Golgi-to-ER retrograde trafficking is largely supported by genetic studies in yeast. These analyses reveal defective Golgi-to-ER transport in conditional mutants for yeast COPI subunits sec21p and sec27p, the orthologs of mammalian γ-COP and β'-COP, respectively, and demonstrate the cooperation of other resident ER sorting constituents in this transport.[137,138] In addition, more recent in vitro reconstitutions of Golgi sorting demonstrate COPI-vesicles can mediate the transport of Golgi enzymes from the cis-Golgi to the VTCs.[139] Studies in yeast and mammalian systems have also suggested a role for COPI-coated vesicles in anterograde sorting from VTCs to the Golgi and within the Golgi stacks, though these functions for COPI are the subject of much debate.[4,140-142] The relative importance of COPI to retrograde versus anterograde sorting in the ER-Golgi interface thus remains to be established.

An endosomal-specific COPI coat apparently lacking the γ and δ subunits has been identified in association with vesicles trafficking from early to late endosomes in a manner dependent on the acidic pH of these compartments.[143-147] In addition, endosomal COPI is involved in the biogenesis of multivesicular bodies (MVBs), also known as endosomal carrier vesicles (ECVs), in both mammalian cells and yeast.[135,144,148] MVBs/ECVs appear to represent intermediate compartments in sorting from early to late endosomes and/or late endosomes in the process of maturing into lysosomes.[3,135]

To maintain selective sorting, COPI, like other protein coats, must distinguish appropriate cargo, such as proteins to be recycled back to the ER. To accomplish this COPI recognizes a dilysine retention/retrieval signal with the consensus sequence KKXX (where K is lysine and

X is any residue) in the cytoplasmic tail of a number of ER-resident membrane proteins.[137,149] A major cargo of COPI vesicles is the p24 family, a conserved group of membrane proteins implicated in regulating vesicle formation.[150] A subgroup of the p24 family, including the p23 protein, contains the KKXX sorting motif in their cytosolic tails, while all p24 proteins carry a double-phenylalanine (FF) sorting motif that is also recognized by COPI. Though the exact requirements for individual subunits in binding membrane cargo are unclear, a model for COPI-cargo interactions has been proposed.[140] In this model the KKXX motif first contacts γ-COP followed by a shift in binding to an α-/β'-/ε-COP subcomplex, while a β/γ/ζ subcomplex selectively interacts with the FF motif. COPI also appears to participate in recycling of some soluble ER proteins containing the carboxy-terminal H/KDEL (where H is histidine/K is lysine, D is glutamic acid, E is lysine, and L is leucine) retention/retrieval signal when bound to the multi-spanning membrane protein Erd2p, which acts as the intracellular H/KDEL-receptor.[151]

As with numerous other protein coats, the small GTPase ARF is critical for COPI-mediated vesicle formation. This initially requires ARF GEF-mediated ARF1 activation (i.e., GDP→ GTP exchange) and membrane recruitment in a BFA sensitive reaction.[152] COPI is subsequently recruited to donor membrane sites through interactions with ARF1•GTP.[153] ARF1-COPI association at the membrane provides kinetically stable sites needed for cargo recruitment with coatomer apparently remaining after ARF1 dissociation.[154] Recent studies have revealed an interplay between the activation state of ARF1 and positive and negative selection of cargo by COPI.[155,156] In one proposed model, interactions between specific sorting signals (e.g., RRXX, where R is arginine, as found in some p24 proteins) and COPI at the membrane induce COPI conformational changes that prevent GTP hydrolysis.[155] This presumably results in COPI-ARF1•GTP remaining membrane-associated long enough for "productive" assembly of COPI-cargo vesicles. In contrast, in the so termed "discard pathway", other sorting signals (e.g., the KKXX and FF motifs, as found in some p24 proteins) do not prevent GTP hydrolysis of ARF1•GTP. This allows GTP hydrolysis by ARF-GAP and disassociation of COPI, ARF1•GDP, and cargo, thus blocking vesicle formation. These models suggest that competing sorting signals can act positively or negatively during COPI vesicle budding with specificity conferred by GTP hydrolysis. ARF1 also appears to be involved in recruitment of COPI in the endosomal pathway.[157] This recruitment is pH-dependent suggesting that cytosolic ARF1 is able to sense the acidic luminal environment of endosomal compartments and MVBs, probably indirectly via associations with an endosomal membrane protein(s). These findings, thus explain the observed pH-dependence of COPI association with endosomes/MVBs.[143,144] Inhibition of COPI/ARF1 by dominant-negative ARF1 mutants and BFA results in abberant Golgi and endosomal morphology.[158-160] In addition, disassociation of COPI from membranes with BFA results in Golgi disorganization and redistribution of Golgi contents to the ER.[161] These and numerous other studies suggest a fundamental role for COPI/ARF1 in the biogenesis of a number of secretory/endocytic organelles.[4,161]

COPII

The COPII coat was initially identified using genetic approaches in yeast and in vitro reconstitutions of ER-to-Golgi transport.[162] Subsequent purification of factors required for vesicle budding from the yeast ER revealed COPII coats to be composed of the Sec23p/Sec24p and Sec13p/Sec31p complexes and the small GTPase Sar1p (Fig. 4).[163,164] Like COPI proteins, constituents of COPII coats are largely conserved from yeast to humans.[6,40]

Electron microscopy and 3-dimensional reconstructions in yeast reveal that COPII coat assembly at membranes proceeds orderly with cytosolic Sar1p•GDP initially binding to lipids.[130,165] Here Sar1p•GDP associates with a membrane-bound GEF (yeast Sec12p) to produce activated Sar1p•GTP. Sar1p•GTP then recruits Sec23p/Sec24p, which probably aids in cargo selection/sequestration, followed by Sec13/Sec31p, which appears to act in a structural role.[166] Multiple "bow-tie"-shaped Sec23p/Sec24p heterodimers and elongated, flexible Sec13p/Sec31p heterotetramers (two each of Sec13p and Sec31p) appear to associate laterally and horizontally to form a flexible, curved COPII basket.[167]

Live-cell imaging and immunoflourescence techniques have localized assembled COPII coats to ER TEs.[132,168] Sorting from TEs appears to involve two steps, COPII-mediated concentration of newly synthesized secretory proteins at ER exit sites and a "hand-off" to COPI for sorting via VTCs to the Golgi.[169] Visualization of the dynamics of ER exit sites using Sec13 and sec24 proteins tagged with the green fluorescent protein (GFP) reveal COPII associates with hundreds of relatively immobile TE exit sites that do not appear to be consumed by anterograde ER sorting.[169,170] COPII appears to dissociate prior to vesicle fusion with ER/Golgi intermediate compartments in a reaction mediated, at least in part, by the Sar1p GAP, COPII component Sec23p. Sec23p promotes GTP hydrolysis of Sar1p•GTP thus destabilizing Sar1p/COPII-lipid interactions.[171] The requirement of COPII in ER-to-Golgi biosynthetic sorting is also revealed in genetic studies in which conditional mutants of yeast COPII subunits (e.g., Sec23p, Sec13p, Sec31p, Sec24p), Sar1p, and the Sar1p GEF Sec12p display phenotypes consistent with defective ER exit.[172-174]

Evidence suggests that proteins exit the ER through bulk flow as well as a selective mechanism(s) involving specific ER-sorting signals.[130,165] Interestingly, selective and efficient anterograde ER export in mammalian cells and yeast appears to be mediated by a variety of such ER-exit motifs. For mammalian ERGIC-53,[175] the vesicular stomatitis virus glycoprotein (VSV-G),[176] yeast Sys1p,[177] and a mammalian potassium channel[178] the respective motifs KKFF, DXE, DXE, and EXD & EXE (where K is lysine, F is phenylalanine, D is aspartate, E is glutamic acid, and X is any residue) facilitate ER-exit through apparent interactions with COPII. A FF motif present in the cytosolic tails of p24 proteins has also been shown to function in ER-sorting.[179] A recent study revealed a FXXXFXXXF signal in cytosolic domain of the dopamine D1 receptor is recognized by the newly described ER-membrane protein DRiP78 during ER exit.[180] Together, such reports suggest an as yet fully defined specificity exists for ER anterograde sorting, possibly involving accessory factors acting with COPII coats at the level of signal-recognition/cargo recruitment.

Adaptor-Related Proteins Define Novel Coats of the Secretory and Endocytic Pathways

The diversity of identified sorting-motifs and intricate trafficking routes between late-secretory and endocytic organelles and the plasma membrane suggest a need for a variety of protein coats with diverse adaptor components. Some variety is obtained through the expression of AP complex adaptin isoforms.[40] As described above, adaptin isoforms, some of which show cell/tissue-specific expression, can associate in AP complexes involved in specialized sorting events, such as basolateral sorting (e.g., AP-1B)[63-65] and SV endocytosis (e.g., AP-3 containing β3/βNAP and μ3B).[104] However, the small number of AP complexes, even with isoforms, seems insufficient to provide selectivity for all late-secretory and endocytic transport steps. Furthermore, genetic studies show that removal of one or more AP complexes does not completely abolish sorting in the respective pathway(s).[181] Indeed, deletion of all AP genes in yeast does not eliminate biosynthetic sorting to the vacuole, block endocytosis, eliminate clathrin assembly on coats, or result in an apparent growth defect.[36,37,96] These results imply the presence of additional adaptor proteins that can function redundantly with AP complexes in the late-secretory and endocytic pathways.

Database mining and genomics approaches used to identify many adaptin isoforms have more recently revealed novel adaptor-related proteins. Classification as adaptor-related is often based on sequence similarity to known adaptors (or adaptin subunits) and/or a functional similarity to know adaptors, such as the ability to recognize sorting signals and recruit clathrin to forming transport vesicles. Two families of such adaptor-related proteins, the GGAs and the Stoned B family, define novel protein coats involved in late-secretory and endocytic trafficking. These proteins have been the subject of a number of recent investigations and are described in the following sections.

The GGA Family of Late-Secretory Adaptors

A number of independent studies employing database searches for proteins bearing homology to select adaptin domains and two-hybrid screens for proteins interacting with activated ARF identified the GGA (for Golgi-localized, γ ear-containing, ARF-binding) family of adaptor-related coat proteins.[182-186] This family comprises three members in mammals (GGA1, GGA2, and GGA3), two members in *S. cerevisiae* and *S. pombe* (Gga1p and Gga2p), and one member each in Drosophila and *C. elegans*.[40] Interestingly, the GGAs display a unique modular arrangement of domains that bear homology to proteins and/or functional domains known to be involved in protein trafficking. This organization consists of an amino-terminal VHS (for Vps27p, Hrs, STAM homology) domain; a GAT (for GGA and TOM homology) domain; a variable, nonconserved linker region; and a carboxy-terminal GAE domain (for γ-adaptin ear homology) (for details on above factors bearing homology to the GGAs see ref. 3) (Fig. 5A). Though they bear some homology to AP-1 subunit γ-adaptin, the GGAs appear to exist as monomers in vivo.[182,183] Immunofluorescence and electron microscopy studies demonstrate the mammalian GGAs localize to coated buds and vesicles at or near the TGN (Fig. 1).[182-185] At the TGN, the GGAs colocalize with AP-1 and possibly physically associate with AP-1 through interactions of the GGA hinge and the γ-adaptin ear domains.[187] The GGAs are recruited to membranes by ARF1•GTP in a reaction sensitive to BFA and blocked by overexpression of dominant-negative ARF1 mutants.[182,184] The GGAs also interact with activated ARF3.[184]

Rapid advances in our understanding of mammalian GGA function have come from analyses of individual GGA domains (ref. 41 and Fig. 5A). The GGA VHS domain is homologous to the amino-terminal VHS domains of several proteins implicated in sorting including mammalian Hrs (hepatocyte growth factor regulated tyrosine kinase substrate) and its yeast homolog Vps27p, both of which function in endosomal trafficking.[3] The crystal structures of the VHS domains from Hrs and TOM1 (target of myb1) suggest the presence of multiple sites for protein-protein and protein-membrane interactions.[188,189] Functional analyses of the mammalian GGAs' VHS domains demonstrate interactions with the cytoplasmic tails of: CD- and CI-M6PR; sortilin and sorLA, two intracellular sorting-receptors that share homology with the yeast carboxypeptidase Y (CPY) sorting receptor Vps10p; low density lipoprotein receptor-related protein 3 (LRP3); and β-secretase, a protease involved in the production of β-amyloid in the brain.[74,190-194] Mapping of these interactions through two-hybrid and in vitro-binding experiments show the GGA VHS domain binds an acidic cluster-dileucine sorting signal located in the cytosolic tails of the M6PRs and the sortilin receptor.[74,90,91] Interactions between the GGAs and M6PRs appear to be partially regulated by the phosphorylation state of a serine within an acidic-dileucine signal.[195] Recent crystallographic analyses of GGA1 and GGA3 VHS domains in complex with a peptide corresponding to the carboxyl-terminus of the CI- and CD-M6PRs identified the residues that bind the acidic cluster-dileucine signal DXXLL (where D is aspartic acid, X is any residue, and L is leucine).[196,197] These GGA VHS residues are poorly conserved in other VHS-containing proteins like TOM1, Hrs, and STAM (signal-transducing adaptor molecule), none of which interact with dileucine signals.[196,197] Interestingly, the GGA VHS domain appears to bind a novel sorting motif in SorLA conforming to the consensus ΨΨXXØ (where Ψ is an acidic residue, X is any residue, and Ø is a bulky hydrophobic residue).[194] The GAT domain interacts with ARF1•GTP and ARF3•GTP, while overexpression of the GAT displaces ARF1-regulated protein coats AP-1, AP-3, AP-4 from the TGN.[182,184] More detailed examinations of GAT activity reveal that GAT binding interferes

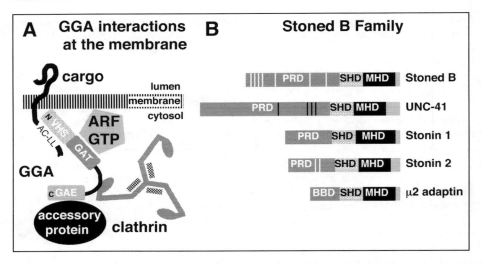

Figure 5. Schematic representation of adaptor-related coat proteins. A) At sites of transport vesicle formation, monomeric GGA proteins recruit cargo through interactions of the amino-terminal VHS domain with
acidic cluster-dileucine (AC-LL) motifs in the cytosolic domains of membrane proteins, such as some
intracellular sorting receptors. GGA proteins are themselves recruited to membranes through interactions
of the GAT domain with membrane bound ARF1•GTP. Interactions between the GGAs and clathrin have
been localized to clathrin-binding motifs in the hinge domain, though other sites of clathrin-binding have
also been reported (see text for details). The carboxyl-terminal GAE domain has been suggested to play a
role in recruitment of accessory proteins. B) Members of the Stoned B family of monomeric adaptor-related
proteins are presented. Family members are characterized by the presence of an amino-terminal proline-rich
domain (PRD) (except for μ2-adaptin), an internal stonin-homology domains (SHD), and a μ-homology
domain (MHD) proximal to the amino-terminus. In addition, Drosophila Stoned B and mammalian
Stonin 2 contain seven and two NPF motifs (indicated by white bars), respectively. *C. elegans* UNC-41
contains four DPF motifs (indicated by black bars). Neither mammalian Stonin 1 nor μ2-adaptin contains
NPF or DPF motifs. The β-adaptin-binding domain (BBD) of μ2-adaptin is also indicated. See text for
additional abbreviations and relevant references.

with ARF's interactions with ARF GAP, which probably blocks hydrolysis of ARF1•GTP to
ARF1•GDP and ARF1 release from the membrane (for a review of ARF cycling see ref. 5).[127]
GAT-ARF interactions thus result in transient stabilization of ARF1•GTP and, by extension,
the GGAs on membranes.[127] Stabilization of the GGAs probably allows recruitment of additional GGA-coat constituents required for vesicle formation. Puertollano et al[127] have also
shown the nonconserved hinge region of all three human GGAs interact with clathrin in vitro
and GGA1 can recruit clathrin to the TGN in vivo. As with the γ-adaptin subunit of AP-1, in
vitro binding experiments demonstrate GGA1 and GGA2 interact with γ-synergin, and possibly several other unidentified proteins, via the GGA carboxyl-terminal γ-adaptin ear (GAE)
domain.[183] Interactions between all three mammalian GGAs and γ-synergin were also demonstrated using a two-hybrid approach.[185] These findings suggest the GAE domain may play a
role in recruitment of accessory factors to the site of forming coated-vesicles, a function also
proposed for the γ-adaptin subunit of AP-1.[49]

Investigations in yeast have added to our understanding of GGA function in vivo through
new discoveries and elaborations on insights from mammalian studies. An important and redundant role for yeast Gga1p and Gga2p in biosynthetic sorting to the yeast vacuole was
shown in a mutant yeast strain (*gga1Δ gga2Δ*) deleted for both *GGA* genes.[182,183,198] This

mutant, while not defective for growth, displays a myriad of sorting phenotypes including defective vacuolar sorting and mislocalization of a number of vacuolar hydrolases usually transported via the "CPY-pathway", an alternative biosynthetic pathway to the aforementioned ALP-pathway;[182,183,198,199] defective processing of the yeast mating pheromone α-factor,[38,199,200] probably due to mislocalization of Golgi-resident protease Kex2p;[199] defective sorting of the syntaxin Pep12p from the Golgi to late endosome/vacuolar membranes;[201] and defective vacuolar biogenesis.[183,199] Combining the *gga2Δ* mutation with a temperaturesensitive clathrin mutation or deletions of the genes encoding AP-1 subunits β1 and γ-adaptin results in severe sorting and growth defects,[38,200] suggesting a functional association of the GGAs with clathrin and AP-1 in vivo. However, a direct association between the GGAs and AP-1 in mammals is controversial.[200] Detailed structure-function studies of individual GGA domains in yeast revealed a functional importance of the VHS, GAT and hinge domains in vivo; interactions between clathrin-binding motifs in Gga1p and Gga2p hinge domains and clathrin in vitro; and a functional cooperation, probably in clathrin binding, between the GAE and the hinge in vivo.[199] As with the mammalian orthologs, yeast Gga1p and Gga2p interact with activated ARF1 and ARF2 proteins via sequences within the conserved GAT domain.[198] However, evidence of interactions between the yeast GGA VHS domains and intracellular sorting receptors is still lacking.

The Stoned B Family of Endocytic Adaptors

Early genetic analyses in Drosophila identified the *stoned* locus and showed it to be required for normal neuronal function.[202] The dicistronic *stoned* gene encodes two proteins, stoned A (STNA) and stoned B (STNB).[203] Both STNA and STNB are localized to the presynaptic plasma membrane (or "plasmalemma") of central and peripheral neurons, suggesting a role in SV formation and endocytosis.[204]

Sequence analysis suggest STNA is a novel protein. However, STNB appears to be an adaptor-related protein based on homology between its carboxyl-terminal region and the signal-binding domain of μ2-adaptin, also termed the μ-homology domain (Fig. 5B). Fine analyses of synapses in the Drosophila paralytic mutant *stoned* demonstrates a large decrease in SV numbers; an accumulation of SV recycling intermediates; and a mislocalization and increased degradation of synaptotagmin, a presynaptic membrane protein that interacts with AP-2 in coated-pit formation.[204] Interestingly, the μ2-homology domain of STNB appears to be important for STNB-synaptotagamin interactions and the *stnB* mutation genetically interacts with a synaptotagamin mutation (*sytI*).[205] Also, overexpression of synaptotagamin restores SV formation and viability in *stnB* flies.[206] These findings implicate STNB in the plasma membrane-recruitment of synaptotagamin, which may in turn recruit other factors required for coated-vesicle formation such as AP-2.[94] A STNB homologue, termed UNC-41, has also been identified in *C. elegans* and is also implicated in SV cycling.[207]

STNB, like "stoned B family" members UNC-41 and the mammalian stonins (described below), contains an amino-terminal PRD (proline-rich domain) region enriched in proline and serine residues followed by a SHD (stonin-homology domain) region (Fig. 5B).[41] Stoned B protein μ2-adaptin also contains a SHD, but does not contain a PRD sequence (Fig. 5B).[41] The PRD of STNB contains seven NPF (asparagine (N)- proline (P)-phenylalanine(F)) motifs, which interact with EH domains of various proteins implicated in endocytosis.[28,29] Thus, STNB, perhaps in cooperation with synaptotagamin, may act as an adaptor protein at the site of endocytic vesicle formation. The role of the SHD is yet to be determined.

Recently two mammalian stoned B family members, stonin 1 and stonin 2, were identified in mice and humans through searches of sequence databases (Fig. 5B).[208,209] The stonins exhibit the same modular organization and μ2-homology as other members of the stoned B family and, like STNB, exist as monomers in both cytosolic and membrane-associated cellular fractions.[208,209] Unlike Drosophila STNB, which is enriched in neural tissues, the mammalian stonins appear to be expressed in nearly all tissues examined.[208,209] Stonin 2, but not stonin 1, contains two NPF motifs in its PRD, suggesting possible associations with proteins containing EH domains. Two-hybrid and in vitro binding analyses reveal such cooperative interactions of the NPFs of stonin 2 with the EH domains of Eps15 and intersectin 1.[208] In vitro experiments also reveal that stonin 2 associates with AP-2 (Fig. 1),[208] possibly indirectly through interactions between DPF motifs in Eps15 bound to stonin 2 and α-adaptin.[208] In addition, stonin 2, like STNB, is capable of interacting with synaptotagmin via its μ2-homology domain.[208,209] This stonin domain does not, however, bind tyrosine-sorting signals, as does the homologous domain in μ2-adaptin. Importantly, overexpression of stonin 2 inhibits internalization from the cell surface, further implicating stonin 2 as a key component of the coated-vesicle biogenesis machinery.[208] Results from in vitro vesicle-uncoating assays suggest a specific role for stonin 2 in the removal of AP-2/clathrin coats in mammalian neuronal cells.[209]

Conclusions and Future Prospects

The hard work of countless researchers has clearly demonstrated that protein coats play an essential role in protein sorting and organelle biogenesis across eukaryotic species. The observed diversity of coats reflects the cell's need for selective and regulated protein trafficking critical for functional and spatial compartmentalization of secretory/endocytic organelles and cell membrane. The widely studied protein coats composed of multi-subunit AP complexes, often with help from the scaffolding protein clathrin, serve these functions within the late-secretory and endocytic pathways, while the COP complexes act in the early secretory pathway. This traditional model of protein coat-mediated sorting became more complex following recent identification of novel adaptor-related coat proteins, such as the GGAs and Stoned B family.

Though many of the basic principles of protein coat-mediated intracellular transport and endocytosis have been elucidated, unanswered questions persist. Numerous coat and accessory proteins, and their interplay with the identified sorting machinery, remain to be discovered. This is evident from the wealth of novel factors and isoforms of known factors found in nearly every new broad-based genetic or database search. Efforts to further characterize these factors and the processes to which they contribute will add new, and hopefully unforeseen, dimensions to our understanding of eukaryotic cellular biology. In addition, gaps persist in our descriptions of known coat and accessory proteins and the mechanics of specific sorting steps. For example, how are proteins so efficiently selected for transport by one coat-complex, or analogous factor, over another at a common donor compartment when such promiscuity is observed in coat-signal interactions? What is the role of the monomeric adaptor-related proteins in sorting relative to the AP complexes? What are the molecular mechanisms at work in the highly complex, individual transport steps of vesicle fission, uncoating, and fusion? How and to what extent does protein coat-mediated trafficking truly contribute to the maintenance, biogenesis, and function of cellular organelles in vivo? And perhaps the most important question, what is the physiological relevance of intracellular and endocytic sorting to human health and disease?

Acknowledgements

I would like to thank Dr. Josephine Briggs and Dr. Juan S. Bonifacino for their support during the conception and development of this project. I would also like to thank Dr. Rosa Puertollano, Dr. Markus Boehm and Dr. Erik Snapp for critical reading of the manuscript. This work was supported in part by a National Research Council Associateship. Due to space limitations it was not possible to describe all relevant findings, so I would like to apologize to all those whose work may have been omitted from this discussion.

References

1. Delahunty M, Bonifacino JS. Disorders of intracellular protein trafficking in human disease. Connective Tissue Research 1995; 31:283-286.

2. Dell'Angelica EC, Mullins C, Caplan S et al. Lysosome-related organelles. FASEB 2000; 14:1265-1278.

3. Mullins C, Bonifacino JS. The molecular machinery for lysosome biogenesis. BioEssays 2001; 23:333-343.

4. Lippincott-Schwartz J, Roberts T, Hirschberg K. Secretory protein trafficking and organelle dynamics in living cells. Annu Rev Cell Dev Biol 2000; 16:557-589.

5. Donaldson JG, Jackson CL. Regulators and effectors of the ARF GTPases. Curr Opin Cell Biol 2000; 12:475-482.

6. Kirchhausen T. Three ways to make a vesicle. Nat Rev Mol Cell Biol 2000; 1:182-198.

7. Wu X, Zhao X, Baylor L et al. Clathrin exchange during clathrin-mediated endocytosis. J Cell Biol 2001; 155:291-300.

8. Rodman S, Wandinger-Ness A. Rab GTPases coordinate endocytosis. J Cell Sci 2000; 113:183-192.

9. Pfeffer SR. Transport-vesicle targeting: Tethers before SNAREs. Nat Cell Biol 1999; 1:E17-E21.

10. Simons K, Toomre D. Lipid rafts and signal transduction. Mol Cell Biol 2000; 1:31-39.

11. Nichols BJ, Lippincott-Schwartz J. Endocytosis without clathrin coats. Trends Cell Biol 2001; 11:406-412.

12. Blott EJ, Griffiths GM. Secretory lysosomes. Nat Rev Mol Cell Biol 2002; 3:122-131.

13. Pearse BMF, Smith CJ, Owen DJ. Clathrin coat construction in endocytosis. Curr Opin Struct Biol 2000; 10:220-228.

14. Liu S-H, Towler MC, Chen E et al. A novel clathrin homolog that codistributes with cytoskeletal components functions in the trans-Golgi network. EMBO J 2001; 20:272-284.

15. Ungewickell E, Branton D. Assembly units of clathrin coats. Nature 1981; 289:420-422.

16. ter Haar E, Musacchio A, Harrison SC et al. Atomic structure of clathrin: A β propeller terminal domain joins an α zigzag linker. Cell 1998; 95:563-573.

17. Morgan JR, Prasad K, Hao W et al. A conserved clathrin assembly motif essential for synaptic vesicle endocytosis. J Neurosci 2000; 20:8667-8676.

18. Goodman Jr OB, Krupnick JG, Santini F et al. Beta-arrestin acts as a clathrin adaptor in endocytosis of the β2-adrenergic receptor. Nature 1996; 383:447-450.

19. Krupnick JG, Goodman Jr OB, Keen JH et al. Arrestin/clathrin interaction. Localization of the clathrin binding domain of nonvisual arrestins to the carboxy terminus. J Biol Chem 1997; 272:15011-15016.

20. Pierce KJ, Lefkowitz RJ. Classical and new roles of β-arrestins in the regulation of G-protein-coupled receptors. Nat Rev Neuro 2001; 2:727-733.

21. ter Haar E, Harrison SC, Kirchhausen T. Peptide-in-groove interactions link target proteins to the β-propeller of clathrin. Proc Natl Acad Sci USA 2000; 97:1096-1100.

22. Ramjaun AR, McPherson PS. Multiple amphiphysin II splice variants display differential clathrin binding: Identification of two distinct clathrin-binding sites. J Neurochem 1998; 70:2369-2376.

23. Rosenthal JA, Chen H, Slepnev VI et al. The epsins define a family of proteins that interact with components of the clathrin coat and contain a new protein module. J Biol Chem 1999; 274:33959-33965.

24. Drake MT, Downs MA, Traub LM. Epsin binds to clathrin by associating directly with the clathrin-terminal domain. Evidence for cooperative binding through two discrete sites. J Biol Chem 2000; 275:6479-6489.

25. McPherson PS, Garcia EP, Slepnev VI et al. A presynaptic inositol-5-phosphatase. Nature 1996; 379:353-357.

26. Ungewickell E, Ungewickell H, Holstein SE et al. Role of auxilin in uncoating clathrin-coated vesicles. Nature 1995; 378:632-635.

27. Dell'Angelica EC. Clathrin-binding proteins: Got a motif? Join the network! Trends Cell Biol 2001; 11:315-318.

28. Slepnev VI, De Camilli P. Accessory factors in clathrin-dependent synaptic vesicle endocytosis. Nat Rev Neurosci 2000; 1:161-172.

29. Takei K, Haucke V. Clathrin-mediated endocytosis: Membrane factors pull the trigger. Trends Cell Biol 2001; 11:385-391.
30. Lemmon SK, Jones EW. Clathrin requirements for normal growth of yeast. Science 1987; 238:504-509.
31. Payne GS, Baker D, van Tuinen E et al. Protein transport to the vesicle and receptor-mediated endocytosis by clathrin heavy chain-deficient yeast. J Cell Biol 1988; 106:1453-1461.
32. Payne GS, Schekman R. Clathrin: A role in the intracellular retention of a Golgi membrane protein. Science 1989; 245:1358-1365.
33. Chu DS, Pishvaee B, Payne GS. The light chain subunit is required for clathrin function in Saccharomyces cerevisiae. J Biol Chem 1996; 271:33123-33130.
34. Seeger M, Payne GS. Selective and immediate effects of clathrin heavy chain mutations on Golgi membrane protein retention in Saccharomyces cerevisiae. J Cell Biol 1992; 118:531-540.
35. Bensen ES, Costaguta G, Payne GS. Synthetic genetic interactions with temperaturesensitive clathrin in Saccharomyces cerevisiae: Roles for synaptojanin-like Inp53p and dynamin-related Vps1p in clathrin-dependent protein sorting at the trans-Golgi network. Genetics 2000; 154:83-97.
36. Stepp JD, Pellicena-Palle A, Hamilton S et al. A late Golgi sorting function for Saccharomyces cerevisiae Apm1p, but not for Apm2p, a second yeast clathrin AP medium chain-related protein. Mol Biol Cell 1995; 6:41-58.
37. Yeung BG, Phan HL, Payne GS. Adaptor complex-independent clathrin function in yeast. Mol Biol Cell 1999; 10:3643-3659.
38. Costaguta G, Stefan CJ, Bensen ES et al. Yeast Gga coat proteins function with clathrin in Golgi to endosome transport. Mol Biol Cell 2001; 12:1885-1896.
39. Bazinet C, Katzen AL, Morgan M et al. The Drosophila clathrin heavy chain gene: Clathrin function is essential in a multicellular organism. Genetics 1993; 134:1119-1134.
40. Boehm M, Bonifacino JS. Adaptins: The final recount. Mol Biol Cell 2001; 12:2907-2920.
41. Robinson MS, Bonifacino JS. Adaptor-related proteins. Curr Opin Cell Biol 2001; 13:444-453.
42. Gallusser A, Kirchhausen T. The β1 and β2 subunits of the AP complexes are the clathrin coat assembly components. EMBO J 1993; 12:5237-5244.
43. Dell'Angelica EC, Klumperman J, Stoorvogel W et al. Association of the AP-3 adaptor complex with clathrin. Science 1998; 280:431-434.
44. Traub LM, Kornfeld S, Ungewickell S. Different domains of the AP-1 adaptor complex are required for Golgi membrane binding and clathrin recruitment. J Biol Chem 1995; 270:4933-4942.
45. Owen DJ, Vallis Y, Pearse BMF et al. The structure and function of the μ2-adaptin appendage domain. EMBO J 2000; 19:4216-4227.
46. Dell'Angelica EC, Mullins C, Bonifacino JS. AP-4, a novel protein complex related to clathrin adaptors. J Biol Chem 1999; 274:7278-7285.
47. Hirst J, Bright NA, Rous B et al. Characterization of a fourth adaptor-related protein complex. Mol Biol Cell 1999; 10:2787-2802.
48. Page LJ, Robinson MS. Targeting signals and subunit interactions in coated vesicle adaptor complexes. J Cell Biol 1995; 131:619-630.
49. Page LJ, Sowerby PJ, Winnie WY et al. Gamma-synergin: An EH domain-containing protein that interacts with γ-adaptin. J Cell Biol 1999; 146:993-1004.
50. Doray B, Kornfeld S. Gamma subunit of the AP-1 adaptor complex binds clathrin: Implications for cooperative binding in coated vesicle assembly. Mol Biol Cell 2001; 12:1925-1935.
51. Yeung BG, Payne GS. Clathrin interactions with C-terminal regions of the yeast AP-1 β and γ subunits are important for AP-1 association with clathrin coats. Traffic 2001; 2:565-576.
52. Owen DJ, Vallis Y, Noble ME et al. A structural explination for the binding of multiple ligands by the alpha-adaptin appendage domain. Cell 1999; 97:805-815.
53. Bonifacino JS, Marks MS, Ohno H et al. Mechanisms of signal-mediated protein sorting in the endocytic and secretory pathways. Proc Assoc American Phy 1996; 108:285-295.
54. Bonifacino JS, Dell'Angelica EC. Molecular basis for the recognition of tyrosine-based sorting signals. J Cell Biol 1999; 145:923-926.
55. Heilker R, Spiess M, Crottet P. Recognition of sorting signals by clathrin adaptors. BioEssays 1999; 21:558-567.

56. Hofmann MW, Honing S, Rodionov D et al. The leucine-based sorting motifs in the cytoplasmic domain of the invariant chain are recognized by the clathrin adaptors AP-1 and AP-2 and their medium chains. J Biol Chem 1999; 274:36153-36158.
57. Rapoport I, Chen YC, Cupers P et al. Dileucine-based sorting signals bind to the β chain of AP-1 at a site distinct and regulated differently from the tyrosine-based motif binding-site. EMBO J 1998; 17:2148-2155.
58. Takatsu H, Futatsumori M, Yoshino K et al. Similar subunit interactions contribute to assembly of clathrin adaptor complexes and COPI complex: Analysis using yeast three-hybrid system. Biochem Biophys Res Commun 2001; 284:1083-1089.
59. Zhu Y, Traub LM, Kornfeld S. ADP-ribosylation factor 1 transiently activates high-affinity adaptor protein complex AP-1 binding sites on Golgi membranes. Mol Biol Cell 1998; 9:1323-1337.
60. Wagner M, Rajasekaran AK, Hanzel DK et al. Brefeldin A causes structural and functional alterations of the trans-Golgi network of MDCK cells. J Cell Sci 1994; 107:933-943.
61. Ooi CE, Dell'Angelica EC, Bonifacino JS. ADP-ribosylation factor 1 (ARF1) regulates recruitment of the AP-3 adaptor complex to membranes. J Cell Biol 1998; 142:391-402.
62. Ohno H, Tomemori T, Nakatsu F et al. Mu 1B, a novel adaptor medium chain expressed in polarized epithelial cells. FEBS Letts 1999; 449:215-220.
63. Folsch H, Ohno H, Bonifacino JS et al. A novel clathrin adaptor complex mediates basolateral targeting in polarized epithelial cells. Cell 1999; 99:189-198.
64. Folsch H, Pypaert M, Schu P et al. Distribution and function of AP-1 clathrin adaptor complexes in polarized epithelial cells. J Cell Biol 2001; 152:595-606.
65. Sugimoto H, Sugahara M, Folsch H et al. Differential recognition of tyrosine-based basolateral signals by AP-1 subunit μ1B in polarized epithelial cells. Mol Biol Cell 2002; 13:2374-2382.
66. Gan Y, McGraw TE, Rodriguez-Boulan E. The epithelial-specific adaptor AP1B mediates post-endocytic recycling to the basolateral membrane. Nat Cell Biol 2002; 4:605-609.
67. Glickman JN, Conibear E, Pearse BM. Specificity of binding of clathrin adaptors to signals on the mannose-6-phosphate/insulin-like growth factor II receptor. EMBO J 1989; 8:1041-1047.
68. Mauxion F, Le Borgne R, Munier-Lehmann H et al. A casein kinase II phosphorylation site in the cytoplasmic domain of the cation-dependent mannose 6-phosphate receptor determines the high affinity interaction of the AP-1 Golgi assembly proteins with membranes. J Biol Chem 1996; 271:2171-2178.
69. Zhu Y, Traub LM, Kornfeld S. High-affinity binding of the AP-1 adaptor complex to trans-Golgi network membranes devoid of mannose 6-phosphate receptors. Mol Biol Cell 1999; 10:537-549.
70. Le Borgne R, Hoflack B. Mannose 6-phosphate receptors regulate the formation of clathrin-coated vesicles in the TGN. J Cell Biol 1997; 137:335-345.
71. Aguilar RC, Ohno H, Roche KW et al. Functional domain mapping of the clathrin-associated adaptor medium chains μ1 and μ2. J Biol Chem 1997; 272:27160-27166.
72. Ohno H, Aguilar RC, Yeh D et al. The medium subunits of adaptor complexes recognize distince but overlapping sets of tyrosine-based sorting signals. J Biol Chem 1998; 273:25915-25921.
73. Honing S, Sosa M, Hille-Rehfeld A et al. The 46-kDa mannose 6-phosphate receptor contains multiple binding sites for clathrin adaptors. J Biol Chem 1997; 272:19884-19890.
74. Zhu Y, Doray B, Poussu A et al. Binding of GGA2 to the lysosomal enzyme sorting motif of the mannose-6-phosphate receptor. Science 2001; 292:1716-1718.
75. Zizioli D, Meyer C, Gundula G et al. Early Embryonic death of mice deficient in γ-adaptin. J Biol Chem 1999; 274:5385-5390.
76. Meyer C, Zizioli D, Lausmann S et al. Mu1A-adaptin-deficient mice: Lethality, loss of AP-1 binding and rerouting of mannose 6-phosphate receptors. EMBO J 2000; 19:2193-2203.
77. Ohno H, Stewart J, Fournier M-C et al. Interactions of tyrosine-based sorting signals with clathrin-associated proteins. Science 1995; 269:1872-1875.
78. Boll W, Ohno H, Songyang Z et al. Sequence requirements for the recognition of tyrosine-based endocytic signals by clathrin AP-2 complexes. EMBO J 1996; 15:5789-5795.
79. Rapoport I, Miyazaki M, Boll W et al. Regulatory interactions in the recognition of endocytic sorting signals by AP-2 complexes. EMBO J 1997; 16:2240-2250.
80. Fingerhut A, von Figura K, Honing S. Binding of AP-2 to sorting signals is modulated by AP-2 phosphorylation. J Biol Chem 2001; 276:5476-5482.

81. Ricotta D, Conner SD, Schmid SL et al. Phosphorylation of the AP-2 mu subunit by AAK1 mediates high affinity binding to membrane protein sorting signals. J Cell Biol 2002; 156:791-795.

82. Conner SD, Schmid SL. Identification of an adaptor-associated kinase, AAK1, as a regulator of clathrin-mediated endocytosis. J Cell Biol 2002; 156:921-929.

83. Kirchhausen T. Clathrin adaptors really adapt. Cell 2002; 109:413-416.

84. Collins BM, McCoy AJ, Kent HM et al. Molecular architecture and functional model of the endocytic AP2 complex. Cell 2002; 109:523-535.

85. Slepnev VI, Ochoa G-C, Butler MH et al. Tandem arrangement of the clathrin and AP-2 binding domains in amphiphysin 1 and distribution of clathrin coat function by amphiphysin fragments comprising these sites. J Biol Chem 2000; 275:17583-17589.

86. Laporte SA, Oakley RH, Zhang J et al. The beta2-adrenergic receptor/beta-arrestin complex recruits the clathrin adaptor AP-2 during endocytosis. Proc Natl Acad Sci USA 1999; 96:3712-3717.

87. Salcini AE, Chen H, Iannolo G et al. Epidermal growth factor pathway substrate 15, Eps15. Int J Biochem Cell Biol 1999; 31:805-809.

88. Chen H, Fre S, Slepnev VI et al. Epsin is an EH-domain-binding protein implicated in clathrin-mediated endocytosis. Nature 1998; 394:793-797.

89. Umeda A, Meyerholz A, Ungewickell E. Identification of the universal cofactor (auxilin 2) in clathrin coat dissociation. Eur J Cell Biol 2000; 79:336-342.

90. Hao W, Luo Z, Zheng L et al. AP180 and AP-2 interact directly in a complex that cooperatively assembles clathrin. J Biol Chem 1999; 274:22785-22794.

91. Robinson MS, Kreis TE. Recruitment of coat proteins onto Golgi membranes in intact and permeabilized cells: Effects of brefeldin A and G protein activators. Cell 1992; 69:129-138.

92. Zhang JZ, Davletov BA, Sudhof TC et al. Synaptotagmin I is a high affinity receptor for clathrin AP-2: Implications for membrane recycling. Cell 1994; 78:751-760.

93. Chapman ER, Desai RC, Davis AF et al. Delineation of the oligomerization, AP-2 binding, and synprint binding region of the C2B domain of synaptotagmin. J Biol Chem 1998; 273:32966-32972.

94. Haucke V, Wenk MR, Chapman ER et al. Dual interactions of synaptotagmin with $\mu2$- and α-adaptin facilitates clathrin-coated pit nucleation. EMBO J 2000; 19:6011-6019.

95. Rohde G, Wenzel D, Haucke V. A phosphatidylinositol (4,5)-bisphosphate binding site within mu2-adaptin regulates clathrin-mediated endocytosis. J Cell Biol 2002; 158:209-214.

96. Huang KM, D'Hondt K, Riezman H et al. Clathrin functions in the absence of heterotetrameric adaptors and AP180-related proteins in yeast. EMBO J 1999; 18:3897-3908.

97. Rad MR, Phan HL, Kirchrath L et al. Saccharomyces cerevisiae Ap12p, a homologue of the mammalian clathrin AP beta subunit, plays a role in clathrin-dependent Golgi functions. J Cell Sci 1995; 108:1605-1615.

98. Grant B, Hirsh D. Receptor-mediated endocytosis in the Caenorhabditis elegans oocyte. Mol Biol Cell 1999; 10:4311-4326.

99. Shim J, Lee J. Moleular genetic analysis of apm-2 and aps-2, genes encoding the medium and small chains of the AP-2 clathrin-associated protein complex in the nematode Caenorhabditis elegans. Mol Cells 2000; 10:309-316.

100. Gonzalez-Gaitan M, Jackle H. Role of Drosophila α-adaptin in presynaptic vesicle recycling. Cell 1997; 88:767-776.

101. Berdnik D, Torok T, Gonzalez-Gaitan M et al. The endocytic protein α-adaptin is required for numb-mediated asymmetric cell division in Drosophila. Dev Cell 2002; 3:221-231.

102. Nesterov A, Carter RE, Sorkina T et al. Inhibition of the receptor-binding function of clathrin adaptor protein AP-2 by dominant-negative mutant $\mu2$ subunit and its effects on endocytosis. EMBO J 1999; 18:2489-2499.

103. Rous BA, Reaves BJ, Ihrke G et al. Role of adaptor complex AP-3 in targeting wild-type and mutated CD63 to lysosomes. Mol Biol Cell 2002; 13:1071-1082.

104. Blumstein J, Faundez V, Nakatsu F et al. The neuronal form of adaptor protein-3 is required for synaptic vesicle formation from endosomes. J Neuro 2001; 21:8034-8042.

105. Le Borgne R, Alconada A, Bauer U et al. The mammalian AP-3 adaptor-like complex mediates the intracellular transport of lysosomal membrane glycoproteins. J Biol Chem 1998; 273:29451-29461.

106. Storch S, Braulke T. Multiple C-terminal motifs of the 46-kDa Mannose 6-phosphate receptor tail contribute to efficient binding of medium chains of AP-2 and AP-3. J Biol Chem 2001; 276:4298-4303.

107. Drake MT, Zhu Y, Kornfeld S. The assembly of AP-3 adaptor complex-containing clathrin-coated vesicles on synthetic liposomes. Mol Biol Cell 2000; 11:3723-3736.
108. Simpson F, Bright NA, West MA et al. A novel adaptor-related protein complex. J Cell Biol 1996; 133:749-760.
109. Faundez V, Horng JT, Kelly RB. A function for the AP-3 coat complex in synaptic vesivle formation from endosomes. Cell 1998; 93:423-432.
110. Peden AA, Rudge RE, Winnie WY et al. Assembly and function of AP-3 complexes in cells expressing mutant subunits. J Biol Chem 2002; 156:327-336.
111. Cowles CR, Odorizzi G, Payne GS et al. The AP-3 adaptor complex is essential for cargo-selective transport to the yeast vacuole. Cell 1997; 91:109-118.
112. Piper RC, Bryant NJ, Stevens TH. The membrane protein alkaline phosphatase is delivered to the vacuole by a route that is distinct from the VPS-dependent pathway. J Cell Biol 1997; 138:531-545.
113. Stepp JD, Huang K, Lemmon SK. The yeast adaptor protein complex, AP-3, is essential for the efficient delivery of alkaline phosphatase by the alternative pathway to the vacuole. J Cell Biol 1997; 139:1761-1774.
114. Vowels JJ, Payne GS. A dileucine-like sorting signal directs transport into an AP-3-dependent, clathrin-independent pathway to the yeast vacuole. EMBO J 1998; 17:2482-2493.
115. Rehling P, Darsow T, Katzmann DJ et al. Formation of AP-3 transport intermediates requires Vps41p function. Nat Cell Biol 1999; 1:346-353.
116. Ooi CE, Moreira JE, Dell'Angelica EC et al. Altered expression of a novel adaptin leads to defective pigment granule biogenesis in the Drosophila eye color mutant garnet. EMBO J 1997; 16:4508-4518.
117. Mullins C, Hartnell LM, Wassarman DA et al. Defective expression of the μ3 subunit of the AP-3 adaptor complex in the Drosophila pigmentation mutant carmine. Mol Gen Genet 1999; 262:401-412.
118. Mullins C, Hartnell LM, Bonifacino JS. Distinct requirements for the AP-3 adaptor complex in pigment granule and synaptic vesicle biogenesis in Drosophila melanogaster. Mol Gen Genet 2000; 263:1003-1014.
119. Kretzschmar D, Poeck B, Roth H et al. Defective pigment granule biogenesis and aberrant behavior caused by mutations in the Drosophila AP-3 β-adaptin gene ruby. Genetics 2000; 155:213-223.
120. Salem N, Faundez V, Horng JT et al. A v-SNARE participates in synaptic vesicle formation mediated by the AP-3 adaptor complex. Nat Neurosci 1998; 1:551-556.
121. Kantheti P, Qiao X, Diaz ME et al. Mutation in AP-3 δ in the mocha mouse links endosomal transport to storage deficiency in platelets, melanosomes, and synaptic vesicles. Neuron 1998; 21:111-122.
122. Feng L, Seymour AB, Jiang S et al. The β3A subunit gene (Ap3b1) of the AP-3 adaptor complex is altered in the mouse hypopigmentation mutant pearl, a model for Hermansky-Pudlal syndrome and night blindness. Hum Mol Genet 1999; 8:323-330.
123. Dell'Angelica EC, Shotelersuk V, Aguilar RC et al. Altered trafficking of lysosomal proteins in Hermansky-Pudlak syndrome due to mutations in the β3A subunit of the AP-3 adaptor. Mol Cell 1999; 3:11-21.
124. Boehm M, Aguilar RC, Bonifacino JS. Functional and physical interactions of the adaptor protein complex AP-4 with ADP-ribosylation factors (ARFs). EMBO J 2001; 20:6265-6276.
125. Goldberg J. Structural basis for activation of ARF GTPase: Mechanisms of guanine nucleotide exchange and GTP-myristoyl switching. Cell 1998; 95:237-248.
126. Pasqualato S, Menetrey J, Franco M et al. The structural GDP/GTP cycle of human Arf6. EMBO Rep 2001; 2:234-238.
127. Puertollano R, Randazzo PA, Presley JF et al. The GGAs promote ARF-dependent recruitment of clathrin to the TGN. Cell 2001; 105:93-102.
128. Aguilar RC, Boehm M, Gorshkova I et al. Signal-binding specificity of the μ4 subunit of the adaptor protein complex AP-4. J Biol Chem 2001; 276:13145-13152.
129. Simmen T, Honing S, Icking A et al. AP-4 binds basolateral signals and participates in basolateral sorting in epithelial MDCK cells. Nat Cell Biol 2002; 4:154-159.
130. Barlowe C. Traffic COPs of the early secretory pathway. Traffic 2000; 1:371-377.
131. Klumperman J. Transport between ER and Golgi. Curr Opin Cell Biol 2000; 12:445-449.

132. Presley JF, Cole NB, Schroer TA et al. ER-to-Golgi transport visualized in living cells. Nature 1997; 389:81-85.
133. Malhotra V, Serafini T, Orci L et al. Purification of a novel class of coated vesicles mediating biosynthetic protein transport through the Golgi stack. Cell 1989; 58:329-336.
134. Waters MG, Serafina T, Rothman JE. "Coatomer": A cytosolic protein complex containing subunits of nonclathrin-coated Golgi transport vesicles. Nature 1991; 349:248-251.
135. Gu F, Gruenberg J. Biogenesis of transport intermediates in the endocytic pathway. FEBS Letts 1999; 452:61-66.
136. Griffiths G, Pepperkok R, Locker JK et al. Immunocytochemical localization of β-COP to the ER-Golgi boundary and the TGN. J Cell Sci 1995; 108:2839-2856.
137. Letourneur F, Gaynor EC, Hennecke S et al. Coatomer is essential for retrieval of dilysine-tagged proteins to the endoplasmic reticulum. Cell 1994; 79:1199-1207.
138. Lewis MJ, Pelham HRB. SNAREmediated retrograde traffic from the Golgi complex to the endoplasmic reticulum. Cell 1996; 85:205-215.
139. Lin C-C, Love HD, Gushue JN et al. ER/Golgi intermediates acquire Golgi enzymes by brefeldin A-sensitive retrograde transport in vitro. J Cell Biol 1999; 147:1457-1472.
140. Nickel W, Wieland FT. Biogenesis of COPI-coated transport vesicles. FEBS Letts 1997; 413:395-400.
141. Gaynor EC, Emr SD. COPI-independent anterograde transport: Cargo-selective ER to Golgi protein transport in yeast COPI mutants. J Cell Biol 1997; 136:789-802.
142. Pelham HRB. Traffic through the Golgi apparatus. J Cell Biol 2001; 155:1099-1101.
143. Whitney AJ, Gomez M, Sheff D et al. Cytoplasmic coat proteins involved in endosome function. Cell 1995; 83:703-713.
144. Aniento F, Gu F, Parton RG et al. An endosomal β-COP is involved in the pH-dependent formation of transport vesicles destined for late endosomes. J Cell Biol 1996; 133:29-41.
145. Daro E, Sheff D, Gomez M et al. Inhibition of endosome function in CHO cells bearing a temperaturesensitive defect in the coatomer (COPI) component ε-COP. J Cell Biol 1997; 139:1747-1759.
146. Piguet V, Gu F, Foti M et al. Nef-induced CD4 degradation: A diacidic-based motif in Nef functions as a lysosomal targeting signal through the binding of β-COP in endosomes. Cell 1999; 97:63-73.
147. Botelho RJ, Hackman DJ, Schreiber AD et al. Role of COPI in phagosome maturation. J Biol Chem 2000; 275:15717-15727.
148. Gu F, Aniento F, Parton RG et al. Functional dissection of COP-I subunits in the biogenesis of multivesicular endosomes. J Cell Biol 1997; 139:1183-1195.
149. Cosson P, Letourneur F. Coatomer interaction with di-lysine endoplasmic reticulum retention motifs. Science 1994; 263:1629-1631.
150. Stamnes MA, Craighead MW, Hoe MH et al. An integral membrane component of coatomer-coated transport vesicles defines a family of proteins involved in budding. Proc Natl Acad Sci USA 1995; 92:8011-8015.
151. Majoul I, Sohn K, Wieland FT et al. KDEL receptor (Erd2p)-mediated retrograde transport of the cholera toxin A subunit from the Golgi involves COPI, p23, and the COOH terminus of Erd2p. J Cell Biol 1998; 143:601-612.
152. Donaldson JG, Cassel D, Kahn RA et al. ADP-ribosylation factor, a small GTP-binding protein, is required for binding of the coatomre protein β-COP to Golgi membranes. Proc Natl Acad Aci USA 1992; 89:6408-6412.
153. Palmer DJ, Helms JB, Beckers CJ et al. Binding of coatomer to Golgi membranes requires ADP-ribosylation factor. J Biol Chem 1993; 268:12083-12089.
154. Presley JF, Ward TH, Pfeifer AC et al. Dissection of COPI and Arf dynamics in vivo and role in Golgi membrane transport. Nature 2002; 417:187-193.
155. Goldberg J. Decoding of sorting signals by coatomer through a GTPase switch in the COPI coat complex. Cell 2000; 100:671-679.
156. Lanoix J, Ouwendijk J, Stark A et al. Sorting of Golgi resident proteins into different subpopulations of COPI vesicles: A role for ArfGAP1. J Cell Biol 2001; 155:1199-1212.
157. Gu F, Gruenberg J. ARF1 regulates pH-dependent COP functions in the early endocytic pathway. J Biol Chem 2000; 275:8154-8160.

158. Gaynor EC, Chen C-Y, Emr SD et al. ARF is required for maintenance of yeast Golgi and endosome structure and function. Mol Biol Cell 1998; 9:653-670.

159. Rambourg A, Clermont Y, Jackson CL et al. Effects of brefeldin A on the three-dimensional structure of the Golgi apparatus in a sensitive strain of Saccharomyces cerevisiae. Anat Rec 1995; 241:109.

160. Dascher C, Balch WE. Dominant inhibitory mutants of ARF1 block endoplasmic reticulum to Golgi transport and trigger disassembly of the Golgi apparatus. J Biol Chem 1994; 269:1437-1448.164.

161. Lippincott-Schwartz J, Cole NB, Donaldson JG. Building a secretory apparatus: Role of ARF1/COPI in Golgi biogenesis and maintenance. Histochem Cell Biol 1998; 109:449-462.

162. Baker D, Hicke L, Rexach M et al. Reconstitution of SEC gene product-dependent intercompartmental protein transport. Cell 1988; 54:335-344.

163. Barlowe C, d'Enfert C, Schekman R. Purification and characterization of SAR1p, a small GTP-binding protein required for transport vesicle formation from the endoplasmic reticulum. J Biol Chem 1993; 268:873-879.

164. Salama NR, Yeung T, Schekman RW. The Sec13p complex and reconstitution of vesicle budding from the ER with purified cytosolic proteins. EMBO J 1993; 12:4073-4082.

165. Antonny B, Schekman R. ER export: Public transportation by the COPII coach. Cur Opin Cell Biol 2001; 13:438-443.

166. Matsuoka K, Schekman R, Orci L et al. Surface structure of the COPII-coated vesicle. Proc Natl Acad Sci USA 2001; 98:13705-13709.

167. Lederkremer GZ, Cheng Y, Petre BM et al. Structure of the Sec23p/34p and Sec13p/31p complexes of COPII. Proc Natl Acad Sci USA 2001; 98:10704-10709.

168. Scales SJ, Pepperkok R, Kreis TE. Visualization of ER-to-Golgi transport in living cells reveals a sequential mode of action for COPII and COPI. Cell 1997; 90:1137-1148.

169. Stephens DJ, Lin-Marq N, Pagano A et al. COPI-coated ER-to-Golgi transport complexes segregate from COPII in close proximity to ER exit sites. J Cell Sci 2000; 113:2177-2185.

170. Hammond AT, Glick BS. Dynamics of translational endoplasmic reticulum sites in vertebrate cells. Mol Cel Biol 2000; 11:3013-3030.

171. Antonny B, Madden D, Hamamoto S et al. Dynamics of the COPII coat with GTP and stable analogues. Nat Cell Biol 2001; 3:531-537.

172. Novick P, Field C, Schekman R. Identification of 23 complementation groups required for post-translational events in the yeast secretory pathway. Cell 1980; 21:205-215.

173. Barlowe C. COPII: A membrane coat that forms endoplasmic reticulum-derived vesicles. FEBS Letts 1995; 369:93-96.

174. Nakano A, Muramatsu M. A novel GTP-binding protein, Sar1p, is involved in transport from the endoplasmic reticulum to the Golgi apparatus. J Cell Biol 1989; 109:2677-2691.

175. Kappeler F, Klopfenstein DR, Foguet M et al. The recycling of ERGIC-53 in the early secretory pathway. J Biol Chem 1997; 272:31801-31808.

176. Nishimura N, Balch WE. A di-acidic signal required for selective export from the endoplasmic reticulum. Science 1997; 277:556-558.

177. Votsmeier C, Gallwitz D. An acidic sequence of a putative yeast Golgi membrane protein binds COPII and facilitates ER export. EMBO J 2001; 20:6742-6750.

178. Ma D, Zerangue N, Lin Y-F. Role of ER export signals in controlling surface potassium channel numbers. Science 2001; 291:316-319.

179. Fiedler K, Veit M, Stamnes MA et al. Bimodal interaction of coatomer with the p24 family of putative cargo receptors. Science 1996; 273:1396-1399.

180. Bermak JC, Li M, Bullock C et al. Regulation of transport of the dopamine D1 receptor by a new membrane-associated ER protein. Nat Cell Biol 2001; 3:492-498.

181. Boehm M, Bonifacino JS. Genetic analyses of adaptin function from yeast to mammals. Gene 2002; 20:175-186.

182. Dell'Angelica EC, Puertollano R, Mullins C et al. GGAs: A family of ADP ribosylation factor-binding proteins related to adaptors and associated with the Golgi complex. J Cell Biol 2000; 149:81-93.

183. Hirst J, Lui WWY, Bright NA et al. A family of proteins with γ-adaptin and VHS domains that facilitate trafficking between the trans-Golgi network and the vacuole/lysosome. J Cell Biol 2000; 149:67-79.

184. Boman AL, Zhang C-J, Zhu X et al. A family of ADP-ribosylation factor effectors that can alter membrane transport through the trans-Golgi. Mol Biol Cell 2000; 11:1241-1255.

185. Takatsu H, Yoshino K, Nakayama K. Adaptor γ-ear homology domain conserved in γ-adaptin and GGA proteins that interact with γ-synergin. Biochem Biophys Res Comm 2000; 271:719-725.

186. Poussu A, Lohi O, Lehto V-P. Vear, a novel Golgi-associated protein with VHS and γ-adaptin "ear" domains. J Biol Chem 2000; 275:7176-7183.

187. Doray B, Ghosh P, Griffiths J et al. Cooperation of GGAs and AP-1 in packaging MPRs at the trans-Golgi network. Science 2002; 297:1700-1703.

188. Mao Y, Nickitenko A, Duan X et al. Crystal structure of the VHS and FYVE tandem domains of Hrs, a protein involved in membrane trafficking and signal transduction. Cell 2000; 100:447-456.

189. Misra S, Beach BM, Hurley JH. Structure of the VHS domain of human Tom1 (target of myb1): insights into interactions with proteins and membranes. Biochemistry 2000; 19:11282-11290.

190. Puertollano R, Aguilar RC, Gorshkova I et al. Sorting of mannose 6-phosphate receptors mediated by the GGAs. Science 2001; 292:1712-1716.

191. Takatsu H, Katoh Y, Shiba Y et al. Golgi-localizing, γ-adaptin ear homology domain, ADP-ribosylation factor-binding (GGA) proteins interact with acidic dileucine sequences within the cytoplasmic domains of sorting receptors through their Vps27p/Hrs/STAM (VHS) domains. J Biol Chem 2001; 276:28541-28545.

192. Nielsen MS, Madsen P, Christensen EI et al. The sortilin cytoplasmic tail conveys Golgi-endosome transport and binds the VHS domain of the GGA2 sorting protein. EMBO J 2001; 2180-2190.

193. He X, Chang W-P, Koelsch G et al. Memapsin 2 (β-secretase) cytosolic domain binds to the VHS domains of GGA1 and GGA2: Implications on the endocytosis mechanism of memapsin 2. FEBS Letts 2002; 524:183-187.

194. Jacobsen L, Madsen P, Nielsen MS et al. The sorLA cytoplasmic domain interacts with GGA1 and −2 and defines minimum requirements for GGA binding. FEBS Letts 2002; 511:155-158.

195. Kato Y, Misra S, Puertollano R et al. Phosphoregulation of sorting signal-VHS domain interactions by a direct electrostatic mechanism. Nat Struct Biol 2002; 9:532-536.

196. Misra S, Puertollano R, Kato Y et al. Structural basis for acidic-cluster-dileucine sorting-signal recognition by VHS domains. Nature 2002; 415:933-937.

197. Shiba T, Takatsu H, Nogi T et al. Structural basis for recognition of acidic-cluster dileucine sequence by GGA1. Nature 2002; 415:937-941.

198. Zhdankina O, Strand NL, Redmond JM et al. Yeast GGA proteins interact with GTP-bound Arf and facilitate transport through the Golgi. Yeast 2001; 18:1-18.

199. Mullins C, Bonifacino JS. Structural requirements for function of yeast GGAs in vacuolar protein sorting, α-factor maturation, and interactions with clathrin. Mol Biol Cell 2001; 21:7981-7994.

200. Hirst J, Lindsay MR, Robinson MS. GGAs: Roles of the different domains and comparisons with AP-1 and clathrin. Mol Biol Cell 2001; 12:373-3588.

201. Black MW, Pelham HRB. A selective transport route from Golgi to late endosomes that requires the yeast GGA proteins. J Cell Biol 2000; 151:587-600.

202. Grigliatti TA, Hall L, Rosenbluth R et al. Temperaturesensitive mutations in Drosophila melanogaster. XIV. A selection of immobile adults. Mol Gen Genet 1973; 120:107-114.

203. Andrews J, Smith M, Merakovsky J et al. The stoned locus of Drosophila melanogaster produces a dicistronic transcript and encodes two distinct polypeptides. Genetics 1996; 143:1699-1711.

204. Fergestad T, Davis WS, Broadie K. The stoned protein regulates synaptic vesicle recycling in the presynaptic terminal. J Neurosci 1999; 19:5847-5860.

205. Phillips AM, Smith M, Ramaswami M et al. The products of the Drosophila stoned locus interact with synaptic vesicles via synaptotagmin. J Neurosci 2000; 20:8254-8261.

206. Fergestad T, Broadie K. Interactions of stoned and synaptotagmin in synaptic vesicle endocytosis. J Neurosci 2001; 21:1218-1227.

207. Cremona O, De Camilli P. Synaptic vesicle endocytosis. Curr Opin Neurobiol 1997; 7:323-330.

208. Martina JA, Bonangelino CJ, Aguilar RC et al. Stonin 2: An adaptor-like protein that interacts with components of the endocytic machinery. J Cell Biol 2001; 153:1111-1120.

209. Walther K, Krauss M, Diril MK et al. Human stoned B interacts with AP-2 and synaptotagmin and facilitates clathrin-coated vesicle uncoating. EMBO reports 2001; 2:634-640.

CHAPTER 3

The Role of Proteins and Lipids in Organelle Biogenesis in the Secretory Pathway

Thomas F. J. Martin

Abstract

Membrane compartments in the secretory pathway retain their identity in spite of continuous membrane and protein flux through each compartment. A challenge in cell biology is to discover how compartment identity is established and maintained. A related issue is how protein and membrane cargo is sorted from resident molecules in a donor compartment and vectorially delivered to an acceptor compartment without compromise to the integrity of individual compartments. We review accumulating evidence indicating that compartmental identity is conferred combinatorially by members of key protein families (Rabs, ARFs, SNAREs) and lipid constituents (phosphoinositides). These molecules and their effectors participate in assembling exit sites in donor compartments that sort and package cargo, and entry sites in recipient compartments that mediate cargo entry without intermixing compartment constituents.

Introduction

The classical morphological studies on fixed cells of Palade and coworkers[1] defined the organization and distribution of membrane organelles that constitute the secretory pathway of eukaryotic cells. This system, consisting of the endoplasmic reticulum (ER); the Golgi complex with cis, medial and trans cisternae; the trans Golgi network (TGN); endosomes and lysosomes and the plasma membrane, mediates membrane and protein transport between intracellular compartments and the plasma membrane. The static views of the system traditionally depicted in biology text books provides little indication of the dramatic turnover and flux of cargo through this system evident from classical studies and dramatically reemphasized in recent live cell imaging studies using fluorescent cargo.[2] A central challenge of cell biology is to discover how membrane compartments retain their identity in the face of continuous membrane and protein flux through those compartments. Related to this is the issue of how cargo is sorted at a donor compartment and vectorially delivered to an acceptor compartment with sufficient specificity to maintain the integrity of individual compartments. Research over the last decade has revealed that major families of proteins and lipids localize to specific membrane compartments in the secretory pathway and that these function combinatorially in complexes to establish specific exit and entry mechanisms that safeguard compartment identity and provide the machinery to mediate cargo flux out of and into compartments.

The Biogenesis of Cellular Organelles, edited by Chris Mullins. ©2005 Eurekah.com and Kluwer Academic/Plenum Publishers.

Protein Sorting Confers a Transient Nature to Secretory Pathway Organelles

In mammalian cells, the Golgi stack consists of functionally polarized cisternae through which cargo is sequentially conveyed for modification by Golgi-associated enzymes. In anterograde ("forward") trafficking in the secretory pathway, cargo is exported from the ER in tubulovesicular intermediates (also know as intermediate compartments, or ICs) that move on microtubule tracks to the cis Golgi region. The trans side of the Golgi is a key sorting station from which protein cargo (with associated biomolecules such as lipids and carbohydrates) is delivered to multiple intracellular and cell surface destinations, or secreted out of the cell, through the formation and selective trafficking of vesicular or tubulovesicular transport intermedates. Vesicles and tubulovesicular intermediates move along microtubules to endosomal or plasma membrane sites where they fuse for cargo delivery. Extensive retrograde ("reverse") trafficking from the plasma membrane through endosomes to lysosomes and the TGN, and from the Golgi to the ER, also characterize the secretory pathway. Time-lapse imaging studies of cargo proteins tagged with GFP have provided detailed estimates of the flux of membrane and soluble cargo passage through the secretory pathway and Golgi and yielded rate constants of ~3% min[-1].[3] Studies of GFP-tagged Golgi enzymes, in contrast, indicate that Golgi constituents are relatively stably associated with cisternal elements[4] although there is also substantial flux of Golgi constituents between cisternal elements and with the ER.[2]

Cargo trafficking through the ER-Golgi-endosomal-plasma membrane pathway involves at least four distinct, mechanistic steps: (1) formation of vesicular or tubulovesicular intermediates containing cargo for sorting, but not resident donor compartment constituents (i.e., "cargo sorting and vesicle budding"); (2) transport and targeting of transport intermediates to the acceptor compartment (i.e., "targeting"); (3) docking and tethering of donor vesicles at the acceptor compartment (i.e., "docking"); and (4) delivery of cargo to the acceptor compartment via membrane fusion (i.e., "fusion"). These steps must be accomplished with accuracy and specificity to ensure the maintenance of donor and acceptor compartments as well as the vectorial (anterograde or retrograde) delivery of cargo.

A key issue in understanding the biogenesis and maintenance of secretory organelles is determining how membrane compartments are maintained in the face of continuous membrane and protein flux during cargo trafficking, a process that by definition adds a transient quality to donor and acceptor compartments. Many questions relating to compartment maintenance persist. For example, are there protein and/or lipid constituents that characterize a specific compartment and confer its identity? How does cargo exit from one compartment and enter another without compromising the integrity of either compartment? How are transport intermediates conveyed to an acceptor compartment with the targeting specificity required to prevent compartment mixing? Without doubt, many cytosolic and membrane-bound factors are critical in these events. Key among these are the numerous protein and lipid mediators that confer specificity in sorting at exit points on donor compartment and specificity to targeting and fusion of transport vesicles at entry points at acceptor compartments. These factors are the subject of the following sections.

The Molecular Machinery Regulating Compartment Identity

The establishment and maintenance of compartment identity has occupied cell biologists for the last four decades (some excellent reviews addressing our current knowledge in this area include refs. 2, 5-9). Compartmental identity appears to be a combinatorial property established by hierarchies of protein family members and lipid constituents. In mammalian cells, these constituents consist of the six members of the ARF GTPase family, 60 members of the Rab GTPase family and their regulators, at least five isomers of inositol phospholipids (PI(3)P,

PI(4)P, PI(3,5)P$_2$, PI(4,5)P$_2$, and PI(3,4,5)P$_3$), 35 SNARE protein family members and seven Sec1p family accessory factors.[10] Members of the two largest families, the Rabs and SNAREs, are key constituents in targeting and fusion events in virtually all trafficking stations in the secretory pathway. Each of these protein families is sufficiently large to serve as unique identifiers of a membrane compartment and to confer specificity in transport and fusion events.[10-12] Individual Rab proteins are distributed in distinct and overlapping membrane compartments (Fig. 1) with Rab1 on the ER and early Golgi, Rab6 on middle to late Golgi, Rab5 and Rab4 on early endosomes, Rab11 on recycling compartments, Rab 9 on late endosomes and TGN, Rab3 on regulated secretory vesicles, etc.[13-15] Rab proteins cycle between GTP- and GDP-bound states, which regulate membrane binding.[13] Their critical roles as specifiers of compartment

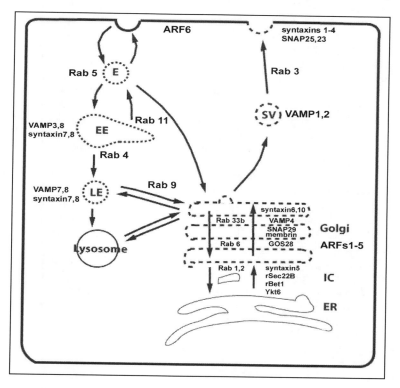

Figure 1. Secretory compartment identity is combinatorial. Individual compartments in the secretory pathway (ER= endoplasmic reticulum; IC= intermediate compartment; cis-medial-trans Golgi cisternae; SV= secretory vesicle; E= endosome; EE= early endosome; LE= late endosome; lysosome) contain specific members of a 35 member SNARE protein family, a 60 member Rab protein family, a six member ARF protein family and one of the four phosphoinositides (PI(4,5)P$_2$, PI(3)P, PI(4)P, and PI(3,5)P$_2$) utilized in trafficking. ARFs, phosphoinositides, cargo signals and coat proteins are assembled at exit points to generate tubulovesicular transport vesicles from a donor compartment. Vesicles are transported and docked for fusion at entry sites in acceptor compartments by the assembly of Rabs, phosphoinositides, tethering complexes and SNAREs. Recycling pathways return membrane constituents to donor compartments. Diagram depicts representative members of the SNARE protein family (from ref. 19), the Rab protein family (from ref. 15) and the ARF protein family (from ref. 44). The distributions of phosphoinositides on representative organelles are indicated: PI(4,5)P$_2$ (solid line), PI(3)P (short-hatch line), PI(4)P (long-hatch line), and PI(3,5)P$_2$ (not shown). Phosphoinostide localization is based on PLCd1-PH-GFP, FYVE$_2$-GFP and OSBP-PH-GFP probes (discussed in refs. 30, 34 and 35).

identity have been revealed by the characterization of multiprotein complexes that Rabs assemble to mediate the specific tethering of donor vesicles to acceptor membranes, which is accompanied by the activation of SNARE protein complexes for fusion.[16,17]

SNARE proteins also exhibit a membrane compartment-specific distribution (Fig. 1).[18,19] Cognate sets of SNAREs distributed between donor and acceptor compartments are involved in fusion between ER and Golgi (rSec22b, rBet1, membrin, ykt6, syntaxin5), within the Golgi (membrin, GOS-28, membrin, syntaxin16), between endosomes (syntaxins 7,8,13; VAMPs 3,8), and between secretory vesicles and plasma membrane (VAMP1,2; syntaxins 1-4; SNAP-25, 23).[18-20] SNARE proteins, originally classified as v- (vesicular) and t- (target membrane) SNAREs to designate donor and acceptor compartment proteins, have been more recently reclassified as R- or Q-SNAREs based on the presence of highly conserved arginine or glutamine residues.[21] The key feature of SNARE proteins is the presence of conserved heptad repeats in their sequences that form coiled-coil structures. A four-helix bundle forms between donor and acceptor membranes that consists of three SNARE helices contributed by Q-SNAREs in one membrane and one helix contributed by an R-SNARE in the other membrane.[22,23] In spite of an ability of soluble SNARE helices to promiscuously engage in complex formation in vitro, recent studies indicate a substantial degree of specificity in complex formation for membrane-associated SNAREs.[20,24] The formation of complexes between particular Q- and R-SNAREs likely imparts specificity to the fusion of particular donor and acceptor membranes. However, this specificity probably operates at a secondary level because SNARE complex formation follows Rab-dependent mechanisms that impart their own specificity for targeting and tethering of donor and acceptor membranes.[11,12]

The most recently defined constituents that impart compartmental identity to membranes consist of phosphorylated inositides (PIs). The inositol headgroup of phosphatidylinositol, a relatively abundant phospholipid of the cytoplasmic leaflet of membranes, undergoes dynamic phosphorylation at the 3-, 4- and 5-hydroxy positions of the ring to yield seven phosphorylated inositide lipids. Three of these, PI(3)P, PI(4)P and PI(4,5)P_2, and possibly a fourth PI(3,5)P_2, are widely employed in membrane trafficking at entry and exit sites.[25-29] Membranes in the secretory pathway contain characteristic PIs (Fig. 1). This was established by the distribution of PI-binding domain-GFP fusion protein chimeras, which has confirmed and extended biochemical studies of PI distribution. PI(4,5)P_2 exhibits a distribution largely restricted to the plasma membrane[30] (see ref. 31 for EM resolution) but can redistribute to endosomes under conditions of overstimulation.[32] PI(3)P is found exclusively in the early endosomal compartment.[33] PI(3,5)P_2 resides on the vesicular contents of multivesicular bodies in the endosomal pathway.[26] PI(4)P, while not as firmly established, is reported to reside mainly on Golgi cisternae.[34] Thus, the PIs demarcate membrane compartments and likely confer part of the identity to a membrane compartment. The localized synthesis of specific PIs through recruitment of lipid kinases establishes membrane domains within compartments as distinct exit and entry sites for vesicle fission and fusion. Phosphoinositide kinase and phosphatase mutants have been found to disrupt trafficking to and from specific organelles in yeast and mammalian cells.[26] A rich array of proteins that participate as effectors in specific stages of vesicle budding, docking/tethering and fusion contain domains that recognize and bind specific membrane PIs (Table 1). Stereoselective specific recognition of the inositol phosphates of the lipid headgroups is achieved through binding interactions with key lysine and arginine residues present in FYVE domains,[35,36] ENTH domains,[37] PX domains,[38] and PH domains.[39,40] GTPases with well-known roles in trafficking frequently have regulators (ARF-GEFs with PH domains) whose activities are controlled by PIs.[41] GTPases (ARFs and Rabs) in turn also regulate PI phosphorylation (see below).

The ARF proteins are fewer in number than the number of membrane compartments yet they implement specific cargo sorting operations essential for exit, and they catalyze vesicle

Table 1. Membrane trafficking proteins with phosphoinositide-binding motifs

Protein	Binding Motif	Lipid Binding	Role in Trafficking
epsin	ENTH[37]	$PI(4,5)P_2$	endocytosis
AP180/CALM	ENTH	$PI(4,5)P_2$	endocytosis
HRS/Vps27	VHS[130]		early to late endosome
	FYVE[36]	$PI(3)P$	
EAST	VHS	$PI(3)P$	endocytosis
GGA	VHS	?	TGN to endosome
EEA1	FYVE	$PI(3)P$	early endosome
Rabip4	FYVE	$PI(3)P$	recycling endosome
PIKfyve/Fab1p	FYVE	$PI(3)P$	multivesicular body formation
Rabenosyn-5	FYVE	$PI(3)P$	early and recycling endosome
Vac1p	FYVE	$PI(3)P$	TGN to endosome
Vam7p	PX[35,38,131,132]	$PI(3)P$	endosome to vacuole (lysosome)
Snx3	PX	$PI(3)P$	early to recycling endosome
Snx7, 16 etc	PX	$PI(3)P$	receptor endocytosis
PLD 1/2	PX	$PI(4,5)P_2$?	Golgi trafficking
	PH	$PI(4,5)P_2$	
Vps5, Vps17	PX	$PI(3)P$	sorting nexins; early, recycling endosomes
dynamin 1/2	PH[40,133]	$PI(4,5)P_2$	Golgi to PM, endocytosis
GRP1	PH	$PI(3,4,5)P_3$	ARF6-GEF
ARNO, cytohesin1	PH	$PI(3,4)P_2$ $PI(3,4,5)P_3$	ARF-GEF
β-spectrin, α-actinin	PH	$PI(4,5)P_2$	Golgi and PM cytoskeletal framework
CAPS	PH	$PI(4,5)P_2$	regulated vesicle exocytosis
Rabphilin3	C2[134]	$PI(4,5)P_2$	regulated vesicle exocytosis
synaptotagmin	C2	$PI(4,5)P_2$	regulated vesicle exocytosis

formation (Fig. 1). Class I ARFs (ARFs 1-3) are generally localized in the Golgi while the class III ARF (ARF6) is located at the plasma membrane and in peripheral endosomes.[41] Specific exit points in a compartment are probably dictated by the localization and regulation of a large number of ARF-GEF and ARF-GAP proteins that regulate the GTP cycle on these GTPases. Low molecular weight ARF-GEFs (ARNO/cytohesin and EFA6 families) functioning in the periphery contain PH domains that mediate their recruitment to sites of $PI(4,5)P_2$ and $PI(3,4,5)P_3$ production at the plasma membrane. Some ARF-GAPs similarly contain PH domains.[41-44] The higher molecular weight family of ARF-GEFs (Gea/GBF/GNOM and Sec7/ BIG families) localize to specific regions of the Golgi by mechanisms that are not clear.[45] ARF function is intimately tied to membrane PIs by the regulation of nucleotide exchange mediated by phospholipids[44] as well as by the fact that phosphoinositide kinases are direct effectors for ARFs[46-48] as are the phospholipase Ds (PLDs), which regulate phosphoinositide kinases through phosphatidic acid (PA) production.[42]

While neither the Rab, SNARE, ARF nor PI families of molecules may individually specify the nature of a compartment, a combinatorial code of these might. Thus, early endosomes are demarcated by Rab5, PI(3)P, FYVE domain-containing effectors that bind PI(3)P, and a specific constellation of SNARE proteins. Studies of trafficking have established that these molecules assemble to form the molecular machinery that controls specific exit from and entry into a compartment. Following a consideration of the general mechanisms employed for compartment exit and entry, specific examples where these molecular constituents are involved in selected aspects of traffic control in the secretory pathway will be discussed below.

General Mechanisms Employed for Cargo Exit and Entry: Fission and Fusion

Mechanisms operating at exit sites sort specific cargo and assemble constituents for vesicle budding and fission (Fig. 2). The class I ARF GTPases play a central role in these processes in the ER, Golgi and endosomal compartments by regulating the assembly of several types of vesicle coat complexes including COPI at the Golgi, AP-1-clathrin at the TGN, GGAs at the TGN, AP-4 at the TGN and AP-3-clathrin on endosomes.[49] Activated ARF-GTP binds membranes then recruits protein coat complexes COPI,[50] AP-1,[51] AP-4,[52] and the GGAs.[53] Adaptor-coat recruitment by ARF is a cooperative process aided by low affinity interactions of individual adaptor proteins with sorting signals on the cytoplasmic tails of transmembrane cargo proteins,[54] thus achieving the sorting of cargo into membrane domains destined for vesicle formation. PIs play an essential and complex role in ARF-dependent budding in the Golgi, as discussed below.

Mechanisms operating at entry sites target vesicles to specific acceptor membrane compartments and assemble the machinery for membrane fusion (Fig. 2). The Rab proteins are the primary determinants of vesicle transport and targeting to a membrane compartment where SNARE complex formation and fusion can occur. The characterization of Rab effector proteins reveals that a diverse array of protein complexes are assembled at the interface between a donor vesicle and an acceptor membrane. These represent an effective combinatorial mechanism for mediating specific membrane tethering interactions that are coupled to the activation of SNAREs for fusion. These Rab effector complexes are highly specialized for specific vesicle trafficking events and thus far exhibit few similarities between Rab systems.[16,17] One of the best-studied of these is a tethering complex for Rab5 involving EEA1 (early endosome antigen 1) on endosomes. The EEA1 complex interacts with Q-SNAREs, a Sec1 family protein and with NSF, all of which are thought to mediate SNARE complex activation for fusion.[15] Rab1 on ER vesicles utilizes p115 as an effector, which binds to GM130, a Golgi matrix component, and to giantin, a protein present on vesicles, to establish ER vesicle tethering to recipient Golgi membranes.[55,56] p115 also interacts with SNARE proteins, which provides a link to fusion.[57] p115 is additionally implicated in vesicle tethering and activation of the SNAREs GOS-28 and syntaxin5 in complex formation at the Golgi.[58] Rab2-mediated transport between the ER and Golgi utilizes golgin-45 as an effector in forming a tethering complex with a medial Golgi matrix protein GRASP55.[59] In yeast vacuolar homotypic fusion, the Rab Ypt7p interacts with Vps41p and Vps39p, which are part of a large complex of at least six proteins (termed the HOPS complex) that tethers vacuolar membranes and associates with a Vam3p-containing SNARE complex via a Sec1p homolog Vps33p.[60] In this case, the HOPS complex functions to activate a Rab, via the Ypt7p nucleotide exchange activity of Vps39p, as well an additional effector role. Both PI(3)P and PI(4,5)P$_2$ are required for priming and fusion steps for vacuolar membranes[60,61] although the binding partners for these lipids has not yet been defined. Sec4p, a yeast Rab on post-Golgi secretory vesicles destined to the plasma membrane, interacts with Sec15p that assembles into a complex of ten proteins (termed the "exocyst") that tethers vesicles

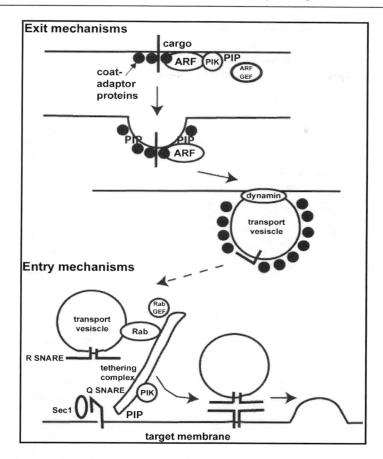

Figure 2. Exit from and entry into compartments utilize core constituents. Exit mechanisms: ARF proteins govern sites of exit from compartments through combinatorial interactions involving direct recruitment of coat and adaptor proteins, which in turn interact with sorting motifs on cargo proteins. ARFs recruit phosphatidylinositol kinases (PIK) that synthesize phosphoinositides (PIP) in membrane domains. Phosphoinositides in turn recruit coat and adaptor proteins and regulate the activity of ARF guanine nucleotide exchange factors (ARF-GEF). Recruitment of accessory factors along with adaptor-coat complexes results in deformation of membrane. Subsequent scission of nascent vesicle is promoted by dynamin. Entry mechanisms: Rab proteins govern transport vesicle targeting and tethering to acceptor membranes by recruiting Rab-binding proteins that serve as tethering complexes. Tethering complexes anchor donor and acceptor membranes, contain regulators of Rab guanine nucleotide exchange (Rab-GEF), and interact with membrane PIPs. Formation of local membrane domains of phosphoinositides is promoted by recruitment of PIK. Interactions of tethering complexes with NSF (not shown), members of the Sec1 protein family, and with Q-SNAREs promote organization of SNARE protein complexes. Fusion between donor and acceptor membranes is initiated by trans complexes formed between R- and Q-SNAREs.

at specific sites containing Sec3p, a spatial landmark on the plasma membrane, in advance of SNARE complex activation.[16] By assembling such unique multiprotein complexes that bridge donor and acceptor membranes, Rab proteins provide a layer of specificity to vesicle targeting. Through interactions with SNAREs, Sec1 family members and NSF, tethering complexes activate the next layer of specificity involving SNARE complex formation for fusion.

Exit Mechanisms in Trafficking

Exit from the Plasma Membrane into the Endosomal Pathway

Clathrin-mediated endocytosis from the plasma membrane is an example of a trafficking exit process that employs combinatorial mechanisms of cargo binding and localized synthesis of a PI to initiate the assembly of a complex of coat and adaptor proteins on a membrane domain. The macromolecular coat complex consisting of clathrin triskelions is thought to contribute to the physical deformation of the membrane that results in budding clathrin-coated vesicles.[62] The assembly of clathrin coats is mediated by a large number of mutually interacting proteins that are recruited to patches on the plasma membrane. Clathrin coat formation is initiated by membrane recruitment of the clathrin adaptor proteins AP-2 and AP180 that bind clathrin to coated pits. Accessory factors such as endophilin, epsin, amphiphysin and dynamin attach to the adaptors and lead to the formation of an invaginated vesicle attached to the membrane by a narrow neck. Amphiphysin and dynamin assemble in a helical array at the neck and the latter catalyzes GTP-dependent scission of the membrane to form a coated vesicle. Clathrin lattice formation is a process that can be nucleated by the binding of AP-2 and AP180 adaptors to membranes and has been reconstituted on artificial monolayer membranes.[63] In a cellular context, AP-2 recruitment to specific membrane sites would be mediated by binding to the cytoplasmic domains of transmembrane proteins that are cargo or receptors for soluble cargo that contain sorting signals for AP-2 binding.[54,62]

PI(4,5)P$_2$ on the plasma membrane plays an essential role in all aspects of clathrin-mediated endocytosis. A PI(4,5)P$_2$-binding PH domain fusion protein from PLCδ1 interferes with both early and late stages of endocytosis in permeable cells.[64] In addition, the inclusion of PI(4,5)P$_2$ in liposomes markedly enhances the formation of clathrin-coated vesicles formed from the liposomes by a collection of cytosolic factors.[65] The clathrin adaptors AP180 and AP2, epsin and dynamin each contain PI(4,5)P$_2$-binding domains[28] that are essential for mediating their recruitment to the membrane (Table 1). Synaptojanin1, a protein with inositol phospholipid 4- and 5-phosphatase activities, which would remove the PI(4,5)P$_2$ underlying the clathrin coat, is implicated in the uncoating of clathrin-coated vesicles.[66] The formation of clathrin lattices mediated by the assembly of a collection of proteins that each specifically binds PI(4,5)P$_2$ suggests that there are PI(4,5)P$_2$-rich plasma membrane domains that form at sites of endocytosis and that the control of PI(4,5P$_2$) synthesis at these sites plays a critical role in regulating the overall process of endocytosis.[29] This begs the question as to what regulates the formation of PI(4,5)P$_2$ at specific sites on the plasma membrane?

The γ isoform of PI(4)P 5-kinase is expressed at high concentrations in the nervous system where extensive endocytic recycling of synaptic vesicles occurs by PI(4,5)P$_2$-dependent mechanisms. This isoform is localized to GTPγS-arrested, clathrin-coated buds in synaptosomes and undergos Ca^{2+} influx-dependent dephosphorylation.[67] Dephosphorylation activates the kinase, which would cause local increases in PI(4,5)P$_2$ synthesis to accelerate the assembly of clathrin adapters and accessory factors for endocytic retrieval of synaptic vesicles following Ca^{2+}-triggered exocytosis.

Another potential mechanism that may accelerate endocytosis via recruitment of a PI(4)P 5-kinase and local activation of PI(4,5)P$_2$ synthesis is mediated by the ARF6 GTPase. ARF6 regulates several distinct pathways of endocytosis and membrane recycling. Overexpression of GTPase-defective ARF6 mutants in some cell types results in a dramatic accumulation of PI(4,5)P$_2$-rich, actin-coated vacuoles derived from endocytic vesicles that are unable to recycle back to the plasma membrane.[32] In other cell types, the same mutants stimulate clathrin-mediated endocytosis.[68] These effects of mutant ARF6 expression on peripheral membrane trafficking are likely mediated by the constitutive activation of PI(4)P 5-kinase, which is a direct effector of ARF6,[46] and the unregulated production of PI(4,5)P$_2$. This is supported by studies showing similar effects result from PI(4)P 5-kinase overexpression.[32] ARF6 has also been shown to be an important participant in β-arrestin-dependent, clathrin-mediated endocytosis of G protein-coupled receptors from the plasma membrane.[69] Activation of the β-adrenergic receptor is associated with β-ARK-mediated phosphorylation of the receptor and the recruitment of β-arrestin, which mediates the assembly of clathrin coats through interactions with clathrin and the β subunit of AP-2.[70] β-arrestin also interacts with ARNO, an ARF6 guanine nucleotide exchange factor, and with ARF6-GDP, likely promoting GTP exchange on ARF6 and its activation.[69] GIT1, an ARF6 GTPase activating protein, interacts with β-ARK.[71] This suggests that receptor occupancy may promote increased local recycling of ARF6. ARF6 activation would promote formation of PI(4,5)P$_2$-rich membrane domains. This in turn may enhance the recruitment of AP-2, β-ARK and other clathrin accessory factors that bind PI(4,5)P$_2$ during formation of clathrin-coated pits and scission of clathrin-coated vesicles.

Exit Points at the Golgi

While ARF6 has been implicated in the regulation of endocytic events relatively recently, the role of class I ARF proteins, especially ARF1, in Golgi trafficking has been studied extensively and is the subject of a number of excellent recent reviews.[14,41,42,44] There is general agreement that a central role of ARF proteins is recruitment of adaptor and/or coat proteins to membranes. An issue of considerable uncertainty for ARF function in the Golgi concerns the exact mechanism by which a diversity of vesicular or tubulovesicular membranes are formed at specific locations within the Golgi. A number of potential direct effectors for ARF have been identified including βCOP of the coatomer complex, the GGA proteins, phospholipase D1 (PLD1), arfaptins, mitotic kinesin-like protein, and phosphoinositide kinases.[41,44,47,48] Recent analysis of ARF1 mutants reveal that regions of the protein essential for COPI recruitment to Golgi membranes are distinct from those mediating activation of PLD1, and that neither effector appears to be essential for mediating the effects of ARF1 on Golgi vesiculation.[72] This suggests that other effector mechanisms were critical for ARF1 function in the Golgi. The discovery that phosphoinositide kinases[46-48] and GGA adaptors[73] are directly regulated by ARFs provides important new insights into the Golgi exit process.

There is considerable evidence that PIs, either PI(4)P or PI(4,5)P$_2$, play essential roles in the formation of transport vesicles for exit from the Golgi. The initial observation that Sec14p in yeast, a protein required for Golgi exit, encodes a PI transfer protein suggests that phospholipid metabolism is somehow coupled to protein trafficking mechanisms in the Golgi.[74] Recent work has establishes that PI(4)P levels decline in *sec14* mutants in which Golgi transit is defective whereas levels are restored in *sac1* mutants that suppress the *sec14* phenotype and restore Golgi transport.[75,76] The Sac1 gene encodes an inositol phospholipid phosphatase that can convert PI(4)P to PI.[77] Thus, defects in PI dephosphorylation (*sac1* mutations) appear to compensate for defects in synthesis (*sec14* mutations). Mutations in Pik1p, one of the yeast PI 4-kinases, also result in defects in Golgi exit of secretory cargo.[75,78,79] Pik1p localizes to the Golgi and is the homologue of PI 4-kinaseβ, which is recruited to the Golgi by ARF proteins in mammalian cells.[47] Recent work suggests that yeast Frq1p, a homologue of the mammalian Ca^{2+}-binding protein frequenin, may play a role in regulating the Pik1 PI 4-kinase in the Golgi.[80] Yeast cells containing *pik1* mutations accumulate Berkeley bodies, a phenotype that indicates a block in Golgi exit similar to that exhibited by cells lacking functional ARF1 or Sec14.[79] Consistent with this, reduced PI(4)P levels are detected in *arf1* mutants.[79] These results indicate that PI(4)P may be an important effector for ARF1 in Golgi exit mechanisms.

It is, however, unclear whether PI(4)P itself is essential or whether it serves as a precursor for PI(4,5)P$_2$, which could play an essential role. That PI(4)P, rather than PI(4,5)P$_2$, is critical is suggested by the fact that mutations in the only identified yeast PI(4)P 5-kinase, Mss4p, do not appear to affect Golgi transit.[79] What may be the effector of PI(4)P in Golgi export mechanisms? A by-pass suppressor of *sec14*, Kes1p, was identified as a yeast oxysterol binding protein that contains a PH domain that binds to PI(4)P.[34,81] Localization of the protein to the Golgi depends on the presence of a functional PH domain and Golgi PI(4)P.[34,81] Genetic studies suggest that Kes1p could function as a regulator or effector of ARF1, though its exact function remains to be determined.[81]

For the mammalian Golgi, there is evidence that PI(4,5)P$_2$ rather than, or in addition to, PI(4)P is an important effector for the role of ARF1 in trafficking. ARF1 recruits both PI-4 kinaseβ and PI(4)P 5-kinase to Golgi membranes in vitro to catalyze the sequential phosphorylation of PI to PI(4,5)P$_2$.[47] ARF1 directly activates the type I PI(4)P 5-kinase.[46,48] Although PI(4,5)P$_2$ principally resides in the plasma membrane, it is also detected in the Golgi.[31] The structure of the Golgi is highly dynamic and is ARF-dependent as indicated by its rapid disassembly induced by brefeldin A, a fungal antibiotic that inhibits certain ARF-GEF proteins.[82] There is also rapid disassembly and reassembly during and following mitosis.[6] Recent studies find that primary alcohols that inhibit PLD induce reversible Golgi fragmentation in vitro. These effects of alcohols are correlated with decreased PI(4,5)P$_2$ synthesis presumably resulting from decreased PA production by PLD, which might result in decreased PI(4)P 5-kinase activity.[83,84] Golgi fragmentation may result from disassembly of a spectrin-ankyrin-actin network like that characterized at the erythrocyte membrane and believed to serve as a structural scaffold.[85] A specific spectrin isoform (βIII) may constitute part of the foundation for anchoring an actin meshwork that structures the Golgi.[86] Spectrin recruitment to Golgi membranes depends upon ARF and PI(4,5)P$_2$ but not COPI or PLD, and is likely mediated in part by a carboxy-terminal PH domain in spectrin. Other studies show that actin recruitment to Golgi membranes is regulated by ARF, that actin is associated with budded vesicles, and that cytochalasin D inhibition of actin assembly altered the association of budded vesicles with the Golgi.[87] Evidence that the actin cytoskeleton and myosin motors are important for Golgi function has been reviewed recently[88,89] and it is suggested that vesicle fission, tethering, release or transport away from the Golgi could be mediated by the Golgi cytoskeleton. The central roles of ARF1 and PI(4,5)P$_2$ in the assembly of a Golgi actin skeleton and their involvement in Golgi vesicle budding may be analogous to the recently emergent role of ARF6 at the plasma membrane in recruiting PI(4)P 5-kinase for PI(4,5)P$_2$ synthesis,[46] clathrin-dependent and clathrin-independent endosome formation,[90] and actin cytoskeletal nucleation.[91]

How different protein cargoes are selected in the Golgi and packaged into vesicles or tubulovesicular compartments for transport to a variety of distinct destinations (endosomes, lysosomes, plasma membrane) remains a question of considerable interest. Each of several sorting and budding events is ARF-dependent and direct interactions between Golgi ARFs and COPI as well as the clathrin adapters are reported. Recent work on the GGA protein adapters provides considerable new insight into the sorting and budding of late endosome-directed vesicles, the formation of which results from a combinatorial set of interactions in the TGN between ARF, cargo, clathrin and other molecules. Three mammalian and two yeast genes encode the GGA proteins (Golgi-localized γ-ear-containing ARF binding proteins). The GGAs were discovered in yeast two-hybrid screens for ARF3 interacting proteins[92] or as proteins homologous to the clathrin-binding ear domain of γ-adaptin, a large subunit of AP-1.[93,94] These modular coat proteins link clathrin to ARF at exit sites in the TGN (for references see ref. 73). The GGA proteins are recruited to membranes through direct interactions with activated ARF-GTP (i.e., activated, membrane-bound ARF) and contain clathrin-box motifs that interact with the amino-terminal domain of clathrin. In addition, the GGA amino-terminal VHS domain interacts with acidic cluster-dileucine sorting signals in the cytoplasmic tails of mannose-6-phosphate receptors (M6PRs), whose luminal domains are required for sorting lysosomal hydrolases to late endosomal/lysosomal compartments.[95,96] Combinatorial interactions of the GGA proteins with ARF, clathrin and M6PR sorting motifs provides an elegant mechanism for coupling cargo selection with vesicle formation at Golgi exit sites.

The placement of ARF-GEFs and their regulation likely contribute to the localization of the above processes to specific sites at the TGN. In addition, the localized synthesis of $PI(4,5)P_2$ at sites on the Golgi may also play an important role in this localization.[44] The PIs, $PI(4)P$ or $PI(4,5)P_2$, could contribute to adaptor recruitment at the Golgi similarily to their recruitment of AP-2 and AP180 to the plasma membrane. PIs might interact with GGA proteins, although this has yet to be directly tested. The structure of the amino-terminal VHS domain in GGA proteins is remarkably similar to that of the structurally conserved amino-terminal ENTH domains present in AP180 and epsin that serves in $PI(4,5)P_2$ interaction.[63,97] Yeast mutants that lack inositol phospholipid phosphatases (i.e., synaptojanins) accumulate $PI(4,5)P_2$ at the plasma membrane and on intracellular organelles and they exhibit defects in trafficking out of the TGN to endosomes.[98] Interactions of adaptors and coats with $PI(4)P$ and $PI(4,5)P_2$ would help to specify membrane compartment identity as part of the combinatorial process for establishing the budding site.

Entry Mechanisms in Trafficking: Tethering, Priming and Fusion

Rab3 and the Entry of Secretory Vesicles into the Plasma Membrane by Exocytic Fusion

Because of its importance for integrated function and signaling in the nervous system, mechanisms responsible for the transport, tethering/docking and fusion of post-Golgi vesicles of the Ca^{2+}-regulated secretory pathway have been intensively studied.[18] Rab3 proteins are thought to play a central organizing role in directing vesicles into a regulated fusion pathway. However, the mechanisms involved have been difficult to identify. The membrane fusion mechanism for vesicle exocytosis is relatively well understood and is mediated by the vesicle SNARE protein VAMP2 and the plasma membrane SNAREs SNAP-25 and syntaxin1. These proteins are thought to "zipper" together to form trans complexes that mediate close membrane apposition and initiate fusion.[19]

The mechanisms responsible for targeting and tethering vesicles and for initiating SNARE complex assembly are not as well understood as those for vesicle fusion during exocytosis. Several accessory factors that interact with SNAREs are thought to have critical roles in targeting/tethering. Munc18/n-Sec1, a Sec1p family member, prevents SNARE complex formation by sequestering syntaxin1 in a closed conformation that fails to interact with SNAP-25 and VAMP2.[99,100] In recent studies, overexpression of munc18 in chromaffin cells increased the number of primed docked vesicles and enhanced exocytosis.[101] Conversely, vesicle docking and exocytosis are strongly decreased in chromaffin cells from *munc18* knockout mice.[101] This work suggests that munc18-bound syntaxin may be a platform for vesicle docking or tethering, and that vesicle arrival may initiate a transition to the open form of syntaxin competent for SNARE complex formation and fusion. In other membrane compartments (e.g., endosomes), Rab effectors and their partners function in vesicle tethering coupled to SNARE complex priming by interacting with members of the Sec1p family and/or with acceptor compartment SNAREs.[102] Secretory vesicles in neurons and endocrine cells contain Rab3 proteins. Thus, Rab3 or one its effectors could promote munc18 dissociation from syntaxin at the time of vesicle tethering or docking. There is evidence that Rab3 is involved in the processes of targeting and tethering secretory vesicles to the plasma membrane.[103-105]

Rabphilin3, a Rab3-binding protein that is peripherally bound to vesicles, is a potential Rab3 effector protein. Rabphilin3 contains an amino-terminal Rab3-binding domain[106] and tandem carboxy-terminal C2 domains that specifically bind $PI(4,5)P_2$ in a Ca^{2+}-dependent manner.[107] $PI(4,5)P_2$ on the plasma membrane is essential for the Ca^{2+}-dependent exocytosis of dense-core vesicles.[108] Also, Rabphilin3 is proposed to be one of the effectors of PIs that may mediate vesicle tethering.[107] Rab3A-deficient mice exhibit deficiencies in synaptic vesicle recruitment to synapses that are not evident in Rabphilin3 knockout mice.[109] However, there may be redundancies in vesicle tethering mechanisms that could account for this. A Rab3-binding protein with a domain organization similar to Rabphilin3, granulophilin, is expressed in certain endocrine cells in lieu of Rabphilin3 and binds munc18.[110] A protein with these properties could potentially activate syntaxin by munc18 displacement, though this remains to be investigated. While there is little evidence that Rabphilin3 actually functions as an effector of Rab3, aside from its ability to bind Rab3, it may nonetheless function as a vesicle-bound tethering protein that interacts with plasma membrane $PI(4,5)P_2$ and activates SNARE protein function. This model is supported by genetic interaction studies in *Caenorhabditis elegans*.[111] The carboxy-terminus of Rabphilin3 interacts with SNAP-25 and could play a role in SNARE activation.

Another potential Rab3 effector is Rim1 (Rab3-interacting molecule), which localizes to the active zone of synapses and is tethered in the presynaptic cytoskeletal matrix.[112] Rim1 is a multidomain protein that contains an amino-terminal Rab3-binding domain and PDZ and C2 domains. Rim1 interacts with a number of proteins including the plasma membrane SNARE, SNAP-25, the Ca^{2+} sensor synaptotagmin, and other presynaptic constituents (Ca^{2+} channels and α-liprins), thus indicating it may tether synaptic vesicles to the plasma membrane via interactions with vesicle Rab3 and plasma membrane proteins.[113,114] Rim1 also interacts with munc13-1, a protein thought to function in the priming of SNARE proteins. Munc13-1 interacts with the amino-terminal domain of syntaxin and may promote formation or stabilization of the open form of syntaxin through competing with munc18 binding.[115] Vesicle priming can be regulated in a Ca^{2+}-dependent manner in a form of synaptic plasticity known as "augmentation". Recent work has indicated this form of plasticity may be mediated through Ca^{2+}-dependent, phospholipase C-catalyzed hydrolysis of $PI(4,5)P_2$ to diacylglycerol (DAG), which can bind to the C1 domain of munc13-1 to enhance its activity in SNARE priming.[116] Thus, Rim1 may be a Rab3 effector that tethers synaptic vesicles and localizes binding partners (such as munc13-1) that act to promote SNARE complex formation for fusion.

Rab5 Governs Entry Points in the Endosomal-Lysosomal Pathway

Fusion in the endosomal trafficking pathway is directed by protein tethering complexes organized by Rab5 and other Rab proteins in the membrane context of PI(3)P. A role for PI(3)P is evident from studies of protein transport to the yeast vacuole in which an essential function for the VPS (vacuolar protein sorting) gene VPS34 was identified.[26] VPS34 encodes a lipid kinase that phosphorylates PIs at the 3- position of the inositol ring. Rab5 is an essential component in the homotypic fusion of early endosomes, which can be reconstituted in a cell-free assay.[117] Rab5-GTP interacts with a large (> 20) number of potential effector proteins in affinity chromatography experiments.[117] Two of the Rab5-binding proteins, Rabex-5 and Rabaptin-5, form a complex that acts to activate GDP for GTP exchange on Rab5. The importance of EEA1 as a Rab5 effector required for endosome fusion is shown through endosome fusion assays. Here EEA1 is found to be the major constituent of the required cytosol fraction. EEA1 contains amino- and carboxy-terminal Rab5-GTP binding domains that mediate tethering of endosomes in preparation for fusion. Endosome tethering is reinforced by a carboxy-terminal FYVE domain in EEA1 that interacts with PI(3)P on the endosome.[118] EEA1 also binds hVPS34, a PI 3-kinase, whose recruitment to the endosomal membrane could promote additional synthesis of PI(3)P and lead to the formation of membrane microdomains in the endosome.[119] EEA1 also interacts with the SNARE syntaxin 13, which is required for homotypic endosome fusion, and with NSF, which may prime SNARE complexes for fusion.[120] In yeast, a Rab5/

Ypt21p effector containing a FYVE domain, Vac1p, interacts with Vps45p, a Sec1 homolog, as well as with Pep12p, an endosomal SNARE.[26,121] EEA1, as a major component of a Rab5 effector complex, may function to couple membrane tethering to SNARE protein activation for fusion. Overall, the mechanisms elucidated for Rab5-mediated endosomal entry illustrates the operation of a heirarchy of membrane-specific protein and lipid constituents that interact to assemble complexes governing the fusion specificity of homologous membrane compartments.

Rab4, 5 and 11 are present in overlapping as well as distinct membrane regions in endosomal compartments.[122] A second FYVE domain-containing Rab5 effector, Rabenosyn-5, was recently identified[102] and shown to also interact with Rab4.[123] Rabenosyn-5 binds hVPS45, a Sec-1 family protein that interacts with early endosomal SNARE proteins syntaxins 13, 6 and 4. Rabaptin-5 also interacts with Rab4 in a similar manner.[123] Dual effectors for these Rabs are proposed to mediate the assembly of segregated but adjacent Rab5 and Rab4 domains on endosomal membranes. Rab4 also has an identified potential effector, Rab4ip. Rab4ip contains a FYVE domain, indicating that it too operates within PI(3)P-containing membrane domains in the endosomal system.[124] Recycling membrane proteins such as the transferin receptor are believed to enter the endosomal pathway through Rab5-containing endosomes and transit to recycling endosomes marked by Rab4. Hybrid Rab5/Rab4-containing compartments represent intermediates in the internalization and recycling pathway, and the dual Rab effectors such as Rabenosyn-5 and Rabaptin-5 function to coordinate neighboring membrane domains. Rabaptin-5 also interacts with Rabphilin-3, an effector for Rab3 (see above), thus suggesting Rab5-containing membrane domains coordinate endocytosis that follows exocytosis of Rab3-containing membrane domains in synaptic vesicles.[125]

While PI(3)P-containing membranes characterize the early and recycling endosomal pathway, a distinct PI, PI(3,5)P_2, plays an important role in the late endosomal pathway. The Fab1 gene in yeast encodes a FYVE finger domain protein with PI(3)P 5-kinase activity and a characterized mammalian counterpart, PIKfyve.[126-128] Cells containing *fab1* mutations exhibit enlarged vacuoles[126] and overexpression of a dominant negative PIKfyve in mammalian cells results in vacuolization of endosomal compartments.[129] It is thought that PI(3,5)P_2 plays an essential permissive role in membrane budding into or out of multivesicular bodies that enables sorting of endosomal cargo into the lumen of this compartment or back to earlier endosomal compartments. The factors regulating Fab1p/PIKfyve activity or mediating the essential role of PI(3,5)P_2 remain to be discovered. Nonetheless, this represents an intriguing switch for shutting down PI(3)P-dependent Rab function in the early endosomal pathway while activating late endosomal membrane trafficking events.[26]

Future Prospects

The last decade has witnessed dramatic progress in the discovery of protein and lipid constituents that control trafficking in the secretory pathway. New technologies for protein study and the wealth of information gained from genome sequencing projects are rapidly driving the identification and characterization of the most critical factors. At the key nodes in trafficking, the sorting of cargo into assembled transport intermediates and the targeting of transport intermediates to their correct destinations for fusion, the ARF and Rab GTPases, respectively, govern the assembly of macromolecular machines that control exit and entry specificity. Thus, future challenges will involve discoveries of the precise composition of these machineries, the interactions that mediate their assembly, and the biophysical basis by which they interface with membranes to promote fission and fusion.

References

1. Palade G. Intracellular aspects of the process of protein synthesis. Science 1975; 189:347-358.
2. Lippincott-Schwartz J, Roberts TH, Hirschberg K. Secretory protein trafficking and organelle dynamics in living cells. Annu Rev Cell Dev Biol 2000; 16:557-589.
3. Hirschberg K, Miller CM, Ellenberg J et al. Kinetic analysis of secretory protein traffic and characterization of Golgi to plasma membrane transport intermediates in living cells. J Cell Biol 1998; 143:1485-1503.
4. Scaiky N, Presley J, Smith C et al. Golgi tubule traffic and the effects of brefeldin A visualized in living cells. J Cell Biol 1997; 139:1137-1155.
5. Rothman JE, Wieland FT. Protein sorting by transport vesicles. Science 1996; 272:227-234.
6. Warren G, Malhotra V. The organization of the Golgi apparatus. Curr Opin Cell Biol 1998; 10:493-498.
7. Jamieson JD. The Golgi complex: Perspectives and prospectives. Biochim Biophys Acta 1998; 1404:3-7.
8. Pelham HRB. Getting through the Golgi complex. Trends Cell Biol 1998; 8:45-49.
9. Glick BS. Organization of the Golgi apparatus. Curr Opin Cell Biol 2000; 12:450-456.
10. Bock JB, Matern HT, Peden AA et al. A genomic perspective on membrane compartment organization. Nature 2001; 409:839-841.
11. Pelham HRB. SNAREs and the specificity of membrane fusion. Trends Cell Biol 2001; 11:99-101.
12. Scales SJ, Bock JB, Scheller RH. The specifics of membrane fusion. Nature 2000; 407:144-146.
13. Novick P, Zerial M. The diversity of Rab proteins in vesicle transport. Curr Opin Cell Biol 1997; 9:496-504.
14. Takai Y, Sasaki T, Matozaki T. Small GTP-binding proteins. Physiological Reviews 2001; 81:153-208.
15. Zerial M, McBride H. Rab proteins as membrane organizers. Nature Rev Cell Mol Biol 2001; 2:107-119.
16. Guo W, Sacher M, Barrowman J et al. Protein complexes in transport vesicle targeting. Trends Cell Biol 2000; 10:251-255.
17. Pfeffer SR. Rab GTPases: Specifying and deciphering organelle identity and function. Trends Cell Biol 2001; 11:487-491.
18. Jahn R, Sudhof TC. Membrane fusion and exocytosis. Annu Rev Biochem 1999; 68:863-911.
19. Chen YA, Scheller RH. SNAREmediated membrane fusion. Nature Rev Cell Mol Biol 2001; 2:98-106.
20. McNew JA, Parlati F, Fukuda R et al. Compartmental specificity of cellular membrane fusion encoded in SNARE proteins. Nature 2000; 407:153-159.
21. Fasshauer D, Sutton RB, Brunger AT et al. Conserved structural features of the synaptic fusion complex: SNARE proteins reclassified as Q- and R-SNAREs. Proc Natl Acad Sci USA 1998; 95:15781-15786.
22. Sutton RB, Fasshauer D, Jahn R et al. Crystal structure of a SNARE complex involved in synaptic exocytosis at 2.4 angstrom resolution. Nature 1998; 395:347-353.
23. Parlati F, McNew JA, Fukuda R et al. Topological restriction of SNAREdependent membrane fusion. Nature 2000; 407:194-198.
24. Scales SJ, Chen YA, Yoo BY et al. SNAREs contribute to the specificity of membrane fusion. Neuron 2000; 26:457-464.
25. Martin TFJ. Phosphoinositide lipids as signaling molecules: Common themes for signal transduction, cytoskeletal regulation and membrane trafficking. Annu Rev Dev Biol 1998; 14:231-264.
26. Odorizzi G, Babst M, Emr SD. Phosphoinositide signaling and the regulation of membrane trafficking in yeast. Trends Biochem Sci 2000; 25:229-235.
27. Simonsen A, Wurmser AE, Emr SD et al. The role of phosphoinositides in membrane transport. Curr Opin Cell Biol 2001; 13:485-492.
28. Cremona O, DeCamilli P. Phosphoinositides in membrane traffic at the synapse. J Cell Sci 2001; 114:1041-1052.
29. Martin TFJ. PI(4,5)P$_2$ regulation of surface membrane traffic. Curr Opin Cell Biol 2001; 13:493-499.

30. Balla T, Bondeva T, Varnai P. How accurately can we image inositol lipids in living cells? Trends Pharmacol. Sci 2000; 21:238-241.

31. Watt SA, Kular G, Fleming IN et al. Subcellular localization of phosphatidylinositol 4,5-bisphosphate using the pleckstrin homology domain of phospholipase C d1. Biochem J 2002; 363:657-666.

32. Brown FD, Rozelle AL, Yin HL et al. Phosphatidylinositol 4,5-bisphosphate and ARF6-regulated membrane traffic. J Cell Biol 2001; 154:1007-1017.

33. Gillooly DJ, Morrow IC, Lindsay M et al. Localization of phosphatidylinositol 3-phosphate in yeast and mammalian cells. EMBO J 2000; 19:4577-4588.

34. Levine TP, Munro S. Targeting of Golgi-specific pleckstrin homology domains involves both PI 4-kinase-dependent and –independent components. Curr Biol 2002; 12:695-704.

35. Gillooly DJ, Simonsen A, Stenmark H. Cellular functions of phosphatidylinositol 3-phosphate and FYVE domain proteins. Biochem J 2001; 355:249-258.

36. Stenmark H, Aasland R, Driscoll PC. The phosphatidylinositol 3-phosphate binding FYVE finger. FEBS Lett 2002; 513:77-84.

37. DeCamilli P, Chen H, Hyman J et al. The ENTH domain. FEBS Lett 2002; 513:11-18.

38. Sato TK, Overduin M, Emr SD. Location, location, location: Membrane targeting directed by PX domains. Science 2001; 294:1881-1885.

39. Blomberg N, Baraldi E, Nilges M et al. The PH superfold: A structural scaffold for multiple functions. Trends Biochem Sci 1999; 24:441-445.

40. Lemmon MA, Ferguson KM. Signal-dependent membrane targeting by pleckstrin homology (PH) domains. Biochem J 2000; 350:1-18.

41. Donaldson JG, Jackson CL. Regulators and effectors of the ARF GTPases. Curr Opin Cell Biol 2000; 12:475-482.

42. Roth MG. Lipid regulators of membrane traffic through the Golgi complex. Trends Cell Biol 1999; 9:174-179.

43. Jackson CL, Casanova JE. Turning on ARF: The sec7 family of guanine nucleotide exchange factors. Trends Cell Biol 2000; 10:60-66.

44. Randazzo PA, Nie Z, Miura K et al. Molecular aspects of the cellular activities of ADP-ribosylation factors. Science 2000; STKE.

45. Zhao X, Lasell TKR, Melancon P. Localization of large ADP-ribosylation factor-guanine nucleotide exchange factors to different Golgi compartments: Evidence for distinct functions in protein traffic. Mol Biol Cell 2002; 13:119-133.

46. Honda A, Nogami M, Yokozeki T et al. Phosphatidylinositol 4-phosphate 5-kinase alpha is a downstream effector of the small G protein ARF6 in membrane ruffle formation Cell 1999; 99:521-532.

47. Godi A, Pertile P, Meyers R et al. ARF mediates recruitment of PI 4-kinaseb and stimulates synthesis of PI(4,5)P2 on the Golgi complex. Nature Cell Biol 1999; 1:280-287.

48. Jones DH, Morris JB, Morgan CP et al. Type I phosphatidylinositol 4-phosphate 5-kinase directly interacts with ADP-ribosylation factor 1 and is responsible foro phosphatidylinositol 4,5-bisphosphate in the Golgi compartment. J Biol Chem 2000; 275:13963-13966.

49. Robinson MS, Bonifacino JS. Adaptor-related proteins. Curr Opin Cell Biol 2001; 13:444-453.

50. Zhao L, Helms JB, Brugger B et al. Direct and GTP-dependent interaction of ADP ribosylation factor 1 with coatomer subunit beta. Proc Natl Acad Sci USA 1997; 94:4418-4423.

51. Austin C, Hinners I, Tooze SA. Direct and GTP-dependent interaction of ADP-ribosylation factor 1 with clathrin adaptor protein AP-1 on immature secretory granules. J Biol Chem 2000; 275:21862-21869.

52. Boehm M, Aguilar RC, Bonifacino JS. Functional and physical interactions of the adaptor protein complex AP-4 with ADP-ribosylation factors (ARFs). EMBO J 2001; 20:6265-6276.

53. Puertollano R, Randazzo PA, Presley JF et al. The GGAs promote ARF-dependent recruitment of clathrin to the TGN. Cell 2001; 105:93-102.

54. Kirchhausen T Adaptors for clathrin-mediated traffic. Annu Rev Cell Dev Biol 1999; 15:705-532.

55. Moyer BD, Allan BB, Balch WE. Rab1 interaction with a GM130 effector complex regulates COPII vesicle Golgi tethering. Traffic 2001; 2:268-276.

56. Weide T, Bayer M, Koster M et al. The Golgi matrix protein GM130: A specific interaction partner of the small GTPase Rab1b. EMBO Rep 2001; 2:336-341.

57. Allan BB, Moyer BD, Balch WE. Rab1 recruitment of p115 into a cis-SNARE complex: Programming budding COPII vesicles for fusion. Science 2000; 289:444-448.

58. Shorter J, Beard MB, Seemann J et al. Sequential tethering of Golgins and catalysis of SNAREpin assembly by the vesicle-tethering protein p115. J Cell Biol 2002; 157:45-62.

59. Short B, Preisinger C, Korner R et al. A GRASP55-rab2 effector complex linking Golgi structure to membrane traffic. J Biol Chem 2001; 155:877-883.

60. Wickner W. Yeast vacuoles and membrane fusion pathways. EMBO J 2002; 21:1241-1247.

61. Mayer A. What drives membrane fusion in eukaryotes? Trends Biochem. Sci 2001; 26:717-723.

62. Schmid SL. Clathrin-coated vesicle formation and protein sorting: An integrated process. Annu Rev Biochem 1997; 66:511-548.

63. Ford MGJ, Pearse BMF, Higgins MK et al. Simultaneous binding of PtdIns(4,5)P_2 and clathrin by AP180 in the nucleation of clathrin lattices on membranes. Science 2001; 291:1051-1055.

64. Jost M, Simpson F, Kavran JM et al. Phosphatidylinositol 4,5-bisphosphate is required for endocytic coated vesicle formation. Curr Biol 1998; 8:1399-1402.

65. Kinuta M, Yamada H, Abe T et al. Phosphatidylinositol 4,5-bisphosphate stimulates vesicle formation from liposomes by brain cytosol. Proc Natl Acad Sci USA 2002; 99:2842-2847.

66. Cremona O, DiPaolo G, Wenk MR et al. Essential role of phosphoinositide metabolism in synaptic vesicle recycling. Cell 1999; 99:179-188.

67. Wenk MR, Pellegrini L, Klenchin VA et al. PIP kinase Ig is the major PI(4,5)P_2 synthesizing enzyme at the synapse. Neuron 2001; 32:79-88.

68. Altshuler Y, Liu S, Katz L et al. ADP ribosylation factor 6 and endocytosis at the apical surface of Madin-Darby canine kidney cells. J Cell Biol 1999; 147:7-12.

69. Claing A, Chen W, Miller WE et al. b-arrestin-mediated ADP-ribosylation factor 6 activation and b-adrenergic receptor endocytosis. J Biol Chem 2001; 276:42509-42513.

70. Perry SJ, Lefkowitz RJ. Arresting developments in heptahelical receptor signaling and regulation. Trends Cell Biol 2002; 12:130–138.

71. Vitale N, Patton WA, Moss J et al. GIT proteins, a novel family of phosphatidylinositol 3,4,5-trisphosphate-stimulated GTPase-activating proteins for ARF6. J Biol Chem 2000; 275:13901-13906.

72. Kuai J, Boman AL, Arnold RS et al. Effects of activated ADP-ribosylation factors on Golgi morphology require neither activation of phospholipase D1 nor recruitment of coatomer. J Biol Chem 2000; 275:4022-4032.

73. Boman AL. GGA proteins: New players in the sorting game. J Cell Science 2001; 114:3413-3418.

74. Huijbregts RPH, Topalof L, Bankaitis VA. Lipid metabolism and regulation of membrane trafficking. Traffic 2000; 1:195-202.

75. Hama H, Schnieders EA, Thorner J et al. Direct involvement of phosphatidylinositol 4-phosphate in secretion in the yeast Saccharomyces cerevisiae. J Biol Chem 1999; 274:34294-34300.

76. Foti M, Audhya A, Emr SD. Sac1 lipid phosphatase and Stt4 phosphatidylinositol 4-kinase regulate a pool of phosphatidylinositol 4-phosphate that functions in the control of the actin cytoskeleton and vacuole morphology. Mol Biol Cell 2001; 12:2396-2411.

77. Guo S, Stolz LE, Lemrow SM et al. Sac1-like domains of yeast SAC1, INP52 and INP53 and of human synaptojanin encode polyphosphoinositide phosphatases. J Biol Chem 1999; 274:12990-12995.

78. Walch-Solimena C, Novick P. The yeast phosphatidylinositol 4-kinase Pik1 regulates secretion at the Golgi. Nature Cell Biol 1999; 1:523-525.

79. Audhya A, Foti M, Emr SD. Distinct roles for the yeast phosphatidylinositol 4-kinases, Stt4p and Pik1p, in secretion, cell growth and organelle membrane dynamics. Mol Biol Cell 2000; 11:2673-2689.

80. Hendricks KB, Wang BQ, Schnieders EA et al. Yeast homologue of neuronal frequenin is a regulator of phosphatidylinositol 4-kinase. Nature Cell Biol 1999; 138:234-241.

81. Li X, Rivas MP, Fang M et al. Analysis of oxysterol binding protein homologue Kes1p function in regulation of Sec14p-dependent protein transport from the yeast Golgi complex. J Cell Biol 2002; 157:63-77.

82. Donaldson JG, Klausner R. ARF: A key regulatory switch in membrane traffic and organelle structure. Curr Opin Cell Biol 1994; 6:527-531.

83. Siddhanta A, Backer JM, Shields D. Inhibition of phosphatidic acid synthesis alters the structure of the Golgi apparatus and inhibits secretion in endocrine cells. J Biol Chem 2000; 275:12023-12031.

84. Sweeney DA, Siddhanta A, Shields D. Fragmentation and reassembly of the Golgi apparatus in vitro. J Biol Chem 2002; 277:3030-3039.

85. DeMatteis MA, Morrow JS. The role of ankyrin and spectrin in membrane transport and domain formation. Curr Opin Cell Biol 1998; 10:542-549.

86. Godi A, Santone I, Pertile P et al. ADP ribosylation factor regulates spectrin binding to the Golgi complex. Proc Natl Acad Sci USA 1998; 95:8607-8612.

87. Fucini RV, Navarrete A, Vadakkan C et al. Activated ADP-ribosylation factor assembles distinct pools of actin on Golgi membranes. J Biol Chem 2000; 275:1882-18829.

88. Holleran EA, Holzbauer EL. Speculating about spectrin: New insights into the Golgi-associated cytoskeleton. Trends Cell Biol 1998; 8:26-29.

89. Stow JL, Heimann K. Vesicle budding on Golgi membranes: Regulation by G proteins and myosin motors. Biochim Biophys Acta 1998; 1404:161-171.

90. Nichols BJ, Lippincott-Schwartz J. Endocytosis without clathrin coats. Trends Cell Biol 2001; 11:406-412.

91. Schafer DA, D'Souza-Schorey C, Cooper JA. Actin assembly at membranes controlled by ARF6. Traffic 2000; 1:892-903.

92. Boman AL, Zhang C, Zhu X et al. A family of ADP-ribosylation factor effectors that can alter membrane transport through the trans Golgi. Mol Biol Cell 2000; 11:1241-1255.

93. Dell'Angelica EC, Puertollano R, Mullins C et al. GGAs: A family of ADP-ribosylation factor-binding proteins related to adaptors and associated with the Golgi complex. J Cell Biol 2000; 149:81-94.

94. Hirst J, Lui WW, Bright NA et al. A family of proteins with g-adaptin and VHS domains that facilitate trafficking between the trans-Golgi network and the vacuole/lysosome. J Cell Biol 2000; 149:67-80.

95. Misra S, Beach BM, Hurley JH. Structure of the VHS domain of human TomI: Insights into interactions with proteins and membranes. Biochemistry 2000; 39:11282-11290.

96. Shiba T, Takatsu H, Nogi T et al. Structural basis for recognition of acidic cluster dileucine sequence by GGA1. Nature 2002; 415:937-941.

97. Itoh T, Koshiba S, Kigawa T et al. Role of the ENTH domain in phosphatidylinositol 4,5-bisphosphate binding and endocytosis. Science 2001; 291:1047-1051.

98. Stefan CJ, Audhya A, Emr SD. The yeast synaptojanin-like proteins control the cellular distribution of phosphatidylinositol 4,5-bisphosphate. Mol Biol Cell 2002; 13:542-557.

99. Dulubova I, Sugita S, Hill S et al. A conformational switch in syntaxin during exocytosis: Role of munc18. EMBO J 1999; 18:4372-4382.

100. Yang B, Steegmaier M, Gonzalez LC et al. nSec1 binds a closed conformation of syntaxin1A. J Cell Biol 2000; 148:247-252.

101. Voets T, Toonen RF, Brian EC et al. Munc18-1 promotes large dense-core vesicle docking. Neuron 2001; 31:581-591.

102. Nielsen E, Christoforidis S, Uttenweiler-Joseph S et al. Rabenosyn-5, a novel Rab5 effector, is complexed with hVPS45 and recruited to endosomes through a FYVE finger domain. J Cell Biol 2000; 151:601-612.

103. Geppert M, Bolshakov VY, Siegelbaum SA et al. The role of Rab3A in neurotransmitter release. Nature 1994; 369:493-497.

104. Nonet ML, Staunton JE, Kilgard MP et al. Caehorhabditis elegans rab-3 mutant synapses exhibit impaired function and are partially depleted of vesicles. J Neurosci 1997; 17:8061-8073.

105. Martelli AM, Baldini G, Tabellini G et al. Rab3A and Rab3D control the total granule number and the fraction of granules docked at the plasma membrane in PC12 cells. Traffic 2000; 1:976-986.

106. Ostermeier C, Brunger AT. Structural basis of rab effector specificity: Crystal structure of the small G protein rab3A complexed with the effector domain of rabphilin-3A. Cell 1999; 96:363-374.

107. Chung SH, Song WJ, Kim K et al. The C2 domains of Rabphilin3A specifically bind phosphatidylinositol 4,5-bisphosphate containing vesicles in a Ca^{2+}-dependent manner. J Biol Chem 1998; 273:10240-10248.

108. Hay JC, Fisette PL, Jenkins GH et al. ATP-dependent inositide phosphorylation required for Ca^{2+}-activated secretion. Nature 1995; 374:173-177.
109. Schluter OM, Schnell E, Verhage M et al. Rabphilin knock-out mice reveal that rabphilin is not required for Rab3 function in regulating neurotransmitter release. J Neurosci 1999; 19:5834-5846.
110. Coppola T, Frantz C, Perret-Menoud V et al. Pancreatic b-cell protein granulophilin binds Rab3 and Munc18 and controls exocytosis. Mol Biol Cell 2002; 13:1906-1915.
111. Staunton J, Ganetzky B, Nonet ML. Rabphilin potentiates soluble N-ethylmaleimide sensitive factor attachment protein receptor function independently of rab3. J Neurosci 2001; 21:9255-9264.
112. Wang Y, Okamoto M, Schmitz F et al. Rim is a putative rab3 effector in regulating synaptic vesicle fusion. Nature 1997; 388:593-598.
113. Coppola T, Magnin-Luthi S, Perret-Menoud V et al. Direct interaction of the Rab3 effector RIM with Ca^{2+} channels, SNAP-25 and synaptotagmin. J Biol Chem 2001; 276:32756-32762.
114. Schoch S, Castillo PE, Jo T et al. Rim1a forms a protein scaffold for regulating neurotransmitter release at the active zone. Nature 2002; 415:321-326.
115. Brose N, Rosenmund C, Rettig J. Regulation of transmitter release by Unc-13 and its homologues. Curr Opin Neurobiol 2000; 10:303-311.
116. Rosenmund C, Sigler A, Augustin I et al. Differential control of vesicle priming and short-term plasticity by Munc13 isoforms. Neuron 2002; 33:411-424.
117. Christoforidis S, McBride HM, Burgoyne RD et al. The Rab effector EEA1 is a core component of endosome docking. Nature 1999; 397:621-625.
118. Stenmark H, Aasland R, Toh BH et al. Endosomal localization of the autoantigen EEA1 is mediated by a zinc-binding FYVE finger. J Biol Chem 1996; 271:24048-24054.
119. Christoforidis S, Miaczynska M, Ashman K et al. Phosphatidylinositol 3-kinases are Rab5 effectors. Nature Cell Biol 1999; 1:249-252.
120. McBride HM, Rybin V, Murphy C et al. Oligomeric complexes link Rab5 effectors with NSF and drive membrane fusion via interactions between EEA1 and syntaxin 13. Cell 1999; 98:377-386.
121. Peterson MR, Burd CG, Emr SD. Vac1p coordinates Rab and phosphatidylinositol 3-kinase signaling in Vps45p-dependent vesicle docking/fusion at the endosome. Curr Biol 1999; 9:159-162.
122. Sonnichsen B, DeRenzis S, Nielsen E et al. Distinct membrane domains on endosomes in the recycling pathway visualized by multicolor imaging of Rab4, Rab5 and Rab11. J Cell Biol 2000; 149:901-914.
123. DeRenzis S, Sonnichsen B, Zerial M. Divalent Rab effectors regulate the sub-compartmental organization and sorting of early endosomes. Nature Cell Biol 2002; 4:124-133.
124. Cormont M, Mari M, Galmiche A et al. A FYVE finger-containing protein, Rabip4, is a Rab4 effector involved in early endosomal traffic. Proc Natl Acad Sci USA 2001; 98:1637-1642.
125. Ohya T, Sasaki T, Kato M et al. Involvement of Rabphilin3 in endocytosis through interaction with Rabaptin5. J Biol Chem 1998; 273:613-617.
126. Gary JD, Wurmser AE, Bonangelino CJ et al. Fab1p is essential for PI(3)P 5-kinase activity and the maintenance of vacuolar size and membrane homeostasis. J Cell Biol 1998; 143:65-79.
127. Cooke FT, Dove SK, McEwen RK et al. The stress-activated phosphatidylinositol 3-phosphate 5-kinase Fab1p is essential for vacuole function in S. cerevisiae. Curr Biol 1998; 8:1219-1222.
128. Sbrissa D, Ikonomov OC, Shisheva A. PIKfyve, a mammalian ortholog of yeast Fab1p lipid kinase, synthesizes 5-phosphoinositides. J Biol Chem 1999; 274:21589-21597.
129. Ikonomov OC, Sbrissa D, Shisheva A. Mammalian cell morphology and endocytic membrane homeostasis require enzymatically active phosphoinositide 5-kinase PIKfyve. J Biol Chem 2001; 276:26141-26147.
130. Lohi O, Poussu A, Mao Y et al. VHS domain- a longshoreman of vesicle lines. FEBS Lett 2002; 513:19-23.
131. Xu Y, Seet L-F, Hong W. The Phox homology (PX) domain, a new player in phosphoinositide signaling. Biochem J 2001; 360:513-530.
132. Simonsen A, Stenmark H. PX domains: Attracted by phosphoinositides. Nature Cell Biol 2001; 3:E179-E182.
133. Rebecchi MJ, Scarlata S. Pleckstrin homology domains: A common fold with diverse functions. Annu Rev Biophys Biomol Struct 1998; 27:503-528.
134. Rizo J, Sudhof TC. C2 domains- structure and function of a universal Ca^{2+}-binding domain. J Biol Chem 1998; 273:15879-15882.

CHAPTER 4

Endoplasmic Reticulum Biogenesis:
Proliferation and Differentiation

Erik Snapp

Abstract

The endoplasmic reticulum (ER) adopts a number of structural forms that correlate with distinct functions. The differentiation, maintenance, and proliferation of these forms are only beginning to be understood. Differentiation and proliferation can be induced in the normal course of cell differentiation and by cellular stresses. Recent studies suggest that ER forms arise by a combination of self-organization and highly interconnected signaling and synthetic pathways. This review describes a number of ER ultrastructure forms, associated functions, and some of the potential mechanisms of their biogenesis.

Introduction

The endoplasmic reticulum (ER) is arguably the most dynamic and morphologically variable of all membranous organelles. The ER utilizes a cytoskeleton scaffold, associated motor proteins, and less well characterized mechanisms to undergo constant rearrangement while maintaining the characteristic forms of a continuous network of interconnected tubules, cisternae, and highly organized lamellar sheets. These basic structures form the building blocks of the subdomains of the ER, which include rough (RER), smooth (SER), transitional (tER or exit sites), sinusoidal, crystalloid, sarcoplasmic reticulum (SR), karmellae, myeloid bodies, and the nuclear envelope (NE) (Fig. 1).

In many eukaryotic cells, the ER consists of a series of interconnected branching tubular membranes that protrude from the NE and extend to the periphery of the plasma membrane (Fig. 3A). The ER tubules intersect with each other often at 120° angles in a series of three-way junctions that form polygons (Fig. 1, Branching ER).[1,2] The tubules grow, fuse with other tubules, slide along tubules, retract, and are absorbed into other tubules. These processes occur rapidly, on the order of seconds. The network is in a constant state of flux that ultimately produces a macroscopically stable ER structure that changes dramatically and constantly on the microscopic scale.[3] The ER is by far the largest membranous organelle in most cells. In rat hepatocytes, the surface area of the ER is 38 times larger than the plasma membrane and the ER occupies 15% of the total cell volume.[4]

As with other organelles in the secretory pathway, the ER maintains a relatively constant sized despite a constant flux of lipids and proteins into and out of the compartment. The flux includes importation of newly synthesized membrane and lumenal proteins, synthesis of lipids

The Biogenesis of Cellular Organelles, edited by Chris Mullins. ©2005 Eurekah.com and Kluwer Academic/Plenum Publishers.

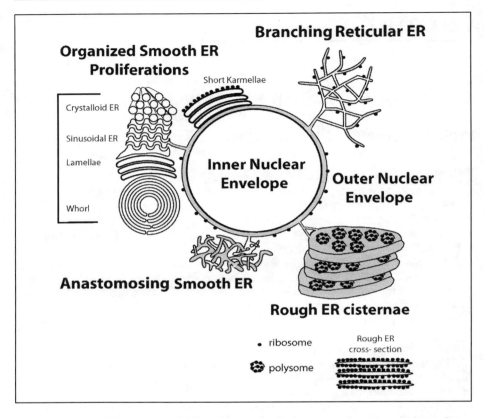

Figure 1. Schematic representation of different forms of endoplasmic reticulum. Gray shading indicates membranous structures. The outer nuclear envelope, branching ER, and rough ER cisternae are all shown with membrane-associated ribosomes. Ribosomes have also been observed on the outermost membranes of some organized smooth ER structures (examples of organized smooth ER structures are depicted). The rough ER depicted at lower right represents the appearance of rough ER in a thinly sliced cell as visualized in an electron micrograph. Typically, only the cross-sections of cisternae with numerous packed ribosomes (polysomes) can be observed. Drawing is not to scale.

for the entire cell, export of secretory cargo of lipids and proteins, and receipt of retrieved and cycling lipids and cargo from the intermediate compartment and the Golgi.[5]

Biogenesis of ER occurs both during the normal course of cell differentiation, as has been observed in newborn rat hepatocytes.[6,7] and activation of immature B-lymphocytes,[8] as well as in response to cellular stress.[9,10] The biogenesis, organization, and maintenance of the ER represent fundamental problems in self-organization. That is, the ER is an energy-dependent, nonequilibrium, steady state organelle arising from multiple complementary and competing processes.[11] Modulation of some processes favors a new steady state, which can create ultra-structure changes and accounts for the morphological plasticity of the ER.

The microtubule cytoskeleton illustrates the concept of self-organization. Similar mixtures of microtubules and motor proteins can organize into distinct assemblies depending on cell type and stage of the cell cycle. Surrey et al used a simple experimental system to demonstrate that varying component ratios, the speed of the motor proteins, their processivity, and their time bound to microtubules strongly influences cytoskeletal patterns generated at steady state.[11] At low motor concentrations, microtubules in solution remain disorganized. However, increasing concentrations of plus ended motors in the presence of ATP and GTP generated "microtubule vortices" and at higher concentrations, "asters." Minus ended motors only formed asters or no structures. By modeling the parameters of their system, the authors identified conditions that produced minimal perturbations of a steady state, while other conditions had dramatic effects.

Recent work has identified similar parameters that modulate the organization and function of ER steady states. The following chapter will review ER functions and how they relate to some exciting recent studies of ER proliferation and differentiation that shed light on its organizing principles.

ER Functions

The functions of the ER are numerous and the reader is referred to ref. 12 for additional ER functions not covered in this chapter. In the following section, some relevant ER functions that illustrate factors that predispose the ER to formation of different structures, and suggest potential relationships between ER morphology and function will be described.

Protein Synthesis, Modification and Quality Control

The ER is the primary site of membrane and secretory protein synthesis, translocation, and maturation in the cell. The two main exceptions are peroxisomes and mitochondria, which have their own protein translocation machinery. Approximately one-third of all cellular protein is translocated into the membrane and/or the oxidizing lumen of the ER.[13] Proteins enter the ER by both co- and post-translational insertion mechanisms. Co-translational insertion occurs through a large multisubunit pore, the translocon.[14-18] Post-translational insertion of tail anchored proteins, such as cytochrome b_5 and bcl-2,[19,20] occurs by an unknown mechanism in multicellular eukaryotes. However, the mechanism has been defined in yeast and requires transmembrane protein components that must enter the ER through translocons.[21] Modifications such as cleavage of the signal sequence and addition of sugar moieties to specific asparagine residues are performed on nascent peptide chains during co-translational insertion into the ER. These functions are performed by translocon-associated proteins such as the signal peptidase and the oligosaccharide transferase complex. A number of components not directly associated with the translocon play essential roles in protein folding and additional post-translational modification of proteins. For example, soluble lumenal ER proteins can be converted into membrane proteins by attachment of a glycosylphosphatidylinositol (GPI) anchor. On the outer leaflet of the ER membrane, cytoplasmic proteins can be prenylated and converted to membrane proteins that can enter the secretory pathway and traffic to the Golgi complex and plasma membrane.[22]

Chaperones serve as the protein folding machines of nascent peptides in the ER. Examples of chaperones include BiP (also referred to as GRP78)(a calcium binding ATPase that binds hydrophobic motifs and belongs to the Hsp70 family),[23] the protein disulfide isomerase family (disulfide bond formation),[24] calnexin (transmembrane) and calreticulin (lumenal)(carbohydrate and peptide binding proteins with additional roles as calcium binding proteins).[25-27] The role of the chaperones does not end after the protein has been synthesized and properly folded. Cellular stresses such as raised temperature or a change in the oxidative state of the ER can induce the misfolding of proteins.[28,29] Chaperones bind misfolded proteins to prevent protein aggregation and in some cases assist the proper refolding of the proteins.[30] In the event that proteins fail to properly fold, either during synthesis or after cellular stress, the cell must prevent accumulation of the space consuming and potentially dangerous.[31] misfolded proteins. ER membrane and lumenal protein destruction occurs by ER associated degradation

(ERAD).[30,32] Chaperones also appear to assist in unfolding proteins to aid in the retro-translocation of proteins through the translocon.[33] and into the cytoplasm where proteins are either assembled into inclusion bodies and aggresomes or degraded by the proteasome.[34] Misfolded lumenal ER proteins that fail to be degraded accumulate in Russell bodies, dilated ribosome-covered ER cisternae or vacuoles containing large lumenal protein aggregates.[35] Russell bodies probably represent a mechanism for sequestering intractably misfolded proteins into discrete regions of the ER.

In the event that misfolded proteins (or even an "overload" of proteins in the ER lumen) accumulate in the ER several distinct stress pathways can become activated. What quantity of misfolded or overexpressed protein constitutes an "overload" remains to be defined and may be surprisingly small (see ER Protein Distribution and Density section). The pathways include the Unfolded Protein Response (UPR),[36] translational control (PERK activated pathway),[37] the ATF6 pathway.[38] and the endoplasmic reticulum overload response (activation of the transcription factor NF-κB).[39] These pathways upregulate transcription levels of ER chaperones, inhibit protein synthesis or even promote cell death.[30]

Lipid Synthesis

Just as the ER is the source of most integral membrane and secretory proteins, the ER, in conjunction with mitochondria (plastids in plants), is also the source of cholesterol and phospholipids, which make up the majority of cellular membranes. The building blocks of phospholipids, fatty acyl CoA and glycerol-3-phosphate, originate in the cytoplasm and are converted into the phosphatidic acid backbone of phospholipids which translocate into the ER outer leaflet.[40] Phosphatidylcholine, phophatidylserine, and ceramide are synthesized by the ER.[40,41] Phosphatidylethanolamine can be synthesized in the ER,[41] however, the major biosynthetic route involves transfer of phosphatidylserine to the inner mitochondrial membrane, where phosphatidylserine decarboxylase converts the substrate to phosphatidylethanolamine.[12,41] To generate phosphatidylcholine, phosphatidylethanolamine must be translocated to the ER, where a methyltransferase performs the conversion.[12] Ceramide is translocated to the cis and medial Golgi for the synthesis of sphingomyelin and glycosphingolipids.[40]

How lipids traffic between the ER and the mitochondria remains poorly understood. It has been observed in many cells, that smooth ER, an ER subdomain associated with lipid synthesis, is found in tight association with mitochondria.[12] Lipid exchange could occur by a form of vesicular traffic, lipid carrier proteins that shuttle between the organelles, direct exchange of lipids by lipid translocating proteins on the faces of the two organelles or potentially by a limited form of membrane hemifusion in which the outer membrane leaflets of both organelles become continuous permitting lipid exchange while preventing exchange of integral membrane proteins. While the actual mechanism remains unknown, several groups have observed regions of close association between ER and mitochondria.[12,42,43] A mitochondria-associated membrane (MAM) fraction appears enriched in phosphatidylserine synthase and phosphatidylethanolamine N-methyltransferase.[12,44] Achleitner et al have observed mitochondria within 9 nm of ER membranes in yeast and found phospholipid transfer between the organelles was rapid and independent of energy or cytoplasmic factors.[45]

Most enzymes of cholesterol biosynthesis are found in both rough and smooth ER, though acyl-CoA-cholesterol transferase is found only in rough ER fraction.[46] As this enzyme esterifies and removes free cholesterol, it is possible that the cholesterol concentration in rough ER is lower than in other ER subdomains and that low cholesterol in the rough ER has a functional relevance. Another potential cholesterol metabolizing enzyme, lamin B receptor is localized and immobilized in the inner NE.[12,47] The physiological relevance of the sterol C_{14} reductase activity in the inner NE remains unclear.

In terms of ER proliferation, much has been learned in the past few years about regulation of lipid synthesis. Cholesterol in vertebrate cells and phosphatidylethanolamine in *Drosophila* are sensed by sterol regulatory element-binding proteins (SREBPs).[48,49] SREBP consists of a leucine zipper transcription factor attached at the carboxyl-terminus to two transmembrane spanning domains and cytosolic regulatory domain at the carboxyl-terminus of the protein. The regulatory domain binds to the cytosolic domain of SCAP, a multi-transmembrane spanning protein with a sterol or lipid-sensing domain. In the presence of SCAP and low sterol levels, SREBP is escorted into the secretory pathway where it traffics to the Golgi complex. There, SCAP activates a protease to cleave SREBP into a form with the transcription factor now bound to a single transmembrane domain. A second proteolytic cleavage within the transmembrane domain releases the transcription factor into the cytoplasm, allowing it to enter the nucleus and promote transcription of sterol synthesis enzymes. Overexpression of the sterol sensing membrane domain of SCAP disregulates the pathway and permits both SCAP and SREBP to transit to the Golgi regardless of sterol levels.[50] The authors interpret this result to mean that an unknown saturable retention protein binds to SCAP to retain it in the ER. It seems likely that similar mechanisms function for phospholipid regulation in vertebrates. In addition, phospholipid synthesis depends on substrate availability, which can also be regulated.

Secretory Traffic

Lipids and proteins (lumenal and integral membrane proteins) are transported to other regions of the cell by the secretory pathway.[5] Proteins (and possibly lipids) are sorted and accumulate at tER exit sites (clusters of tubular membranes), where vesicles and tubules coated with the peripheral protein complex called COPII arise and exit from the center.[51] After releasing their COPII coat, the membrane structures move along microtubule tracks and fuse with the Golgi complex.

The exit rate from the ER of an integral membrane protein (vesicular stomatitis virus G protein fused to green fluorescent protein[52] or VSVG-GFP) was 2.8% of the total ER pool of VSVG-GFP per minute, as assessed using quantitative live cell imaging techniques.[53] This means that a pre-existing pool of VSVG-GFP in the ER will be almost completely emptied within 30 minutes. Export of secretory proteins from the ER is therefore rapid and efficient. Inhibiting secretory traffic from the ER has equally significant consequences for ER structure. Brefeldin A (BFA) is a fungal metabolite that blocks exit from the ER by disrupting the machinery involved in protein sorting at ER exit sites.[54] Prolonged BFA treatment over several hours increases the thickness and density of ER tubules (unpublished personal observation) and dilates tER.[55,56]

To maintain the appropriate distribution of both proteins and their activities in both the ER and the other organelles, the ER makes use of dynamic and static mechanisms. "Dynamic" (retrieval) mechanisms (proteins exit and are returned to the ER) utilize ER retention peptide motifs (-KDEL or -HDEL for lumenal proteins and cytoplasmic di-lysines for integral membrane proteins).[57,58] Retrieval proteins such as the KDEL receptor (Erd2 in yeast)[59] recognize and bind the motifs to return escaped resident ER proteins to the ER by retrograde trafficking pathways from the intermediate compartment and the Golgi.[5] Resident ER proteins that lack these sequences may be retrieved by binding to proteins that contain these motifs or retained by uncharacterized sequences.[60,61] As with anterograde trafficking, retrograde trafficking transport intermediates also contain "escaped" cargo normally retained in the Golgi and intermediate compartments. However, the retrograde trafficking pathways enable the quality control machinery of the ER to sample resident membrane proteins from post-ER compartments and potentially to degrade these proteins by ERAD,[32] when necessary.[62]

The majority of resident ER membrane proteins can be retained by "static" (retention) mechanisms (the proteins do not exit the ER in the first place) such as transmembrane domain length,[63-66] the lack of a positive ER exit signal [67-69] or by being relatively immobilized. There are few examples of the latter mechanism and the best characterized is an inner nuclear envelope protein, lamin B receptor, which is localized by binding to chromatin bound lamin.[47] Many ER lumenal and membrane proteins appear to be highly mobile.[70] The actual mechanism of ER retention of highly mobile transmembrane proteins may involve physical exclusion from ER exit sites. Such a mechanism has been invoked for the retention of misfolded membrane proteins in some cell types.[68,71]

Less is known about lipid sorting from the ER. Some lipids associate with specific membrane proteins that are actively sorted at ER exit sites, while other lipids may enter the secretory pathway by bulk flow. Nonvesicular trafficking pathways are also present.[72-74] Whatever the mechanisms are, they create distinct lipid distributions throughout the secretory pathway, such that the lipid ratios of the ER are readily distinguishable from the Golgi and the plasma membrane.

Drug Detoxification

Some of the enzymes involved in lipid synthesis and the oxidative metabolism of steroids and fatty acids play roles in the detoxification of water insoluble drugs and potentially harmful metabolites that can accumulate in cell membranes.[40] The cytochrome P450 family and other enzymes convert the insoluble compounds into water soluble forms, which allows the cell to excrete the compounds.[40] The conversion process involves addition of hydroxyl groups to water-insoluble hydrocarbons dissolved in membrane using NADPH and NADPH cytochrome P450 reductase.[4] The process generates toxic intermediates, such as free radicals and epoxides, which are metabolized by epoxide hydrolase and glutathione.[75] The cytoplasmic membrane leaflet of the smooth ER (along with cytoplasm and mitochondria)[76] is a major site of drug detoxification and its surface area increases dramatically in response to high levels of drugs such as phenobarbital.[9]

Calcium Storage and Signaling

The "secondary messenger" system of calcium release into the cytoplasm is mediated through either plasma membrane calcium transporters or endoplasmic reticulum calcium channels. The ER is the major calcium storage site in the cell. Regulated calcium release affects stimulation of muscle contraction, stimulation of secretion in secretory cells, the plasticity of neurons, exocytosis and release of transmitters, cell growth, and differentiation, induction of apoptosis, secretory traffic, and oocyte fertilization.[77-79] The amount of calcium in the ER ranges from 5 mM/kg dry wt. for hepatocyte ER[80] to 120 mM/kg dry wt. in terminal cisternae of SR in skeletal muscle.[81] These numbers dramatically differ from measurements of free lumenal calcium, which range from 100 μm to 5 mM.[27] A number of resident ER proteins including calsequestrin and the chaperones calreticulin, calnexin, and BiP bind calcium with varying affinities and capacities and are responsible for the low free lumenal calcium levels.[12]

Calcium is transported into the ER primarily by members of the SERCA (sarco-endoplasmic reticulum Ca^{2+}-ATPase) transporter family.[78] At least one SERCA is directly regulated by one of the calcium binding chaperones, calnexin.[82] Calcium is released from discrete regions of the ER in "sparks" by ryanodine receptors (RyR) and in "puffs" by inositol 1,4,5-triphosphate (IP3) receptors.[12,27] In most cases, the release of calcium is highly localized and this appears to correlate with an inhomogeneous distribution of calcium channels.[12,83,84]

Sites of ER calcium release correlate with discrete subdomains of the ER. In many cell types, sites of ER calcium release form direct interactions (within 80 nm) with mitochondria.

These regions consist of specialized smooth ER domains referred to as AMF-R (autocrine motility factor receptor) tubules.[85,86] AMF-R tubules are physically continuous with the ER, but exhibit different properties including sensitivity to fragmentation induced by ilimaquinone, increased labeling by autocrine motility factor receptor, and decreased labeling of calnexin and calreticulin.[85,86] Calcium released near mitochondria is taken up by mitochondrial ATP-dependent calcium/proton antiporters, such as the NCX transporter.[79] The uptake of calcium by mitochondria stimulates mitochondria metabolism in which the Ca^{2+} responsive matrix dehydrogenases are activated, levels of ATP and NADH increase, and O_2 is consumed.[79] The calcium uptake can also induce opening of the permeability transition pore, which can modulate the release of the proapoptotic effector cytochrome c.[79]

In highly specialized cells, such as skeletal muscles, calcium plays such a critical role in cell function that the ER has been dramatically modified into physically distinct SR subdomains devoted to the modulation of calcium release.[87] The ER of skeletal muscle cells consists of SR wrapped around myofibrils and bound to T-tubules, a subdomain of the plasma membrane.[12,40] The binding of SR and plasma membrane is mediated by direct interactions between dihydropyridine receptors and ryanodine receptors.[12] The structure modulates muscle contraction by creating regulated calcium gradients. Calcium enters into the cytoplasm via the voltage sensitive dihydropyridine receptors and triggers the SR release of calcium through the ryanodine receptors followed by the calcium sensitive release of troponin and tropomyosin from myofibrils.[12] These proteins promote binding of myosin to actin, which leads to skeletal muscle contraction.[40] Excess calcium is rapidly resequestered by the ER by SERCA mediated uptake.[12] In fact, SERCAs accounts for 90% of SR membrane protein.[40]

Building Blocks of the ER

To describe the mechanisms of ER proliferation and differentiation, it is necessary to first introduce the components of the ER, including the cytoskeleton, membrane and lumenal proteins, and membrane lipids. In addition, the sizes, relative proportions, and potential steric effects of the ER's components are illustrated in Figure 2.

Cytoskeleton Scaffold and Motor Proteins

In animal cells, the ER intimately associates with microtubules. Binding to microtubules can be mediated by motor proteins and microtubule associated proteins (MAPs). Klopfenstein et al have identified an ER integral membrane protein (CLIMP-63) that can mediate microtubule association.[88] Overexpression of the protein produced dramatic rearrangements in the ER and altered microtubule distribution. In a follow-up study, Klopfenstein et al investigated the mobility of CLIMP-63 by FRAP (fluorescence recovery after photobleaching) (see ER Biogenesis Methodology section).[89] Not surprisingly, the protein's mobility was low. The unusual finding was that CLIMP-63 mobility and exclusion from the NE were mediated by its lumenal domain. The authors determined that the lumenal domain forms an α-helical 91 nm rod-like structure, which is massive relative to the diameter of the lumen of the ER.

In living cells, a number of studies find clear evidence for a role of microtubules and the motor protein kinesin in formation and breakdown of branching ER tubule polygon networks. Depolymerization of microtubules leads to retraction of the ER from the cell periphery towards the NE.[90] In contrast, depolymerization of actin does not have obvious effects on animal ER morphology, function or motility.[2,91] There are reports in the literature of ER association with spectrin in insect cells.[92]

Curiously, eukaryotic cells that do not have microtubule-associated ER still form triple branched tubular networks of polygon rings (Fig. 3). In both plants and in the budding yeast *Saccharomyces cerevisiae*, the ER associates with the actin cytoskeleton.[93,94] The cortical ER of

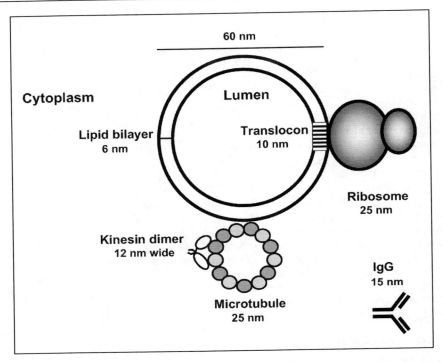

Figure 2. Representation of the relative sizes of ER components. ER tubules range from 40-70 nm in diameter with a circumferences from 125 to 220 nm. The 6 nm membrane bilayer is thinner than the plasma membrane by 1 nm, which likely reflects the differences in the lipid composition between the two membranes.[65,224] The large subunit of the ribosome that characterizes rough ER in electron micrographs measures 25 nm across,[225] the same diameter as a microtubule.[40] The translocon complex (10 nm) that the ribosome binds to is less than half the width of the ribosome and contains an estimated 50-60 transmembrane domains.[16] Kinesin dimers are 12 nm wide, or roughly the width of three tubulin subunits.[226] The shaft is not shown, but this adds an additional 70 nm to the length of kinesin; though kinesin bound membranes are usually less than 40 nm from microtubules, thus suggesting that much of the shaft is folded. For reference, immunoglobulin G (15 nm long and wide) is shown in the lower right corner.[40] Scale bar at lower right = 10 nm.

yeast differs from plants and animals in that the interphase ER does not directly align with actin or microtubules,[94] though ER motility becomes inactivated in the presence of actin depolymerizing drugs and in actin mutants.[94,95] A recent report by Fehrenbacher et al described perinuclear ER association with microtubules during M-phase budding and found that the association is important for inheritance of nuclear ER in yeast.[95] Plant ER morphology and motility also depend on an actin filament scaffold.[93,96-98] Treatment of plants with cytochalasin B[97] or cytochalasin D[99,100] disrupts ER tubule motions.

Despite the very different biochemical and dynamic characteristics of actin and microtubules and their associated motor proteins (myosin for actin and kinesin for microtubules), in plant, fungal, and animal systems the ER forms a dynamic network of triple junction branching tubules. That evolutionarily separated kingdoms would utilize different cytoskeletal elements to achieve similar ER architecture suggests that ER membranes have the inherent capacity to form triple branching tubules and possibly that a dynamic branching ER network is an optimized structure for ER function.

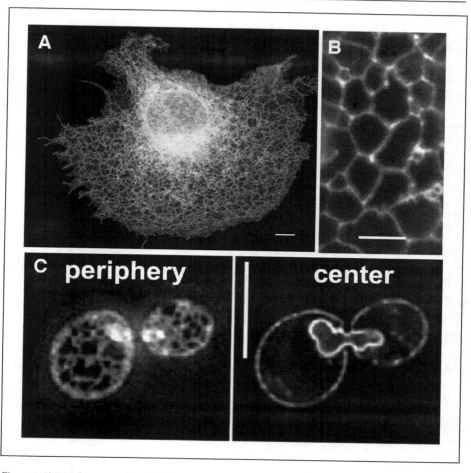

Figure 3. A) ER of a mammalian fibroblast expressing a GFP marker. Scale bar = 5 μm. B) Plant (*Nicotinia tobacum*) ER labeled with an ER-targeted GFP. Scale bar = 5 μm. Image kindly provided by Dr. Federica Brandizzi. C) Yeast (*S. cerevisiae*) expressing Sec63-GFP or signal sequence-GFP-HDEL ER. Images were acquired while focusing on either the center or periphery of the cells. Scale bar = 5 μm. Reprinted with permission from Prinz W et al. J Cell Biol 2000; 150:461-474. © 2000 The Rockefeller University Press. See text for additional details.

Until recently, most research in the ER network formation supported a clear role for the cytoskeleton and its associated motor proteins in stretching out, anchoring, and remodeling branching ER. This paradigm has been challenged by the finding that depolymerization of the microtubule cytoskeleton at low temperatures (below 4°C) or pharmacologically with nocodazole or colchicine does not immediately disrupt the ER network.[90] Instead, over the course of two hours, the ER slowly retracts from the cell periphery towards the nucleus. Moreover, Dreier and Rapoport showed that a tubule network can form in the absence of microtubules.[101] In this study *Xenopus* oocyte-derived ER membrane vesicles (microsomes) were mixed with *Xenopus* oocyte cytosol, ATP, and GTP. Fusion of the microsomes was followed by formation of a branching network of tubules, very similar to branching ER. The study raises the fascinating possibility that the ER has a natural predilection to be a branching network.

Lipid Composition

The ER membrane consists of 80-95% phospholipids and only 5-15% transmembrane or membrane associated proteins (based on calculations described in Appendix 2). The lipid composition of the ER differs significantly from the Golgi and the plasma membrane, which derive much of their lipids from the ER. Rat liver ER is composed of 2.5-5% sphingomyelin, 40-58.4% phosphatidylcholine, 10.1% phosphatidylinositol, 2.9% phosphatidylserine, 17-21.8% phosphatidylethanolamine, and 6-8% cholesterol.[40,102] By comparison, the Golgi contains twice as much cholesterol, three times as much sphingomyelin, and only 49.6% phosphatidylcholine.[102] At the plasma membrane, sphingomyelin increases to 16-19%, phosphatidylcholine is reduced to 17-39.3%, phosphatidylserine drops to 4-9%, and cholesterol increases to 17-38% of total lipid.[40,102]

As previously described, the majority of ER lipid biosynthetic machinery interacts with substrates on the cytoplasmic face of the ER membrane. Yet, cellular membranes are lipid bilayers and lipids must be transferred or flipped from the outer ER membrane leaflet to the inner leaflet. Energy independent and ATP dependent ER flippase activities have been characterized, but the responsible proteins have been elusive.[102-104] However, a yeast flippase, which transfers lipid-linked oligosaccharides from the cytoplasmic face of the ER to the lumen, has been identified.[105] and may aid in a better understanding of ER flippases. The lipid composition of the individual ER leaflets is unknown.[106]

ER Protein Distribution and Density

The lumenal proteins of the ER are present at such high concentrations that they form a gel like matrix.[107] The diffusion of lumenal GFP (5-10 $\mu m^2/s$) is 3-6 times lower than in cytoplasm (25 $\mu m^2/s$) and 9-18 times lower than in water (87 $\mu m^2/s$).[108,109] Dayel et al hypothesized that increased frequency of collision with other proteins accounts for the reduced diffusion coefficient. The majority of lumenal resident ER proteins fall into two major classes, chaperones and calcium binding proteins. In fact, many of the lumenal ER proteins simultaneously act as chaperones and bind calcium. High levels of calcium binding proteins sequester calcium in cells and can increase cytosolic Ca^{2+} from 50 nM to 1 μM or higher (see calcium section).[110] A high density of ER chaperones is likely to be important in accommodating and folding up to 13 million new proteins per minute (see Appendix 1).

Protein mobility and organization in the ER membrane differs from the protein enriched viscous ER lumen. FRAP (see ER biogenesis methodology section) of ER targeted GFP-labeled transmembrane proteins in living cells has revealed that many proteins of the ER exhibit a diffusional mobility unimpeded by barriers, anchoring, or immobilization.[47,70,71,108,111-115] Despite the many functions mediated by ER membrane proteins, their general density is comparable to membranes with known protein densities, and ranges from 15% to less than 7% of the total membrane area in BHK and UT-1 CHO cells (see Appendix 2).[116] Concentrations at high and low extremes have been reported for ER morphologically distinct subdomains in different cell types. Ryanodine receptors in Purkinje neurons cluster to a density of 12% of total membrane area (calculations determined from numbers from ref. 84), while the ER of hibernating squirrel Purkinje neurons and epithelial cells contain protein-free domains up to 10 μm wide.[117] These observations demonstrate that ER transmembrane proteins are not homogeneously distributed throughout the ER and that mechanisms must be present to physically exclude transmembrane proteins from some otherwise continuous ER subdomains.

ER Biogenesis

What Is ER Biogenesis?

It is important to distinguish the concepts of de novo creation of the ER from ER biogenesis. In the strictest sense, de novo biogenesis of the ER cannot occur. Cells do not lose the ER at some stage and then reform it. There are examples of reversible fragmentation of the ER (see ER cell cycle and ER breakdown section), but no recorded instance of a cell that lacks an ER or outer NE spontaneously generating a complete ER.

The ER's role in protein translocation accounts for why the ER can only form from preexisting ER. As described previously, protein insertion in the ER occurs co- and post-translationally. Most protein insertion into the ER membrane and lumen occurs cotranslationally via the translocon. Many essential translocon components, such as Sec 61α and the signal recognition particle receptor α subunit (SRP receptor), are co-translationally inserted into the ER membrane through preexisting translocons.[16] The requirement of preexisting translocons to form translocons is the critical factor that renders de novo ER biogenesis impossible. In practical terms, ER "biogenesis" refers to proliferation and differentiation of existing ER.

ER Biogenesis Methodology

Current studies of ER biogenesis utilize a variety of methods and assays. In many of these studies, the ER is labeled either with a dye, such as DiOC$_6$(3),[1,91,101,118-120] or by expressing an ER-localized GFP-chimera.[94,121] Fluorescence imaging is performed by confocal or fluorescence video microscopy.

The two primary approaches to studying ER proliferation and dynamics are analysis of live cells and the use of mechanically sheared vesicles or microsomes. Live cell studies offer the distinct advantage of observing the dynamics of the ER in its native context. Live cells can be probed with drugs, expression of mutant proteins, and microinjection of antibodies. However, the difficulty lies with assessing whether changes in the ER are the result of a specific perturbation or a secondary effect resulting from perturbation of some other aspect of the cell.

To deconstruct the ER into its essential components, several groups have created in vitro systems consisting of ER-derived mechanically sheared vesicles (microsomes) and mixtures of cytosol, energy (ATP and GTP), and cytoskeletal components. Microsome assembly assays follow membrane tubule and network formation usually in flow chambers with fluorescence, differential interference contrast,[122] or darkfield illumination microscopy.[123] Morphological features of ER subdomains including tER, organized smooth ER structures, and rough ER cisternae are smaller than light microscope resolution (200 nm in the x-y plane)[124] and require electron microscopy (maximum resolution from to 0.1 nm to 20 nm depending on the sample)[40] to classify morphological changes. The major caveat of in vitro ER assays is that they may not necessarily reflect what occurs in living cells.

While the above approaches can investigate overall ER morphology, the technique of fluorescence recovery after photobleaching (FRAP) provides a way to study ER continuity and protein mobility within this membrane system. In FRAP, one can deplete fluorescence in a discrete region of a fluorescently labeled living cell with an intense laser beam and then follow exchange of unbleached molecules into the bleached region with low intensity illumination.[70] This provides a means for obtaining the diffusion coefficients of proteins within the ER and for examining conditions (i.e., stress, calcium depletion, protein misfolding) that may perturb them.[70] To examine the continuity of the ER under different conditions, the technique of fluorescence loss in photobleaching (FLIP) has proved useful.[47] In this technique, one repeatedly bleaches the same discrete region and monitors fluorescence loss from the rest of the cell. If a fluorescent protein is completely mobile and localizes to a compartment continuous with the photobleached region, then all fluorescence should be depleted with time. For example, Nehls et al used FRAP to demonstrate that temperature sensitive transmembrane VSVG-GFP chimeras remain completely mobile at the permissive and nonpermissive temperature, which induces protein misfolding.[71] More severe misfolding conditions, such as tunicamycin treatment, which causes global ER stress, did reduce the diffusion coefficient and the mobile fraction of VSVG-GFP. In the same study, FLIP was applied to the ER of VSVG-GFP expressing cells at the nonpermissive temperature to reveal that misfolded membrane proteins remain in the ER and fail to enter tER exit sites.[71]

ER Network Formation

ER network formation consists of two steps, membrane fusion and tubule/network formation. The next two sections will review what is known about these processes.

Fusion Machinery

The basic process of fusion between two ER-derived vesicles requires the same types of protein components used for other cellular membrane fusion events (Fig. 4). These components include receptor proteins, v- and t-SNAREs,[125,126] an ATP dependent NSF,[127,128] and possibly, a Rab protein.[129]

The fusion of ER microsomes generally requires two sources of energy, ATP and GTP. One candidate ATPase activity is NEM-sensitive factor (NSF).[127,130] Several groups agree that an NSF-family (now the AAA ATPase family)[128] member, p97 (Cdc48p in yeast and also VCP in animal cells),[131] is essential for ER membrane fusion.[132-134] A cofactor, p47 complexes tightly to p97 and is essential for fusion of Golgi membranes[135] and at least one type of ER subdomain, tER.[136] A recent report by Uchiyama et al identified an additional cofactor, VCIP135, necessary for the cycling of p97 and p47 on and off membranes for multiple rounds of membrane fusion. Latterich and Schekman demonstrated that yeast microsomes containing mutants of another ATPase, KAR2 (mammalian BiP), were defective in homotypic fusion.[137]

The v- and t-SNAREs for ER membrane fusion appear to be the same protein, the syntaxin homolog Ufe1p, in *S. cerevisiae*.[133,138,139] Patel and colleagues demonstrated that Ufe1p is essential for homotypic fusion of ER membranes from yeast.[138] The putative mammalian equivalent, syntaxin 18 (11.9% sequence identity), localizes primarily to the ER.[140] An overexpressed mutant syntaxin18 impaired protein export from the ER.[140] Another potential player, the Sec1/munc18 protein Sly1, associates with syntaxin 18 and plays a role in ER and Golgi fusion, though a role for homotypic ER fusion has not yet been demonstrated.[141]

Many membrane fusion reactions gain additional specificity from Rab proteins.[129] Turner et al have demonstrated that microsome fusion can be blocked with guanine nucleotide dissociation inhibitor (an inhibitor of Rab activity).[132] The group also found evidence that p97 and Rab activity are sequential during membrane fusion. The Rab in question has not been purified or cloned.

The previous studies focused on the general act of microsome fusion without distinguishing different subdomains of ER (i.e., rough and smooth). Paiement and colleagues have extensively characterized differences in the rates and fusion requirements of distinct ER subdomains.[142] Paiement found that NE fused to rough microsomes in a Tris buffer containing ATP and GTP.[143] ATP alone was insufficient to promote fusion. This result is consistent with a study by Dreier and Rapoport, which found GTP essential for microsome fusion in a buffer lacking cytosol, while ATPγS did not block fusion.[101] Kan et al identified a GTP activity, formation of phosphatidylinositol (PI), that could account for GTP-mediated fusion.[144] When PI or arachidonic acid was added to the microsome fusion assay, they stimulated rough ER fusion in the absence of GTP or ATP. Lavoie et al[145] observed that rough microsomes fused in cytosol with a specific GTP requirement. In contrast, smooth ER required ATP, no cytosol, and proceeded

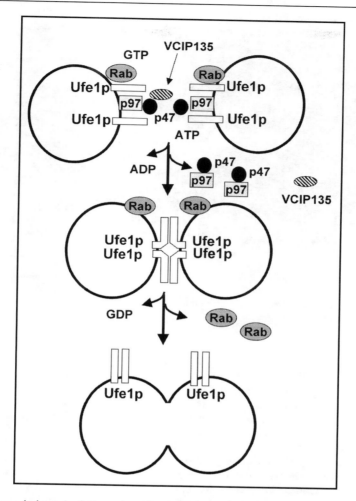

Figure 4. Proposed schematic of ER membrane fusion. Both vesicles depicted contain the identical SNARE, Ufe1p (rectangles). The SNAREs interact with each other in conjunction with several cofactors, including a Rab (oval), p97 (shaded square), p47 (black circle), and VCIP135 (hatched oval). The p97/p47 complex hydrolyzes ATP and brings the vesicles and the SNAREs into closer contact. A GTP hydrolyzing Rab potentially helps mediate the fusion event. See text for additional details.

much more slowly. The conversion of fused smooth microsomes into tER required $\alpha_2 p24$, COPI, syntaxin 5, and a cycle of phosphorylation and dephosphorylation of p97.[133,136] These studies raise intriguing questions. First, why do rough and smooth ER derived microsomes fuse with different kinetics and reaction requirements? The data suggest that rough ER may fuse independently of p97/p47 or NEM. Another question is whether different ER subdomains form and maintain distinct distributions of syntaxin 5, syntaxin 18 or other fusion components. Steegmaier et al have proposed that the smooth ER tubules of steroidogenic cells form a physically distinct subcompartment of the ER and contain a unique syntaxin, syntaxin 17.[146] Fluorescence imaging and photobleaching experiments would be useful here to determine the in vivo distribution and mobility of the various syntaxins and whether they exchange between the two subdomains.

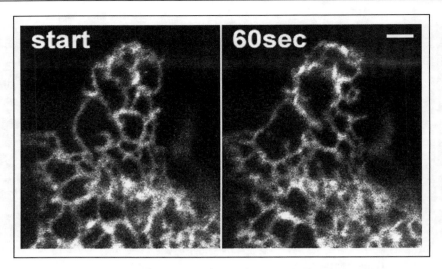

Figure 5. Dynamics of branching ER. The two images are of the same region of a mammalian fibroblast GFP-labeled branching ER at time 0 and after 60 seconds. The tubules have been rearranged into a macroscopically similar structure that bears little similarity to the previous distribution of tubules. Scale bar= 2.5 μm. See text for additional details.

Branching Motions

A seminal paper by Lee and Chen established that the ER is a dynamic structure (Fig. 5) and described the motions of ER tubules in mammalian cells.[3] ER tubules perform three basic motions (tubule elongation, sliding, and ring closure) (Fig. 6), which account for the formation of linear tubules, triple junctions, and a polygonal reticulum. The motions promote branching ER proliferation and polygon breakdown. ER network growth and proliferation is accomplished by tubule extension (Fig. 6A). Increasing the amount of tubules increases ER network density.[3] However, the relative density of the ER network does not vary significantly throughout interphase for many cells because of ER polygon breakdown, which occurs by sliding and closure of polygon rings (Fig. 6B,C). The motions cease in the absence of microtubules in cells.[91] Cytoplasmic streaming occurs within plant cells when ER membranes bind and slide along stationary actin cables and sweep ER, mitochondria, glycosomes, and other small cytoplasmic organelles in the process.[98]

Tubule Formation

In many eukaryotic cells, the ER is composed of cisternae or tubules. Unfortunately, little information is available on the dynamics of cisternal ER formation. The ER within many tissue culture cells, yeast, and plant cells consists of branching tubule networks. Network formation and maintenance has been extensively studied in vivo and in vitro.[12,93,94,147,148]

What drives tubule formation? The simplest model is that microsomes are deformed by some form of mechanical shearing force. Vale and Hirokawa converted artificial liposomes into tubular structures by repeated pipetting.[123] These tubules maintained their shape in the absence of any proteins indicating that once a vesicle is deformed into a tubule, it does not necessarily have an elastic force compelling it to immediately reform into a vesicle. In subsequent studies, model systems have been created that mimic specific aspects of tubule growth and network formation. Most in vitro and in vivo branching network assays using animal cells and components have absolute requirements for a microtubule scaffold and the microtubule plus end motor kinesin.

Branching Network Formation (Cytoskeleton and Motor-Dependent)

Live cell studies and in vitro network formation assays provide clear evidence for a role of microtubules, microtubule-associated motor proteins, and energy (ATP and GTP) in the formation and breakdown of ER networks.[2,123,149] Multiple groups have observed that microtubule depolymerizing drugs halt most ER membrane tubule motions.[90,91,119] Network formation proceeded by pulling of microtubule-bound vesicle membranes, presumably by kinesin, to form tubules. Tubule growth driven by motor protein pulling is referred to as plus-end-directed membrane sliding.[119] New tubules pulled out from existing tubules and as tubules encountered other tubules, rapid fusion events occurred, eventually resulting in networks of tubule-based polygons.

Roux and colleagues performed a similar experiment with ATP, artificial vesicles, Golgi-derived lipid vesicles coated with streptavidin bound to microtubules, and kinesin-coated beads labeled with biotin.[150] They observed network formation in two phases. During the first phase, membrane bound beads moved at the same rate as free beads on microtubules. In the second phase, the tube growth rate decreased and strongly fluctuated possibly reflecting changes in membrane tension. A significant finding of the study was that tubule formation required beads coated with multiple motor proteins. Coating membranes with biotin-labeled kinesin did not result in tubules. The authors proposed that the beads distributed the load among more lipids and motors, resulting in fewer single phospholipid extraction or motor detachment events. Allan and Vale observed large globular domains at the tips of growing in vitro tubules, suggestive of a large complex of microtubule motors.[120] It will be important to determine the in vivo parameters of tubule formation including the number of motors required to form a tubule, the number of attachment sites, and the identity of the attachment sites.

Feiguin et al directly demonstrated a necessary role for kinesin in vivo for maintenance of ER distribution and structure.[151] Kinesin-heavy chain suppression with antisense oligonucleotides restricted the distribution of ER tubules in neurons to the cell center and led to a

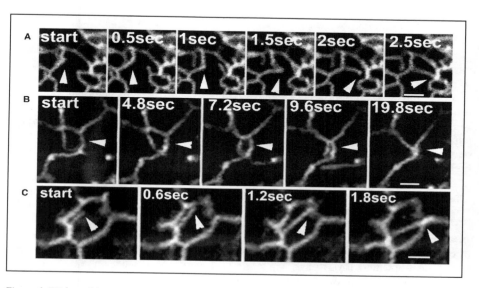

Figure 6. ER branching motions in a mammalian fibroblast expressing an ER-localized GFP. A) Tubule extension (time course of 0 to 2.5 seconds). B) Ring closure (time course of 0 to 19.8 seconds). C) Sliding (time course of 0 to 1.8 seconds). Scale bars= 1.5 μm. Arrows depict respective motions of tublue extension, ring closure, and ER sliding.

disappearance of a reticular network. The mitochondria and microtubule distributions were unaffected. In addition to kinesin, the Allan laboratory found that the primary motor activity during *Xenopus* embryo development corresponded with a minus-end directed dynein.[149,152]

An ER receptor for an ER kinesin remains elusive. A candidate receptor, kinectin, was proposed by Kumar et al,[153] but the *Caenorhabditis elegans* and *Drosophila* genomes contain no evidence of kinectin, indicating that additional receptors must exist.[154] An interesting possibility is that the ER receptor is not a protein, but rather a lipid. Klopfenstein et al identified a kinesin that contains a pleckstrin homology domain that mediates docking with phosphatidylinositol(4,5)-bisphosphate containing vesicles.[155]

Not only do tubules form from motor-driven tension, but they also arise from microtubule dynamics. Waterman-Storer et al characterized tip attachment complexes at the plus end of microtubules that pull tubules as microtubules polymerize in *Xenopus* oocyte membrane network formation assays.[122] When microtubules shortened due to dynamic instability, the tubules also retracted. An additional mechanism of statically attached tubules, which move in a retrograde manner to the cell center by actinomyosin-based retrograde flow, also has been characterized.[119]

Network formation along microtubules appears to be a common solution for the organization of several organelles. Evidence for discontinuous peroxisome[156] (in association with microtubules and dynein/dynactin) and mitochondria[83,157] networks has been observed in living cells.

Branching Network Formation (Cytoskeleton and Motor-Independent)

Based on the studies described in the previous section, it is not intuitive that ER membranes could deform into tubules in the absence of a shearing force. Dreier and Rapoport and Hetzer et al examined network formation using *Xenopus* derived microsomes in the presence of *Xenopus* cytosol and energy (ATP and GTP).[101,158] In the absence of ATP, fusing microsomes increased in size, but did not form tubules. The time required for network formation could be divided into two phases, microsome fusion and tubule network formation. Microsome fusion occurred rapidly within the first ten minutes of the reaction, followed by tubule formation after 20 minutes, and networks developed after 60-90 minutes.

Dreier and Rapoport next attempted forming networks in the presence of either actin or microtubule disrupting drugs.[101] Unexpectedly, branching networks of tubules did form. To confirm the result, the authors depleted cytosol and microsomes of tubulin and still observed network formation. Thus, instead of simply forming successively larger amorphous vesicles, fusing microsomes appear to have the inherent capacity to form tubules and elaborate networks. The main caveat of the Dreier study is that the authors tested several combinations of different sources of microsomes and cytosol. Network formation only occurred for *Xenopus* oocyte microsomes and cytosol and to a lesser degree with other cytosol sources, perhaps reflecting effectors unique to the *Xenopus* oocyte system.

At present the mechanisms of network and tubule formation are not entirely clear. It appears that tubules form from fusing vesicles and elongate into tubules. When the tubules encounter each other, they may fuse at contact points creating a network. Alternatively, microsomes could fuse at discrete sites and form branching tubules along existing tubules.

Studies by others suggest two reasonable mechanisms for tubule formation in the absence of cytoskeletal components and motor proteins. The first possibility involves mechanically deforming the membrane via a physically constricting protein. Studies of endosome formation have identified a protein, dynamin, which pinches and constricts membranes into transient tubules.[40] Incubation of artificial or purified membranes with the soluble ER-associated (and mitochondria[159]) dynamin-like protein-1 (DLP-1)[160] demonstrated that DLP-1, in the presence of GTPγS deforms amorphous membranes into regular tubules, some even forming triple junctions.[161] Unlike ER, the tubules were covered with a dense coat of DLP-1 and were narrower (0.27 nm) than most ER tubules (0.4-0.7 nm). However, microinjected antibodies against DLP-1 appear to disrupt ER structure, which suggests an in vivo role in maintenance of ER structure.[162]

An alternative explanation of Dreier and Rapoport's results involves lipid modification, which can induce tubule formation in the absence of a shearing force. Formation of 50-100 nm tubules from a flat bilayer in the absence of a shearing force requires increasing the area of the outer leaflet of the bilayer without increasing the inner leaflet area.[163] This can be accomplished by flipping lipids from the inner leaflet to the outer leaflet.[164] Other mechanisms include unequal electrostatic screening of the leaflets (multivalent cations on one side and monovalent salt on the other side) or by increasing the effective area of the lipid head groups in the outer leaflet by increasing head group charge by phosphorylation, cleavage of acyl chains by phospholipases,[165,166] or recruiting wedge-shaped lipids to the outer leaflet.[167] Such mechanisms have been observed in vivo for Golgi membranes. Cluett et al induced tubulation of the Golgi complex in the absence of microtubules by releasing beta-COP with BFA or by depleting cytoplasm of ATP.[168] Under similar conditions, tubules up to 7 μm could be formed in vitro with Golgi-derived membranes.

One explanation for the difference in cytoskeleton and motor protein requirements in vitro and in vivo is that while tubule and network formation may be inherent properties of some ER microsomes, a cytoskeleton scaffold and motor proteins can dramatically enhance the rates and efficiency of tubule and network formation in the crowded environment of the cell. The cytoplasm is dense with cytoskeletal components, ribosomes, other organelles, and numerous proteins (see illustrations of the density of cytoplasmic proteins[169]). Motor proteins and microtubule dynamics can provide the force to penetrate the cytoplasm and extend tubules. The microtubule cytoskeleton scaffold appears to anchor ER tubules, allowing them to extend out to the cell periphery.[90,91] The tubule formation mechanism described by Dreier and Rapoport could be important for generating and maintaining ER tubule networks following events that perturb ER continuity.

ER Dynamics During Mitosis and in Response to Calcium Perturbation

The previous sections have described mechanisms of tubule and network formation. Does the ER ever fragment or lose continuity? Zeligs and Wollman observed fragmentation of the ER during mitosis in electron micrographs of rat thyroid epithelial cells.[170] Koch and colleagues made similar observations in fixed 3T3 cells.[171] In light of live cell studies, the results may have been confounded by fixation artifacts.

Photobleaching of GFP containing living cells has demonstrated that the ER remains continuous during mitosis. FLIP studies reveal that the ER remains continuous through at least metaphase.[47,112] By demonstrating in cells that a lipid dye and a GFP-tagged membrane protein labeling mitotic ER diffused with different diffusion coefficients, Zaal et al provided strong evidence against ER (and Golgi) vesiculation. The diffusion coefficients would have been the identical for the two fluorescent probes in a vesiculated ER, because the diffusion of fluorescent vesicles would dominate fluorescence recovery after photobleaching. Thus, the ER remains continuous during mitosis. The continuity and organization of the ER may be important for regenerating other organelles, such as the NE, during cell division.[47]

In contrast to mitosis, fertilization of oocytes does fragment the ER. In starfish eggs, Terasaki and colleagues have observed fragmentation of the ER during fertilization, which corresponds to a calcium wave, and is followed by a rapid reforming of the network.[172] Other groups have reported that mammalian ER networks reversibly fragment in response to calcium ionophores, or high (200 μM and higher) levels of calcium in cytoplasm.[108,121,171] Similar results have been reported in in vitro assembly assays.[101] Continuity was assayed by visual inspection of fluorescently labeled ER, by FRAP, or by EM, revealing an interconnected network of blobs and tubule-based polygons.[101,173] The mechanism for calcium-induced ER fragmentation or constriction is unknown. However, biophysical studies of phospholipids and calcium support a mechanism in which the divalent calcium cations bind to and neutralize the negative charge of phospholipid headgroups and alter the curvature properties of the membrane to favor the formation of vesicles or other structures.[174-176]

ER Subdomains

Heterogeneities exist at multiple levels of ER organization. In the following section, the term "subdomains" will be used to refer to morphologically distinct structures (i.e., cisternae and tubules) and "microdomains" will refer to discrete complexes of proteins and lipids that could differ from similar complexes due to the absence or addition of another protein or different lipid environments that surround identical protein complexes (i.e., the whorl structure of translocon-ribosome complexes strung together by a single mRNA in rough ER.[177] In this section, the distinguishing characteristics of ER subdomains will be described.

Branching and Nonbranching ER

In many adherent tissue culture cells, the ER appears as a branching network of tubules arranged in a polygonal pattern (see tubule and network formation sections). Branching ER contains both rough and smooth ER markers (personal unpublished observation).

In more differentiated cells, the ER adopts several nonbranching forms including cisternae and lamellar sheets. Branching ER can also be modified through association with other organelles such as mitochondria (AMF-R tubules) or plasma membrane (T-tubules). Interaction with nonmembranous structures also can generate nonbranching structures (i.e., binding lamins to form nuclear envelope). Finally, failure to bind the cytoskeleton may also contribute to the formation of nonbranching structures. For example, organized smooth ER structures do not associate with microtubules.[10]

Rough and Smooth ER

The distinction between rough and smooth ER is both functional and morphological. Rough ER (granular ER in earlier literature) refers to ribosome-coated ER and includes tubular, branching, cisternal shapes and the outer NE (Fig. 1). Cells with high rates of protein synthesis such as pancreatic islets, activated B cells, and hepatocytes are packed with ribosome covered rough ER cisternae.[8,40,178] The ribosomes tightly associate with translocon proteins[179-181] and the association is essential to translocate proteins into the membrane and the lumen of the ER.

Rolls et al used FRAP to measure the mobility of GFP-tagged ribosomes, rough, and general ER proteins in *C. elegans* neurons.[114] Though rough and general ER associated proteins were all highly mobile, the rough ER proteins were concentrated in the cell body, while general ER proteins were found throughout the cell body and neurites. Ribosomes were concentrated in the cell body and were immobile on the time scale observed. The authors postulated that the binding of rough ER proteins to the immobile ribosomes reduced their mobility and restricted the mobile rough ER proteins to the cell body, possibly through a bind and release mechanism.

Smooth or agranular ER is not simply rough ER membranes devoid of ribosomes. The morphology of the smooth ER membranes can be readily distinguished from rough ER. Smooth ER can be organized into a dense concentration of tubules or into exotic lamellar sheet structures that range from whorls to stacks to micelle tubes of crystalloid.[40,178,182] Hepatocytes and cells specializing in steroid synthesis (i.e., ovary, testis, and adrenal cortex cells) contain large quantities of smooth ER.[4,40] Smooth ER is enriched in lipid detoxification enzymes such as cytochrome b_5, epoxide hydrolase, and cytochrome P450, cholesterol synthesis proteins

(HMG-CoA reductase), and other proteins including syntaxin 17 and glucose-6-phosphatase.[75,146,183]

The smooth ER is also where tER exit sites form. In vertebrate cells tER sites are long-lived.[184] These sites function in the export of proteins and lipids out of the ER. Peripheral proteins including the COPII coat machinery dynamically associate with these sites to form transport vesicles. In yeast tER sites are near the NE in *Pichia pastoris*, while in *S. cerevisiae* they form throughout the ER network.[185] The mechanisms defining tER formation and stability are an area of active investigation.

ER Differentiation

The characteristics of ER often differ in different cell types. For example, professional secretory cells are filled with densely packed rough ER cisternae capable of synthesizing large quantities of membrane and secretory proteins. In contrast, immature B-lymphocytes maintain a minimal ER of primarily the outer NE. The following sections will describe some of the mechanisms of ER differentiation.

ER and the Nuclear Envelope

The outer NE is studded with ribosomes and participates in lumenal and membrane protein synthesis and translocation. In interphase cells, the NE and ER are physically continuous and can be qualitatively distinguished by the presence of nuclear pores in the NE, their absence in cortical ER (except for annulate lamellae which are stacked cisternal ER domains continuous with the rest of the ER and contain a substantial number of nuclear pore components,[186] and the distinct population of membrane proteins in the inner NE.

The NE and the ER are highly interrelated. Not only are the two organelles continuous, but the ER is also the source of membrane for the NE. During mitosis in higher eukaryotes, the membranes of the NE are absorbed back into the ER and then reassemble from ER membranes at the end of mitosis.[47] Whether the NE is a specialization of the ER or the ER is an outgrowth of the NE remains unclear. Several groups have reported forming nuclear structures by mixing *Xenopus* oocyte microsomes with cytosol and DNA.[101,158,187] The same membrane and cytosol components also can form ER networks.[101,158]

Organized Smooth ER Biogenesis

In cells ranging from yeast to plants to mammals, highly organized smooth membranes have been observed that appear continuous with the endoplasmic reticulum. Organized smooth ER (OSER) structures encompass a number of potentially related structures including closely apposed lamellar sheets (lamellae) (originally termed myeloid bodies), tightly packed whorls of lamellae (Fig. 7A), stacks of lamellar sheets or karmellae on the outer NE, sinusoidal ER (Fig. 7A), and hexagonal arrangements of tubules potentially of collapsed sinusoidal ER referred to as crystalloid ER (see Fig. 1). Many of the different structures can be observed in the same cell suggests that the structures may represent different stages in OSER formation.[10,188] These OSER structures appear in retinal epithelia,[189,190] marine annelid photocytes,[191] hepatocytes of rats treated with the cholesterol synthesis inhibitor lovastatin,[192] or other drugs,[193] and in yeast,[188,194-199] plants (Z-membranes),[200,201] and mammalian cells.[10,182,202-204] overexpressing a variety of resident ER integral membrane proteins. OSER structures may represent a general structure that can be induced and maintained by a common mechanism and utilized by cells for different needs.

The role of OSER structures remains unclear. Some investigators have suggested that OSER structures serve to concentrate smooth ER associated proteins such as the lipid detoxification enzymes cytochrome P450 and cytochrome b_5 to enhance drug metabolism.[193] OSER structures could also serve as a reservoir for lipids to be used for during ER proliferation or differentiation.

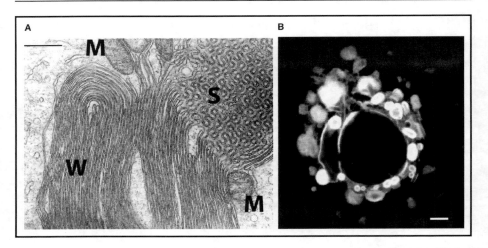

Figure 7. A) Electron micrograph of smooth ER proliferations in a fibroblast. Sinusoidal ER (S) and lamellar whorls (W) are well defined. The outer lamellae are often found closely associated with mitochondria (M). Scale bar in upper left corner represents 0.5 μm. Image was kindly provided by Dr. Francesca Lombardo. B) Confocal fluorescence image of a mammalian fibroblast containing OSER structures. The cell is overexpressing a GFP fusion of an OSER-inducing protein. Scale bar= 5 μm.

A clear role for OSER structures has been described in marine annelids. The worms contain specialized light emitting cells, photocytes, which contain photosomes (structures composed of a mass of sinusoidal ER). The photosome is enwrapped by "intermediate ER," a less organized form of sinusoidal ER, which associates with "dyadic ER", a pair of saccules separated by a tubule of plasma membrane, similar to the arrangement of SR.[191] The saccules and intermediate ER remain dissociated until a stimulatory signal induces them to fuse, which stimulates oxygen radical activation of the chemiluminescent photoprotein polynoidin, resulting in a rapid flash of light. How the intermediate ER and the dyadic ER partition and what triggers the fusion event have not been determined. The OSER most likely enhances the intensity of the chemiluminescent signal by concentrating a large amount of polynoidin into a discrete space.

When OSER structures are labeled with a GFP-chimera or a fluorescent dye, the OSER structures are dramatically brighter than surrounding branching ER (Fig. 7B). To produce a similar intensity of light in branching ER, the cell would have to express substantially higher levels of polynoidin and a much higher density of branching ER. A similar effect could be achieved by producing a sphere the same size as the photosome. The ER's tendency to form lamellar sheets or branching tubules may preclude such a structure.

Proposed mechanisms of OSER formation include "zippering" of opposing membranes by association of the cytoplasmic domains of specific integral membrane proteins.[182,197,200,202,203] or restriction of OSER-inducing proteins to discrete regions within the cell followed by enhanced synthesis of membrane lipid at these sites.[205] Overexpression of proteins with long half-lives appears to be a requirement to induce OSER structures.[206] Enyzmatic activity or other protein function is not required for OSER formation. Vergeres et al found that enzymatically inactive forms of cytochrome b₅ still induce membrane proliferation and that the amino acids in the transmembrane domain influence the efficiency of OSER formation.[196] Different domains of OSER-inducing proteins correlate with OSER formation and the site of OSER localization possibly reflecting sites of function.[188,204,207] Protein mutagenesis and deletion studies provide compelling evidence for protein-protein zippering of membranes in vivo.[182,197,200,202,203]

OSER-like structures can be formed in vitro with protein-free mixtures of lipids. The structures form in a continuous process of intersection-free membrane unfolding.[208-210] It seems likely that the tendency of phospholipids towards such structures is important for OSER formation.

Rough ER Cisternae Differentiation

Professional secretory cells often contain dilated ER membranes heavily decorated with ribosomes. The cisternae form stacks separated by the width of two apposed ribosomes. Important insights into pathways that stimulate differentiation of yeast ER into cisternae have come from David Meyer and colleagues. The Meyer group has studied membrane proliferation in *S. cerevisiae* in response to overexpression of the type I integral membrane protein p180 (the canine ribosome receptor).[181] Overexpressed p180 induces transformation of yeast ER into a series of evenly spaced rough ER membranes throughout the cytoplasm, similar in appearance to the rough ER cisternae of professional secretory cells.[211] Constructs composed of different domains of p180 produce distinct forms of membrane proliferation. Deletion of the carboxy-terminal domain produces closely packed rough ER membranes, while deletion of the ribosomal binding domain results in smooth evenly spaced membranes 80-100 nm apart. Expression of the membrane anchor alone produced karmellae.[211] The authors proposed that ribosome binding in combination with membrane proliferation leads to biogenesis of rough ER cisternae in yeast. It will be interesting to test whether similar processes differentiate the ER in professional secretory cells.

Using microarray analysis and yeast genetics, Block-Alper et al determined that the yeast transcription factor Ino2p (which derepresses phospholipid biosynthetic genes) was essential for all of the forms of membrane proliferation regardless of the expressed protein.[212] Ino2p forms a complex with Ino4p and activates the expression of yeast genes for phospholipid, fatty acid, and sterol biosynthesis.[213] Addition of inositol and choline to media (which rescues Ino2p yeast knockout strains) did not restore the ability to proliferate membranes.

Different groups are divided over the role of ER stress in induction of lipid synthesis and membrane proliferation. Cox et al linked membrane proliferation to the unfolded protein response (UPR) by characterizing IRE1 induced expression of INO1 (a mediator of a phospholipid synthesis pathway).[214] Ire1 and other UPR mutants are inositol auxotrophs.[147] In contrast, others have demonstrated that activation of the UPR was not required for membrane proliferation.[215,216] Menzel et al observed that the UPR was stimulated by the overexpression of a secretory protein or an integral membrane protein and resulted in increased expression of yeast Kar2p (mammalian BiP).[215] IRE1 and the UPR were required to achieve high levels of expression of the secretory protein, but not the integral membrane protein. In plants, Shank et al observed increased expression of phospholipid synthesis enzymes in response to either overexpression of a mutant lumenal protein or treatment with the ER stress inducing drug tunicamycin.[217] A pathway connecting ER stress and lipid synthesis in mammalian cells has not been identified.

Another property recently associated with p180 is that its expression in yeast increases the longevity of SEC61, INO1, and KAR2 mRNAs up to nine-fold by targeting them to the ER membrane.[218] The pathway occurs independently of the UPR, but does require expression of the ribosome binding p180 constructs and the presence of a signal sequence on the mRNA. Whether p180 increases mRNA half-life in mammalian cells and whether the increased mRNA half-life correlates with increased translation of the encoded protein remains to be demonstrated. Still, the result is intriguing and the authors suggest that their results demonstrate how overexpression of a single protein can dramatically increase the complexity and functionality of ER membranes.

A sensing mechanism or direct link between protein levels and membrane proliferation has not been identified. Overexpressed proteins rarely account for more than 5% of total ER membrane protein (see Appendix 2).[10,116] Thus, when considering the effects of overexpressed proteins on ER morphology, proliferation or stress, it is clear that the ER must be very sensitive to detect differences of 0.3-5% in total protein levels.

One mechanism of sensing protein overexpression uses levels of the chaperone BiP as sensors of stress. Inactive Ire1p exists as a monomer and dimerizes when stressed.[219] Bertolotti et al found that Ire1p binds BiP in the monomeric state and releases BiP under conditions of ER stress.[220] They propose a model in which BiP binds with low affinity to the lumenal domain of the stress sensing proteins and when excess folding or misfolding proteins accumulate, BiP releases from the stress sensing protein and binds the unfolded proteins with higher affinity. The unbound stress sensors then dimerize and activate the stress response pathways.

Thus, in the ER lumen, levels of free BiP are tightly regulated such that a small increase in unfolded or misfolded protein could be detected. In addition, the levels of overexpressed protein may increase the lumenal volume and dilate ER tubules, diluting the effective concentration of BiP associated with low affinity sensor proteins and thus induce the UPR and possibly membrane proliferation.

In the ER membrane, a 0.3-5% increase in protein seems unlikely to displace much of the existing lipids and proteins. Furthermore, tail-anchored proteins and some co-translationally inserted membrane proteins have minimal lumenal domains, which precludes interaction with BiP. Yet, tail-anchored proteins readily induce membrane synthesis and OSER formation.[182,196] The ER must have a sensitive probe of the transmembrane protein-lipid ratio, membrane fluidity or ion permeability. Establishing the link between protein expression levels and membrane proliferation in mammalian cells remains an important question in ER biogenesis.

Putting It All Together

The ER is in a nonequilibrium steady-state undergoing constant flux in terms of membrane movement and the loss and gain of proteins and lipids. Within the context of this flux, the ER maintains its composition and general morphology. Perturbations as simple as the overexpression of a single membrane protein or induction of protein misfolding are sufficient to tip this balance and lead to ER proliferation, shrinkage, or gross structural changes.

In the past few years, tools have become available to investigate the idea of dynamic partitioning as a mechanism for forming and maintaining organelle subdomains. In this model, proteins or lipids can accumulate in a nonstatic manner at sites of nucleation.[221] The source of nucleation might include enrichment of an enzymatic substrate, low affinity binding, or subtle changes in the kinetics of the system. For example, the ER forms a calcium responsive interaction with mitochondria to create a new subdomain, the AMF-R tubule. The biophysical properties of the AMF-R tubule are distinct from the otherwise continuous branching ER. One such difference is sensitivity to the sponge metabolite ilimaquinone,[85] which may reflect a difference in the lipid composition of the tubule, due to exchange of phospholipid substrates between ER and mitochondria. In addition, some lumenal proteins (i.e., calreticulin) become depleted from the tubules.[86] Thus, simply altering calcium levels in the regions of close ER and mitochondrial apposition can shift the ER steady state to form or disrupt a subdomain.

The same principle of subtle shifts in the steady state of the ER applies to OSER structures and rough ER cisternae formation, as well. Overexpressing a transmembrane protein to an amount less than 5% of total ER membrane protein triggers stress pathways, lipid synthesis, and membrane reorganization. In several cases, the outcome of these processes is enhanced or altered ER function (i.e., increased secretory protein synthesis capacity for rough ER cisternae in professional secretory cells).

The sensitivity of the ER steady state ultimately reflects the multiple pathways and parameters of the pathways that affect ER morphology and function. An important goal of future studies will be to determine which of the pathways and parameters are physiologically relevant for ER proliferation, differentiation, maintenance, and function. Such information will enable researchers to answer how and why different cells have different ERs. The recent progress in ER studies hints at an exciting future for ER biogenesis research.

Acknowledgements

The author wishes to thank Federica Brandizzi, Francesca Lombardo, and William Prinz for providing images. Thanks to Ramanujan Hegde, Jennifer Lippincott-Schwartz, Federica Brandizzi, Irwin Arias, Nica Borgese, Holger Lorenz, and Sarah Shih for extremely helpful discussions and reviewing the manuscript. The author is supported by a Pharmacology Research and Training (PRAT) Fellowship.

Appendices

Appendix 1: Calculating Amounts of Protein Synthesis in the Endoplasmic Reticulum

Weibel et al estimate the number of ribosomes (and by extension translocons) per μm^2 to be 335.[222] In a liver cell, the rough ER makes up 35% of the total cellular membrane or 38,500 μm.[2,40] This translates to 1.3×10^7 translocons per liver cell. If all translocons are occupied by ribosomes, the rate of protein synthesis is 500 amino acids per minute,[40] and the average protein size is approximately 500 amino acids,[116] then at steady-state, a hepatocyte synthesizes 13 million secretory proteins per minute. Similar calculations for a pancreatic exocrine cell produce a synthesis rate of 2.6 million secretory proteins per minute.[40]

Appendix 2: Calculations of Transmembrane Protein Density

In a freeze fracture electron microscopy study of UT1 cells (a CHO cell derived cell line), each μm^2 of membrane of the ER contained 2000 membrane associated particles that averaged 10 nm in diameter.[10] If most transmembrane domains (TMDs) are alpha helices and the diameter of a TMD is 1.5 nm, then the area occupied by each transmembrane domain is 1.76 nm^2. The densest packing of TMDs possible would place 44 TMDs in a 10 nm diameter particle (78.5 nm^2). For 2×10^3 particles, this would translate to an upper limit of 88,000 TMDs per μm^2 in the ER. In this extreme example, the density of TMDs would be 15.6% of the total surface area of the outer ER membrane face.

However, the authors measured membrane-associated domains, not discrete proteins or even necessarily transmembrane proteins. A number of resident ER membrane proteins are known to contain more than one TMD (i.e., the translocon proteins Sec61α and TRAM contains 10 and 5 TMDs respectively). The measurements also do not distinguish between TMD proteins with large globular cytoplasmic domains or minimal cytoplasmic domains. The estimate does not distinguish peripherally associated proteins (i.e., proteins with GPI or prenyl anchors or cytoplasmic proteins that bind to the ER). Therefore, the number of TMDs and transmembrane proteins in the ER is likely to be substantially less than 8.8×10^5 per μm^2.

An independent estimate of ER transmembrane protein density by Quinn, Griffiths, and Warren estimates a maximum density of 4×10^5 transmembrane proteins per μm^2 of ER.[116,223] The authors assessed the total amount of protein in carbonate washed isolated ER membranes and determined the volume and surface area of the ER in BHK cells. By determining relative amounts of protein at various molecular weights on a polyacrylamide gel, the authors estimated the average molecular weight of transmembrane proteins in the ER at 50 kD. The authors noted that the determined density was likely to be an overestimate due to uncontrolled proteolysis during membrane preparation, incomplete removal of peripherally associated proteins, and the contribution of membrane proteins to the actual surface area. The authors' high estimate of the total surface area of the ER would be ≤ 7% transmembrane proteins. Thus, estimates by this author using the Anderson study data provides an upper limit to transmembrane protein density on the ER surface and the actual number is more likely to be similar to or even lower than the estimate of Quinn et al.[116,223]

References

1. Terasaki M, Song J, Wong JR et al. Localization of endoplasmic reticulum in living cells and glutaraldehyde-fixed cells with fluorescent dyes. Cell 1984; 38:101-108.
2. Dabora SL, Sheetz MP. The microtubule-dependent formation of a tubulovesicular network with characteristics of the ER from cultured cell extracts. Cell 1988; 54:27-35.
3. Lee C, Chen LB. Dynamic behavior of endoplasmic reticulum in living cells. Cell 1988; 54:37-46.
4. DePierre JW, Andersson G, Dallner G. Endoplasmic reticulum and Golgi complex. In: Arias IM, Jakoby WB, Popper H et al, eds. The liver: Biology and pathobiology. New York: Raven Press, 1988:165-188.
5. Lippincott-Schwartz J, Roberts TH, Hirschberg K. Secretory protein trafficking and organelle dynamics in living cells. Annu Rev Cell Dev Biol 2000; 16:557-589.
6. Dallner G, Siekevitz P, Palade GE. Biogenesis of endoplasmic reticulum membranes I. Structural and chemical differentiation in developing rat hepatocyte. J Cell Biol 1966; 30:73-96.
7. Dallner G, Siekevitz P, Palade GE. Biogenesis of endoplasmic reticulum membranes II. Synthesis of constitutive microsomal enzymes in developing rat hepatocyte. J Cell Biol 1966; 30:97-117.
8. Rush JS, Sweitzer T, Kent C et al. Biogenesis of the endoplasmic reticulum in activated B lymphocytes: Temporal relationships between the induction of protein N-glycosylation activity and the biosynthesis of membrane protein and phospholipid. Arch Biochem Biophys 1991; 284:63-70.
9. Remmer H, Merker HJ. Drug-induced changes in the liver endoplasmic reticulum: Association with drug-metabolizing enzymes. Science 1963; 142:1657-1658.
10. Anderson RGW, Orci L, Brown MS et al. Ultrastructural analysis of crystalloid endoplasmic reticulum in UT-1 cells and its disappearance in response to cholesterol. J Cell Sci 1983; 63:1-20.
11. Surrey T, Nedelec F, Leibler S et al. Physical properties determining self-organization of motors and microtubules. Science 2001; 292:1167-1171.
12. Baumann O, Walz B. Endoplasmic reticulum in animal cells and its organization into structural and functional domains. Intern Rev Cytol 2001; 205:149-215.
13. Ellgaard L, Molinari M, Helenius A. Setting the standards: Quality control in the secretory pathway. Science 1999; 286:1882-1888.
14. Crowley KS, Liao S, Worrell VE et al. Secretory proteins move through the endoplasmic reticulum membrane via an aqueous, gated pore. Cell 1994; 78:461-471.
15. Simon SM, Blobel G. A protein-conducting channel in the endoplasmic reticulum. Cell 1991; 65:371-380.
16. Johnson AE, van Waes MA. The translocon: A dynamic gateway at the ER membrane. Annu Rev Cell Biol 1999; 7:90-95.
17. Rapoport TA, Jungnickel B, Kutay U. Protein transport across the eukaryotic endoplasmic reticulum and bacterial inner membranes. Annu Rev Biochem 1996; 65:271-303.
18. Matlack KES, Mothes W, Rapoport TA. Protein translocation: Tunnel vision. Cell 1998; 92:381-390.
19. Wattenberg B, Lithgow T. Targeting of C-terminal (tail)-anchored proteins: Understanding how cytoplasmic activities are anchored to intracellular membranes. Traffic 2001; 2:66-71.
20. Borgese N, D'Arrigo A, De Silvestris M et al. NADH-Cytochrome b_5 reductase and cytochrome b_5: The problem of posttranslational targeting to the endoplasmic reticulum. In: Borgese NaH JR, eds. Endoplasmic Reticulum. New York: Plenum Press, 1993:313-341.

21. Rapoport TA, Rolls MM, Jungnickel B. Approaching the mechanism of protein transport across the ER membrane. Curr Op Cell Biol 1996; 8:499-504.
22. Choy E, Chiu VK, Silletti J et al. Endomembrane trafficking of ras: The CAAX motif targets proteins to the ER and Golgi. Cell 1999; 98:69-80.
23. Munro S, Pelham HRB. An Hsp70-like protein in the ER: Identity with the 78 kd glucose-regulated protein and immunoglobin heavy chain binding protein. Cell 1986; 46:291-300.
24. Noiva R, Lennarz WJ. Protein disulfide isomerase: A multifunctional protein resident in the lumen of the endoplasmic reticulum. J Biol Chem 1992; 267(6):3553-3556.
25. Helenius A, Trombetta ES, Hebert DN et al. Calnexin, calreticulin and the folding of glycoproteins. Trends Cell Biol 1997; 7:193-200.
26. Danilczyk UG, Williams DB. The lectin chaperone calnexin utilizes polypeptide-based interactions to associate with many of its substrates in vivo. J Biol Chem 2001; 276(27):25532-25540.
27. Meldolesi J, Pozzan T. The endoplasmic reticulum Ca^{2+} store: A view from the lumen. TIBS 1998; 23:10-14.
28. Lepock JR, Frey HE, Ritchie KP. Protein denaturation in intact hepatocytes and isolated cellular organelles during heat shock. J Cell Biol 1993; 122(6):1267-1276.
29. Helenius A, Braakman I, Helenius J. Role of ATP and disulfide bonds during protein folding in the endoplasmic reticulum. Nature 1992; 356:260-262.
30. Chevet E, Cameron PH, Pelletier MF et al. The endoplasmic reticulum: Integration of protein folding, quality control, signaling, and degradation. Curr Opin Struct Biol 2001; 11:120-124.
31. Bucciantini M, Giannoni E, Chiti F et al. Inherent toxicity of aggregates implies a common mechanism for protein misfolding diseases. Nature 2002; 416:507-511.
32. Lippincott-Schwartz J, Bonafacino JS, Yuan LC et al. Degradation from the endoplasmic reticulum: Disposing of newly synthesized proteins. Cell 1988; 54:209-220.
33. Nishikawa SI, Fewell SW, Kato Y et al. Molecular chaperones in the yeast endoplasmic reticulum maintain the solubility of proteins for retrotranslocation and degradation. J Cell Biol 2001; 153(5):1061-70.
34. Kopito RR. Aggresomes, inclusion bodies and protein aggregation. Trends Cell Biol 2000; 10:524-530.
35. Valetti C, Grossi CE, Milstein C et al. Russell bodies: A general response of secretory cells to synthesis of a mutant immunoglobulin which can neither exit from, nor be degraded in, the endoplasmic reticulum. J Cell Biol 1991; 115:983-994.
36. Sidrauski C, Chapman R, Walter P. The unfolded protein response: An intracellular signalling pathway with many surprising features. Trends Cell Biol 1998; 8:245-250.
37. Harding HP, Zhang Y, Bertolotti A et al. Perk is essential for translational regulation and cell survival during the unfolded protein response. Mol Cell 2000; 5:897-904.
38. Chen X, Shen J, Prywes R. The luminal domain of ATF6 senses endoplasmic reticulum (ER) stress and causes translocation of ATF6 from the ER to the Golgi. J Biol Chem 2002; 277(15):13045-52.
39. Pahl HL, Baeuerle PA. The ER-overload response: Activation of NF-kB. TIBS 1997; 22:63-67.
40. Alberts B, Bray D, Lewis J et al. Molecular Biology of the Cell. 3rd ed. New York: Garland Publishing, 1994.
41. Voelker DR. Organelle biogenesis and intracellular lipid transport in eukaryotes. Microbio Rev 1991; 55(4):543-560.
42. Meier PJ, Spycher MA, Meyer UA. Isolation and characterization of rough endoplasmic reticulum associated with mitochondria from normal rat liver. Biochim Biophys Acta 1981; 646:283-297.
43. Montisano D, Cascarano J, Pickett CB et al. Association between mitochondria and rough endoplasmic reticulum in rat liver. Anat Rec 1982; 203:441-450.
44. Vance JE, Shiao Y. Intracellular trafficking of phospholipids: Import of phosphatidylserine into mitochondria. Anticancer Res 1996; 16:1333-1340.
45. Achleitner G, Gaigg B, Krasser A et al. Association between the endoplasmic reticulum and mitochondria of yeast facilitates interorganelle transport of phospholipids through membrane contact. Eur J Biochem 1999; 264:545-553.
46. Reinhart MP, Billheimer JT, Faust JR et al. Subcellular localization of the enzymes of cholesterol biosynthesis in rat liver. J Biol Chem 1987; 262:9649-9655.

47. Ellenberg J, Siggia ED, Moreira JE et al. Nuclear membrane dynamics and reassembly in living cells: Targeting of an inner nuclear membrane protein in interphase and mitosis. J Cell Biol 1997; 138(6):1193-1206.
48. Sakai J, Rawson RB. The sterolregulatory element-binding protein pathway: Control of lipid homeostasis through regulated intracellular transport. Curr Opin Lipidology 2001; 12:261-266.
49. Dobrosotskaya IY, Seegmiller AC, Brown MS et al. Regulation of SREBP processing and membrane lipid production by phospholipids in Drosophila. Science 2002; 296:879-883.
50. Yang T, Goldstein JL, Brown MS. Overexpression of membrane domain of SCAP prevents sterols from inhibiting SCAP-SREBP exit from endoplasmic reticulum. J Biol Chem 2000; 275(38):29881-29886.
51. Barlowe C, Orci L, Yeung T et al. COPII: A membrane coat formed by Sec proteins that drive vesicle budding from the endoplasmic reticulum. Cell 1994; 77(6):895-907.
52. Tsien RY. The green fluorescent protein. Annu Rev Biochem 1998; 67:509-544.
53. Hirschberg K, Miller CM, Ellenberg J et al. Kinetic analysis of secretory protein traffic and characterization of Golgi to plasma membrane transport intermediates in living cells. J Cell Biol 1998; 143:1485-1503.
54. Klausner RD, Donaldson JG, Lippincott-Schwartz J. Brefeldin A: Insights into the control of membrane traffic and organelle structure. J Cell Biol 1992; 116(5):1071-80.
55. Ulmer JB, Palade GE. Effects of brefeldin A on the Golgi complex, endoplasmic reticulum and viral envelope glycoproteins in murine erythroleukemia cells. Eur J Cell Biol 1991; 54:38-54.
56. Orci L, Perrelet A, Ravazzola M et al. "BFA bodies": A subcompartment of the endoplasmic reticulum. Proc Natl Acad Sci 1993; 90:11089-11093.
57. Pelham HRB. The retention signal for soluble proteins of the endoplasmic reticulum. Trends Biochem Sci 1990; 15(12):483-486.
58. Munro S, Pelham HRB. A C-terminal signal prevents secretion of luminal ER proteins. Cell 1987; 48:899-907.
59. Semenza JC, Hardwick KG, Dean N et al. ERD2, a yeast gene required for the receptor-mediated retrieval of luminal ER proteins from the secretory pathway. Cell 1990; 61:1349-1357.
60. Hammond C, Helenius A. Quality control in the secretory pathway: Retention of a misfolded viral membrane glycoprotein involves cycling between the ER, intermediate compartment, and Golgi apparatus. J Cell Biol 1994; 126(1):41-52.
61. Sonnichsen B, Fullekrug J, Nguyen VP et al. Retention and retrieval: Both mechanisms cooperate to maintain calreticulin in the endoplasmic reticulum. J Cell Sci 1994; 107:2705-2717.
62. Cole NB, Ellenberg J, DiEuliis D et al. Retrograde transport of Golgi-localized proteins to the ER. J Cell Biol 1998; 140:1-15.
63. Pedrazzini E, Villa A, Borgese N. A mutant cytochrome b5 with a lengthened membrane anchor escapes from the endoplasmic reticulum and reaches the plasma membrane. Proc Natl Acad Sci 1996; 93:4207-4212.
64. Pedrazzini E, Villa A, Longhi R et al. Mechanism of residence of cytochrome b(5), a tail-anchored protein, in the endoplasmic reticulum. J Cell Biol 2000; 148(5):899-913.
65. Bretscher MS, Munro S. Cholesterol and the Golgi apparatus. Science 1993; 261:1280-1281.
66. Yang MY, Ellenberg J, Bonifacino JS et al. The transmembrane domain of a carboxyl-terminal anchored protein determines localization to the endoplasmic reticulum. J Biol Chem 1997; 272(3):1970-1975.
67. Nishimura N, Balch WE. A di-acidic signal required for selective export from the endoplasmic reticulum. Science 1997; 277:556-558.
68. Pentcheva T, Spiliotis ET, Edidin M. Cutting Edge: Tapasin is retained in the endoplasmic reticulum by dynamic clustering and exclusion from endoplasmic reticulum exit sites. J Immunol 2002; 168:1538-1541.
69. Belden WJ, Barlowe C. Role of Erv29p in collecting soluble secretory proteins into ER-derived transport vesicles. Science 2001; 294:1528-1531.
70. Lippincott-Schwartz J, Snapp E, Kenworthy A. Studying protein dynamics in living cells. Nat Rev Molec Cell Biol 2001; 2:444-456.
71. Nehls S, Snapp E, Cole N et al. Dynamics and retention of misfolded proteins in native ER membranes. Nature Cell Biology 2000; 2:288-295.

72. Kok JW, Babia T, Klappe K et al. Ceramide transport from endoplasmic reticulum to Golgi apparatus is not vesicle-mediated. Biochem J 1998; 333(Pt 3):779-86.

73. Moreau P, Rodriguez M, Cassagne C et al. Trafficking of lipids from the endoplasmic reticulum to the Golgi apparatus in a cell-free system from rat liver. J Biol Chem 1991; 266(7):4322-8.

74. Hao M, Lin SX, Karylowski OJ et al. Vesicular and non-vesicular sterol transport in living cells. The endocytic recycling compartment is a major sterol storage organelle. J Biol Chem 2002; 277(1):609-17.

75. Lippincott-Schwartz J. The endoplasmic reticulum-Golgi membrane system. In: Arias IM, Boyer JL, Fausto N et al, eds. The Liver: Biology and Pathobiology. 3rd ed. New York: Raven Press, 1994:215-228.

76. Ziegler DM. Detoxification: Oxidation and reduction. In: Arias IM, Boyer JL, Fausto N et al, eds. The liver: Biology and pathobiology. 3rd ed. New York: Raven Press, 1994:415-427.

77. Periz G, Fortini ME. Ca^{2+}-ATPase function is required for intracellular trafficking of the Notch receptor in Drosophila. EMBO 1999; 18(21):5983-5993.

78. Niggli E. Localized intracellular calcium signaling in muscle: Calcium sparks and calcium quarks. Annu Rev Physiol 1999; 61:311-335.

79. Carafoli E. Calcium signaling: A tale for all seasons. Proc Natl Acad Sci 2002; 99(3):1115-1122.

80. Somlyo AP, Bond M, Somlyo AV. Calcium content of mitochondria and endoplasmic reticulum in liver frozen rapidly in vivo. Nature 1985; 314:622-625.

81. Somlyo AV, Gonzalez-Serratos HG, Shuman H et al. Calcium release and ionic changes in the sarcoplasmic reticulum of tetanized muscle: An electro-probe study. J Cell Biol 1981; 90(3):577-594.

82. Roderick HL, Lechleiter JD, Camacho P. Cytosolic phosphorylation of calnexin controls intracellular Ca^{2+} oscillations via an interaction with SERCA2b. J Cell Biol 2000; 149(6):1235-1247.

83. Rizzuto R, Pinton P, Carrington W et al. Close contacts with the endoplasmic reticulum as determinants of mitochondrial Ca^{2+} responses. Science 1998; 280:1763-1766.

84. Meldolesi J, Pozzan T. The heterogeneity of ER Ca^{2+} stores has a key role in nonmuscle cell signaling and function. J Cell Biol 1998; 142:1395-1398.

85. Wang H, Benlimame N, Nabi IR. The AMF-R tubule is a smooth ilimaquinone-sensitive subdomain of the endoplasmic reticulum. J Cell Sci 1997; 110:3043-3053.

86. Wang H, Guay G, Pogan L et al. Calcium regulates the association between mitochondria and a smooth subdomain of the endoplasmic reticulum. J Cell Biol 2000; 150(6):1489-1497.

87. Mesaeli N, Nakamura K, Opas M et al. Endoplasmic reticulum in the heart, a forgotten organelle? Mol Cell Biochem 2001; 225:1-6.

88. Klopfenstein DRC, Kappeler F, Hauri H. A novel direct interaction of endoplasmic reticulum with microtubules. EMBO 1998; 17:6168-6177.

89. Klopfenstein DR, Klumperman J, Lustig A et al. Subdomain-specific localization of CLIMP-63 (p63) in the endoplasmic reticulum is mediated by its luminal a-helical segment. J Cell Biol 2001; 153(6):1287-1299.

90. Terasaki M, Chen LB, Fujiwara K. Microtubules and the endoplasmic reticulum are highly interdependent structures. J Cell Biol 1986; 103:1557-1568.

91. Lee C, Ferguson M, Chen LB. Construction of the endoplasmic reticulum. J Cell Biol 1989; 109.

92. Baumann O. Association of spectrin with a subcompartment of the endoplasmic reticulum in honeybee photoreceptor cells. Cell Motil Cytoskel 1998; 41:74-86.

93. Staehelin LA. The plant ER: A dynamic organelle composed of a large number of discrete functional domains. Plant J 1997; 11(6):1151-1165.

94. Prinz WA, Grzyb L, Veenhuis M et al. Mutants affecting the structure of the cortical endoplasmic reticulum in Saccharomyces cerevisiae. J Cell Biol 2000; 150:461-474.

95. Fehrenbacher KL, Davis D, Wu M et al. Endoplasmic reticulum dynamics, inheritance, and cytoskeletal interactions in budding yeast. Mol Biol Cell 2002; 13:854-865.

96. Hepler PK, Palevitz BA, Lancelle SA et al. Cortical endoplasmic reticulum in plants. J Cell Sci 1990; 96:355-373.

97. Williamson RE. Filaments associated with the endoplasmic reticulum in the streaming cytoplasm of Chara corallina. Eur J Cell Biol 1979; 20(2):177-183.

98. Kachar B, Reese TS. The mechanism of cytoplasmic streaming in characean algal cells: Sliding of endoplasmic reticulum along actin filaments. J Cell Biol 1988; 106:1545-1552.

99. Menzel D. Dynamics and pharmacological perturbations of the endoplasmic reticulum in the unicellular green alga Acetabularia. Eur J Cell Biol 1994; 64(1):113-119.

100. Liebe S, Menzel D. Actinomyosin-based motility of endoplasmic reticulum and chloroplasts in Vallisneria mesophyll cells. Biol Cell 1995; 1995(2-3):207-222.

101. Dreier L, Rapoport TA. In vitro formation of the endoplasmic reticulum occurs independently of microtubules by a controlled fusion reaction. J Cell Biol 1999; 148(5):883-898.

102. van Meer G, van Genderen IL. Intracellular lipid distribution, transport, and sorting: A cell biologist's need for physicochemical information. New York: Plenum Press, 1994.

103. Gummadi SN, Menon AK. Transbilayer movement of dipalmitoylphosphatidylcholine in proteoliposomes reconstituted from detergent extracts of endoplasmic reticulum. Kinetics of transbilayer transport mediated by a single flippase and identification of protein fractions enriched in flippase activity. J Biol Chem 2002; 277(28):25337-25343.

104. Backer JM, Dawidowicz EA. Reconstitution of a phospholipid flippase from rat liver microsomes. Nature 1987; 327:341-343.

105. Helenius J, Ng DTW, Marolda CL et al. Translocation of lipid-linked oligosaccharides across the ER membrane requires Rft1 protein. Nature 2002; 415:447-450.

106. van Meer G. The lipid bilayer of the ER. TIBS 1986; 11:194-195.

107. Koch GL. The endoplasmic reticulum. Fundamentals of medical cell biology, membranology and subcellular organelles. Greenwich, UK: JAI Press Inc., 1992; 4:397-420.

108. Dayel MJ, Hom EFY, Verkman AS. Diffusion of green fluorescent protein in the aqueous-phase lumen of endoplasmic reticulum. Biophys J 1999; 76:2843-2851.

109. Swaminathan R, Hoang CP, Verkman AS. Photobleaching recovery and anisotropy decay of green fluorescent protein GFP-S65T in solution and cells: Cytoplasmic viscosity probed by green fluorescent protein translational and rotational diffusion. Biophys J 1997; 72:1900-1907.

110. Yu R, Hinkle PM. Rapid turnover of calcium in the endoplasmic reticulum during signaling: Studies with cameleon calcium indicators. J Biol Chem 2000; 275(31):23648-23653.

111. Szczesna-Skorupa E, Chen C, Rogers S et al. Mobility of cytochrome P450 in the endoplasmic reticulum membrane. Proc Natl Acad Sci USA 1998; 95:14793-14798.

112. Zaal KJM, Smith CL, Polishchuk RS et al. Golgi membranes are absorbed into and reemerge from the ER during mitosis. Cell 1999; 99:589-601.

113. Cole NB, Smith CL, Sciaky N et al. Diffusional mobility of Golgi proteins in membranes of living cells. Science 1996; 273:797-801.

114. Rolls MM, Hall DH, Victor M et al. Targeting of rough endoplasmic reticulum membrane proteins and ribosomes in invertebrate neurons. Mol Biol Cell 2002; 13(5):1778-1791.

115. Marguet D, Spiliotis ET, Pentcheva T et al. Lateral diffusion of GFP-tagged H2Ld molecules and of GFP-TAP1 reports on the assembly and retention of these molecules in the endoplasmic reticulum. Immunology 1999; 11:231-240.

116. Quinn P, Griffiths G, Warren G. Density of newly synthesized plasma membrane proteins in intracellular membranes. II. Biochemical studies. J Cell Biol 1984; 98:2142-2147.

117. Azzam NA, Hallenbeck JM, Kachar B. Membrane changes during hibernation: Organelle lipids undergo rapidly reversible rearrangement as body temperature drops. Nature 2000; 407:317.

118. Terasaki M, Reese TS. Interactions among endoplasmic reticulum, microtubules, and retrograde movements of the cell surface. Cell Motil Cytoskel 1994; 29:291-300.

119. Waterman-Storer CM, Salmon ED. Endoplasmic reticulum in membrane tubules are distributed by microtubules in living cells using three distinct mechanisms. Curr Biol 1998; 8:798-806.

120. Allan V, Vale R. Movement of membrane tubules along microtubules in vitro: Evidence for specialised sites of motor attachment. J Cell Sci 1994; 107:1885-1897.

121. Subramanian K, Meyer T. Calcium-induced restructuring of nuclear envelope and endoplasmic reticulum calcium stores. Cell 1997; 89:963-971.

122. Waterman-Storer CM, Gregory J, Parsons SF et al. Membrane/microtubule tip attachment complexes (TACs) allow the assembly and dynamics of plus ends to push and pull membranes into tubulovesicular networks in interphase Xenopus egg extracts. J Cell Biol 1995; 130(5):1161-1169.

123. Vale RD, Hotani H. Formation of membrane networks in vitro by kinesin-driven microtubule movement. J Cell Biol 1988; 107(6):2233-2241.

124. Hecht E. Optics. 2nd ed. Reading, MA: Addison-Wesley; 1987.

125. Pelham HRB. SNAREs and the specificity of membrane fusion. Trends Cell Biol 2001; 11(3):99-101.
126. Chen YA, Scheller RH. SNARE-mediated membrane fusion. Nat Rev Molec Cell Biol 2001; 2:98-106.
127. Malhotra V, Orci L, Glick BS et al. Role of an N-ethylmaleimide-sensitive transport component in promoting fusion of transport vesicles with cisternae of the Golgi stack. Cell 1988; 54:221-227.
128. Patel S, Latterich M. The AAA team: Related ATPases with diverse functions. Trends Cell Biol 1998; 8:65-71.
129. Zerial M, McBride H. Rab proteins as membrane organizers. Nat Rev Mol Cell Biol 2001; 2:107-118.
130. Haas A. NSF- fusion and beyond. Trends Cell Biol 1998; 8:471-473.
131. Egerton M, Ashe OR, Chen D et al. VCP, the mammalian homolog of cdc48, is tyrosine phosphorylated in response to T cell antigen receptor activation. EMBO 1992; 11:3533-3540.
132. Turner MD, Plutner H, Balch WE. A Rab GTPase is required for homotypic assembly of the endoplasmic reticulum. J Biol Chem 1997; 272(21):13479-13483.
133. Roy L, Bergeron JJM, Lavoie C et al. Role of p97 and syntaxin 5 in the assembly of transitional endoplasmic reticulum. Mol Biol Cell 2000; 11:2529-2542.
134. Latterich M, Frolich K, Schekman R. Membrane fusion and the cell cycle: Cdc48p participates in the fusion of ER membranes. Cell 1995; 82:885-893.
135. Kondo H, Rabouille C, Newman R et al. p47 is a cofactor for p97-mediated membrane fusion. Nature 1997; 388:75-8.
136. Lavoie C, Chevet E, Roy L et al. Tyrosine phosphorylation of p97 regulates transitional endoplasmic reticulum assembly in vitro. Proc Natl Acad Sci 2000; 97(25):13637-13642.
137. Latterich M, Schekman R. The karyogamy gene KAR2 and novel proteins are required for ER-membrane fusion. Cell 1994; 78:87-98.
138. Patel SK, Indig FE, Olivieri N et al. Organelle membrane fusion: A novel function for the syntaxin homolog Ufe1p in ER membrane fusion. Cell 1998; 92:611-620.
139. Hay JC, Klumperman J, Oorschot V et al. Localization, dynamics, and protein interactions reveal distinct roles for ER and Golgi SNAREs. J Cell Biol 1998; 141(7):1489-1502.
140. Hatsuzawa K, Hirose H, Tani K et al. Syntaxin 18, a SNAP receptor that functions in the endoplasmic reticulum, intermediate compartment, and cis-Golgi vesicle trafficking. J Biol Chem 2000; 275:13713-13720.
141. Yamaguchi T, Dulubova I, Min S et al. Sly1 binds to Golgi and ER syntaxins via a conserved N-terminal peptide motif. Dev Cell 2002; 2:295-305.
142. Paiement J, Bergeron J. The shape of things to come: Regulation of shape changes in endoplasmic reticulum. Biochem Cell Biol 2001; 79:587-592.
143. Paiement J. Physiological concentrations of GTP stimulate fusion of the endoplasmic reticulum and the nuclear envelope. Exp Cell Res 1984; 151:354-366.
144. Kan FWK, Jolicoeur M, Paiement J. Freeze-fracture analysis of the effects of intermediates of the phosphatidylinositol cycle on fusion of rough endoplasmic reticulum membranes. Biochim Biophys Acta 1992; 1107:331-341.
145. Lavoie C, Lanoix J, Kan FWK et al. Cell-free assembly of rough and smooth endoplasmic reticulum. J Cell Sci 1996; 109:1415-1425.
146. Steegmaier M, Oorschot V, Klumperman J et al. Syntaxin 17 is abundant in steroidogenic cells and implicated in smooth endoplasmic reticulum membrane dynamics. Mol Biol Cell 2000; 11:2719-2731.
147. Powell KS, Latterich M. The making and breaking of the endoplasmic reticulum. Traffic 2000; 1:689-694.
148. Voeltz GK, Rolls MM, Rapoport TA. Structural organization of the endoplasmic reticulum. EMBO Rep 2002; 3(10):944-50.
149. Lane JD, Allan V. Microtubule-based endoplasmic reticulum motility in Xenopus laevis: Activation of membrane associated kinesin during development. Mol Biol Cell 1999; 10:1909-1922.
150. Roux A, Cappello G, Cartaud J et al. A minimal system allowing tubulation with molecular motors pulling on giant liposomes. Proc Natl Acad Sci 2002; 99(8):5394-5399.
151. Feiguin F, Ferreira A, Kosik KS et al. Kinesin-mediated organelle translocation revealed by specific cellular manipulations. J Cell Biol 1994; 127(4):1021-1039.

152. Allan V. Protein phosphatase 1 regulates the cytoplasmic dynein-driven formation of endoplasmic reticulum networks in vitro. J Cell Biol 1995; 128:879-891.

153. Kumar J, Yu H, Sheetz MP. Kinectin, an essential anchor for kinesin-driven vesicle motility. Science 1995; 267-:1834-1837.

154. Klopfenstein DR, Vale R, Rogers SL. Motor protein receptors: Moonlighting on other jobs. Cell 2000; 103:537-540.

155. Klopfenstein DR, Tomishige M, Stuurman N et al. Role of phosphatidylinositol(4,5)bisphosphate organization in membrane transport by the Unc104 kinesin motor. Cell 2002; 109:347-358.

156. Schrader M, King SJ, Stroh TA et al. Real time imaging reveals a peroxisomal reticulum in living cells. J Cell Sci 2000; 113:3663-3671.

157. Collins TJ, Berridge MJ, Lipp P et al. Mitochondria are morphologically and functionally heterogeneous within cells. EMBO 2002; 21(7):1616-1627.

158. Hetzer M, Meyer HH, Walther TC et al. Distinct AAA-ATPase p97 complexes function in discrete steps of nuclear assembly. Nat Cell Biol 2001; 3:1086-1091.

159. Smirnova E, Shurland D, Ryazantsev SN et al. A human dynamin-related protein controls the distribution of mitochondria. J Cell Biol 1998; 143(2):351-358.

160. Yoon Y, Pitts KR, Dahan S et al. A novel dynamin-like protein associates with cytoplasmic vesicles and tubules of the endoplasmic reticulum in mammalian cells. J Cell Biol 1998; 140(4):779-793.

161. Yoon Y, Pitts KR, McNiven MA. Mammalian dynamin-like protein DLP1 tubulates membranes. Mol Biol Cell 2001; 12:2894-2905.

162. Pitts KR, Yoon Y, Krueger EW et al. The dynamin-like protein DLP1 is essential for normal distribution and morphology of the endoplasmic reticulum and mitochondria in mammalian cells. Mol Biol Cell 1999; 10:4403-4417.

163. Sciaky N, Presley J, Smith C et al. Golgi tubule traffic and the effects of brefeldin A visualized in living cells. J Cell Biol 1997; 139(5):1137-1155.

164. Mui BL, Dobereiner HG, Madden TD et al. Influence of transbilayer area asymmetry on the morphology of large unilamellar vesicles. Biophys J 1995; 69(3):930-41.

165. de Figueiredo P, Drecktrah D, Katzenellbogen JA et al. Evidence that phospholipase A2 activity is required for Golgi complex and trans Golgi network membrane tubulation. Proc Natl Acad Sci USA 1998; 95(15):8642-7.

166. de Figueiredo P, Polizotto RS, Drecktrah D et al. Membrane tubule-mediated reassembly and maintenance of the Golgi complex is disrupted by phospholipase A2 antagonists. Mol Biol Cell 1999; 10(6):1763-82.

167. Chou T, Jaric MV, Siggia ED. Electrostatics of lipid bilayer bending. Biophys J 1997; 72(5):2042-55.

168. Cluett EB, Wood SA, Banta M et al. Tubulation of Golgi membranes in vivo and in vitro in the absence of brefeldin A. J Cell Biol 1993; 120(1):15-24.

169. Goodsell DS. The machinery of life. New York: Springer-Verlag, 1993.

170. Zeligs JD, Wollman SH. Mitosis in rat thyroid epithelial cells in vivo. J Ultrastruct Res 1979; 66:53-77.

171. Koch GL, Booth C, Wooding FB. Dissociation and re-assembly of the endoplasmic reticulum in live cells. J Cell Sci 1988; 91(4):511-522.

172. Terasaki M, Jaffe LA, Hunnicutt GR et al. Structural change of the endoplasmic reticulum during fertilization: Evidence for loss of membrane continuity using the green fluorescent protein. Dev Biol 1996; 179:320-328.

173. Ribeiro CMP, McKay RR, Hosoki E et al. Effects of elevated cytoplasmic calcium and protein kinase C on endoplasmic reticulum structure and function in HEK293 cells. Cell Calcium 2000; 27(3):175-185.

174. Boggs JM. Lipid intermolecular hydrogen bonding: Influence on structural organization and membrane function. Biochim Biophys Acta 1987; 906:353-404.

175. Schneider MF, Marsh D, Jahn W et al. Network formation of lipid membranes: Triggering structural transitions by chain melting. Proc Natl Acad Sci 1999; 96(25):14312-14317.

176. Oritz A, Killian JA, Verkleij AJ et al. Membrane fusion and the lamellar-to-inverted-hexagonal phase transition in cardiolipin vesicle systems induced by divalent cations. Biophys J 1999; 77:2003-2014.

177. Palade GE. A small particulate component of the cytoplasm. J Biophys Biochem Cytol 1955; 1:59-61.
178. Fawcett DW. The Cell. 2nd ed. Philadelphia: W.B. Saunders Company, 1981.
179. Kailes K, Gorlich D, Rapoport TA. Binding of ribosomes to the rough endoplasmic reticulum mediated by the Sec61p-complex. J Cell Biol 1994; 126(4):925-934.
180. Gorlich D, Prehn S, Hartmann E et al. A mammalian homolog of Sec61p and SECYp is associated with ribosomes and nascent polypeptides during translocation. Cell 1992; 71:489-503.
181. Wanker EE, Sun Y, Savitz AJ et al. Functional characterization of the 180-kD ribosome receptor in vivo. J Cell Biol 1995; 130:29-39.
182. Yamamoto A, Masaki R, Tashiro Y. Formation of crystalloid endoplasmic reticulum in COS cells upon overexpression of microsomal aldehyde dehydrogenase by cDNA transfection. J Cell Sci 1996; 109:1727-1738.
183. Galteau M, Antoine B, Reggio H. Epoxide hydrolase is a marker for the smooth endoplasmic reticulum in rat liver. EMBO 1985; 4:2793-2800.
184. Hammond AT, Glick BS. Dynamics of transitional endoplasmic reticulum sites in vertebrate cells. Mol Biol Cell 2000; 11:3013-3030.
185. Rossanese OW, Soderholm J, Bevis BJ et al. Golgi structure correlates with transitional endoplasmic reticulum organization in Pichia pastoris and Saccharomyces cerevisiae. J Cell Biol 1999; 145(1):69-81.
186. Kessel RG. Annulate lamellae: A last frontier in cellular organelles. Int Rev Cytol 1992; 133:43-120.
187. Newport J. Nuclear reconstitution in vitro: Stages of assembly around protein-free DNA. Cell 1987; 48:205-217.
188. Koning AJ, Roberts CJ, Wright RL. Different subcellular localization of Saccharomyces cerevisiae HMG-CoA reductase isozymes at elevated levels correspond to distinct endoplasmic reticulum membrane proliferations. Mol Biol Cell 1996; 7:769-789.
189. Porter KR, Yamada E. Studies on the endoplasmic reticulum: V. Its form and differentiation in pigment epithelial cells of the frog retina. J Biophys Biochem Cyt 1960; 8:181-205.
190. Abran D, Dickson DH. Biogenesis of myeloid bodies in regenerating newt (Notophthalmus viridescens) retinal pigment epithelium. Cell Tissue Res 1992; 268:531-538.
191. Bassot JM, Nicola G. An optional dyadic junctional complex revealed by fast-freeze fixation in the bioluminescent system of the scale worm. J Cell Biol 1987; 105:2245-2256.
192. Rebuffat P, Belloni AS, Cavallini L et al. Effect of mevinolin on rat hepatocytes: A morphometric study. Exp Path 1988; 35:133-139.
193. Berciano MT, Fernandez R, Pena E et al. Formation of intranuclear crystalloids and proliferation of the smooth endoplasmic reticulum in Schwann cells induced by tellurium treatment: Association with overexpression of HMG CoA reductase and HMG CoA synthase mRNA. Glia 2000; 29:246-259.
194. Zimmer T, Ogura A, Takewaka T et al. Gene regulation in response to overexpression of cytochrome P450 and proliferation of the endoplasmic reticulum in Saccharomyces cerevisiae. Biosci Biotechnol Biochem 2000; 64(9):1930-1936.
195. Ohkuma M, Park SM, Zimmer T et al. Proliferation of intracellular membrane structures upon homologous overproduction of cytochrome P-450 in Candida maltosa. Biochim Biophys Acta 1995; 1236:163-169.
196. Vergeres G, Yen TSB, Aggeler J et al. A model system for studying membrane biogenesis: Overexpression of cytochrome b5 in yeast results in marked proliferation of the intracellular membrane. J Cell Sci 1993; 106:249-259.
197. Wiedmann B, Silver P, Schunck W et al. Overexpression of the ER-membrane protein P-450 CYP52A3 mimics sec mutant characteristics in Saccharomyces cerevisiae. Biochim Biophys Acta 1993; 1153:267-276.
198. Elgersma Y, Kwast L, Berg M et al. Overexpression of Pex15p, a phosphorylated peroxisomal integral membrane protein required for peroxisome assembly in S. cerevisiae, causes proliferation of the endoplasmic reticulum membrane. EMBO 1997; 16(24):7326-7341.
199. Sandig G, Kargel E, Menzel R et al. Regulation of endoplasmic reticulum biogenesis in response to cytochrome P450 overproduction. Drug Metab Rev 1999; 31:393-410.

200. Gong F, Giddings TH, Meehl JB et al. Z-membranes: Artificial organelles for overexpressing recombinant integral membrane proteins. Proc Natl Acad Sci 1996; 93:2219-2223.
201. Carette JE, Stuiver M, Lent JV et al. Cowpea mosaic virus infection induces a massive proliferation of endoplasmic reticulum but not Golgi membranes and is dependent on de novo membrane synthesis. J Virol 2000; 74(14):6556-6563.
202. Takei K, Mignery GA, Mugnaini E et al. Inositol 1,4,5-triphosphate receptor causes formation of ER cisternal stacks in transfected fibroblasts and in cerebellar Purkinje cells. Neuron 1994; 12:327-342.
203. Fukuda M, Yamamoto A, Mikoshiba K. Formation of crystalloid endoplasmic reticulum induced by expression of synaptotagmin lacking the conserved WHXL motif in the C terminus: Structural importance of the WHXL motif in the C2B domain. J Biol Chem 2001; 276(44):41112-41119.
204. Smith S, Blobel G. Colocalization of vertebrate lamin B and lamin B receptor (LBR) in nuclear envelopes and LBR-induced membrane stacks of the yeast Saccharomyces cerevisiae. Proc Natl Acad Sci 1994; 91:10124-10128.
205. Pathak RK, Luskey KL, Anderson RGW. Biogenesis of the crystalloid endoplasmic reticulum in UT-1 cells: Evidence that newly formed endoplasmic reticulum emerges from the nuclear envelope. J Cell Biol 1986; 102:2158-2168.
206. Jingami H, Brown MS, Goldstein JL et al. Partial deletion of membrane-bound domain of 3-hydroxy-3-methylglutaryl-coenzyme A reductase eliminates sterol-enhanced degradation and prevents formation of crystalloid endoplasmic reticulum. J Cell Biol 1987; 104:1693-1704.
207. Parrish ML, Sengstag C, Rine JD et al. Identification of the sequences in HMG-CoA reductase required for karmellae assembly. Mol Biol Cell 1995; 6:1535-1547.
208. Borovjagin VL, Vergara JA, McIntosh TJ. Morphology of the intermediate stages in the lamellar to hexagonal lipid phase transition. J Membrane Biol 1982; 1982:199-212.
209. Norlen L. Skin barrier formation: The membrane folding model. J Invest Dermatol 2001; 117:823-829.
210. Ball P. The self-made tapestry: Pattern formation in nature. New York: oxford University Press, 1999.
211. Becker F, Block-Alper L, Nakamura G et al. Expression of the 180-kD ribosome receptor induces membrane proliferation and increased secretory activity in yeast. J Cell Biol 1999; 146:273-284.
212. Block-Alper L, Webster P, Zhou X et al. INO2, a positive regulator of lipid biosynthesis, is essential for the formation of inducible membranes in yeast. Mol Biol Cell 2002; 13:40-51.
213. Henry SA, Patton-Vogt JL. Genetic regulation of phospholipid metabolism: Yeast as a model eukaryote. Prog Nucleic Acid Res 1998; 61:133-179.
214. Cox JS, Chapman RE, Walter P. The unfolded protein response coordinates the production of endoplasmic reticulum membrane. Mol Biol Cell 1997; 8:1805-1814.
215. Menzel R, Vogel F, Kargel E et al. Inducible membranes in yeast: Relation to the unfolded-protein response pathway. Yeast 1997; 13:1211-1229.
216. Stroobants AK, Hettema EH, van den Berg M et al. Enlargement of the endoplasmic reticulum membrane in Saccharomyces cerevisiae is not necessarily linked to the unfolded protein response via Ire1p. FEBS Lett 1999; 453:210-214.
217. Shank KJ, Su P, Brglez I et al. Induction of lipid metabolic enzymes during endoplasmic reticulum stress response in plants. Plant Physiol 2001; 126:267-277.
218. Hyde M, Block-Alper L, Felix J et al. Induction of secretory pathway components in yeast is associated with increased stability of their mRNA. J Cell Biol 2002; 156(6):993-1001.
219. Shamu CE, Walter P. Oligomerization and phosphorylation of the Ire1p kinase during intracellular signaling from the endoplasmic reticulum to the nucleus. EMBO 1996; 15(12):3028-3039.
220. Bertolotti A, Zhang Y, Hendershot LM et al. Dynamic interaction of BiP and ER stress transducers in the unfolded- protein response. Nat Cell Biol 2000; 2(6):326-32.
221. Misteli T. The concept of self-organization in cellular architecture. J Cell Biol 2001; 155(2):181-185.
222. Weibel ER, Staubli W, Gnagi HR et al. Correlated morphometric and biochemical studies on the liver cell. I. Morphometric model stereologic methods and normal morphometric data for rat liver. J Cell Biol 1969; 42:68-91.
223. Griffiths G, Warren G, Quinn P et al. Density of newly synthesized plasma membrane proteins in intracellular membranes. I. Stereological studies. J Cell Biol 1984; 98:2133-2141.

224. Tilney LG, Harb OS, Connelly PS et al. How the parasitic bacterium Legionella pneumophila modifies its phagosome and transforms it into rough ER: Implications for conversion of plasma membrane to the ER membrane. J Cell Sci 2001; 114:4637-4650.

225. Menetret JF, Neuhof A, Morgan DG et al. The structure of ribosome-channel complexes engaged in protein translocation. Mol Cell 2000; 6(5):1219-32.

226. Kozielski F, Sack S, Marx A et al. The crystal structure of dimeric kinesin and implications for microtubule-dependent motility. Cell 1997; 91:985-994.

CHAPTER 5

The Golgi Apparatus:
Structure, Function and Cellular Dynamics

Nihal Altan-Bonnet and Jennifer Lippincott-Schwartz

Abstract

The Golgi apparatus is a membrane-bounded organelle comprised of polarized stacks of cisternae and is required for trafficking of proteins and lipids within all eukaryotic cells. The Golgi, which is positioned centrally in the transport route between the endoplasmic reticulum (ER) and plasma membrane, is an organelle whose size, composition and morphology are effected by protein and lipid flux, as well as the cytoskeletal dynamics. The following chapter discusses various aspects of Golgi structure and function and recent insights into the dynamics of Golgi assembly.

Introduction

Growth and division of eukaryotic cells requires the delivery of new proteins and lipids from their site of synthesis in the endoplasmic reticulum (ER) to the cell surface or to other final destinations.[1,2] This process is not accomplished by a single vesicle transport step, but involves continuous membrane transformation and maturation through the activity of the Golgi apparatus, which is situated centrally in the secretory transport route between the ER and plasma membrane (Fig. 1).[3-9] Comprised of polarized stacks of cisternae enriched in processing enzymes, the Golgi serves as a processing and filtering station within the secretory pathway.[4,8] It covalently modifies proteins and lipids received from the ER and then either recycles components back to the ER or packages them into membrane containers that are delivered to destinations within the cell.[6,7,9] This chapter summarizes important aspects of the structure and dynamics of the Golgi apparatus that are essential for its diverse functions and for its ability to maintain itself as a distinct organelle in the face of ongoing membrane traffic.

Golgi Structure and Distribution

Golgi morphology seen at the electron microscopy level varies considerably between different cell types. In higher eukaryotic cells, the Golgi is typically organized as a series of three to ten flattened cisternae (1 μm diameter) arranged as a stack with surrounding tubules and vesicles (Fig. 2).[10-12] The flattened nature of the cisternae produces a large surface-to-volume ratio that is thought to facilitate the activity of resident Golgi enzymes, which include glycosyltransferases, lipases and proteases.[5] These enzymes are heterogeneously distributed within different Golgi cisternae and are all transmembrane proteins that face the lumen of the cisternae.[13,14] Many serve as processing enzymes to catalyze the incorporation of monosaccarides into glycoproteins

The Biogenesis of Cellular Organelles, edited by Chris Mullins. ©2005 Eurekah.com
and Kluwer Academic/Plenum Publishers.

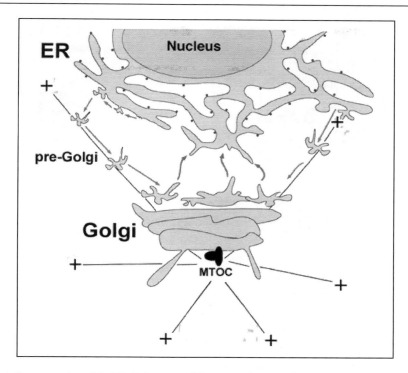

Figure 1. Representation of the ER-Golgi route of the mammalian secretory pathway. The Golgi is often located near the centrosome of the cell (noted by the microtubule-organizing center (MTOC)). Cargo is exported out of the ER, which is contiguous with the nuclear membrane, in membrane carriers (i.e., preGolgi membranes). These carriers track to the Golgi apparatus (arrows pointing from the ER to the Golgi) along microtubules (denoted as straight lines; plus-end orientation of microtubles is noted by the "+"). Membranes are also recycled back to the ER from the Golgi stacks (arrows pointing from the Golgi back to the ER) in a largely microtubule independent pathway.

and glycolipids, and to initiate the biosynthesis of glycolipids, proteoglycans and polysaccharides. The processed products play essential roles in the plasma membrane and extracellular environment of cells.

The stack of cisternae comprising the Golgi exhibits a cis to trans polarity.[3,5,15,16] Newly synthesized membrane and secretory components enter the stack at its cis face, comprised of cisternae and associated tubules/vesicles in close vicinity to the ER. Secretory cargo then passes through cisternae in the middle of the stack. It then leaves the Golgi at the trans face, which is at the opposite end of the stack. How this tight arrangement of cisternae within Golgi stacks is maintained is not clear. One possibility is that the cisternae are cross-linked by matrix proteins,[17,18] which are cytoplasmic proteins having a long coiled-coil region[19] that associate with the Golgi dynamically.[20]

The tubules and vesicles surrounding the Golgi stack are believed to mediate Golgi trafficking events,[4,8] which include transport of molecules into, within and out of this organelle. Continuous binding and dissociation of cytoplasmic coat proteins allows secretory cargo and Golgi enzymes to become enriched within these vesicles/tubules.[21-24] It furthermore activates membrane remodeling machinery that results in forward movement of secretory cargo and retrograde transport of enzymes within the Golgi system.[24] Budding of transport carriers out

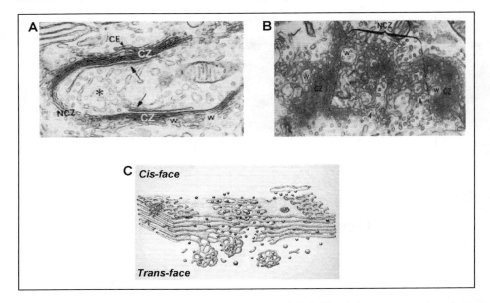

Figure 2. Electron micrographs of the Golgi apparatus in epithelial cells. A) A cross-section through the Golgi apparatus with arrows indicating compact zones (CZ), noncompact zones (NCZ), cis elements (CE), and wells (W). Anastamotic tubules are indicated by the asterisk. B) A face-on view of the Golgi apparatus. Characteristic morphological characteristics are evident, including fenestrated cisternae, anastomozing tubules, sacculo-tubular membranes and vesicles within fenestrations. CZ, NCZ, W, as above. C) Three dimensional illustration of the Golgi apparatus within epithelial cells. Figures reproduced with permission from ref. 11.

from the Golgi and translocation of these carriers through the cytoplasm is mediated by other Golgi-associated peripheral microtubule motor proteins.[25,26]

The membranes that comprise the Golgi are unique in lipid composition. They contain concentrations of lipids that are intermediate between the glycerolipid-rich ER and sterol/sphingolipid-rich plasma membrane.[27,28] The intermediate character of Golgi lipid composition has led to a lipid-sorting model for Golgi protein localization in which Golgi proteins partition into thinner regions of the Golgi bilayer and are excluded from thicker regions that are enriched in sphingolipid and sterols destined from the plasma membrane.[28] The finding that shortening the transmembrane domain of VSVG, a secretory viral glycoprotein, leads to its localization within the Golgi rather than to plasma membrane delivery is consistent with this possibility.[29]

In many animal cells, the Golgi is localized near the microtubule-organizing center (MTOC), which is adjacent to the nucleus (Fig. 3).[30,31] This localization permits Golgi-targeted transport intermediates that bud out from widely dispersed ER export sites to readily converge at one central location by tracking along microtubules. It furthermore allows Golgi-derived intermediates to find microtubules easily for their use to track out to the cell periphery.[25,26,32,33] Interestingly, when microtubules are disrupted with microtubule-disrupting agents (i.e., nocodazole or colchicine) or when the microtubule motor dynein is inhibited, the juxtanuclear localization of the Golgi apparatus is lost.[30] Under these conditions, the Golgi does not simply fragment into small pieces that diffuse within the cytoplasm. Instead, it reforms at ER exit sites as miniature stacks of cisternae that are still capable of receiving, processing and secreting proteins.[34] This reformation occurs as a result of the constitutive cycling of Golgi membrane

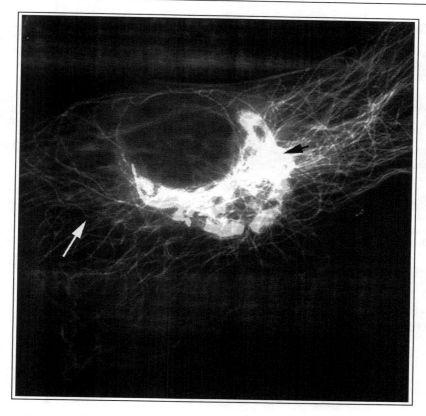

Figure 3. The proximity of the Golgi apparatus (black arrow) to microtubules (white arrow) in a mammalian cell. Golgi appartus and microtubules were labeled with antibodies against the resident enzyme mannosidase II and β-tubulin, respectively. Figure reproduced with permission from ref. 142.

components through the ER (see section on interphase Golgi dynamics).[20,34-36] Thus, when microtubules are disrupted and ER-to-Golgi transport intermediates can no longer translocate to a juxtanuclear site, cycling Golgi enzymes redistribute with ER-to-Golgi transport intermediates to ER exit sites, reforming Golgi membranes at these sites.

Golgi Function and Compartmentalization

The Golgi apparatus serves two primary functions within all eukaryotic cells: the post-translational modification of glycoproteins and glycolipids; and sorting and transport of newly synthesized, ER-derived membrane and proteins destined for the plasma membrane and other final sites. These functions are carried out to differing extents in different regions of the Golgi, which include the cis-, medial- and trans-Golgi.

The cis-Golgi acts to receive incoming transport intermediates derived from the ER and it recycles protein and lipid components back into the ER (Fig. 4).[5] Such recycling serves to resupply the ER with membrane lipid and protein components (including targeting and fusion machinery) necessary for continued export of cargo out of the ER and delivery to the Golgi.[37] Recycling might also serve to inhibit loss of resident ER proteins into the secretory pathway[7] and function as a quality control mechanism to check if secretory cargo is properly folded and

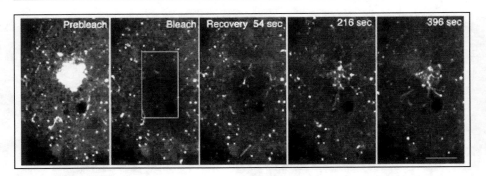

Figure 4. Time lapse of preGolgi structures, so called vesiculo tubule carriers (VTC), carrying the cargo protein VSVG-GFP merging with the Golgi apparatus. COS cells were incubated at 40°C for 12 hours to accumulate the unfolded VSVG-GFP cargo in the ER. Cells were then shifted to 15°C for 3 hours to fold and accumulate VSVG-GFP in VTCs and then further warmed to 32°C to initiate transport of VTCs from the ER region out to the Golgi region. To visualize the merging of VTCs to form the cis- Golgi, VSVG-GFP fluorescence at the Golgi apparatus was photobleached with high intensity laser light (Bleach) and the cell was then imaged with low laser light over a period of 400 seconds. Reproduced with permission from ref. 108. Scale bar represents 9.6 microns.

assembled. Indeed misassembled major histocompatibility complex (MHC) oligomers have been reported to cycle between the Golgi and ER and not be transported to the cell surface.[38,39]

Structurally, the cis-Golgi exists as an array of tubules and associated vesicles (see Fig. 2). These membranes are selectively stained after prolonged osmification and are enriched in several proteins, including ERGIC53, KDEL receptor (KDELR), coatamer (COPI) and Rab2,[40,41] which all are critical for sorting and recycling of proteins between the Golgi and the ER. ERGIC-53 and KDELR are cargo receptors that transport specific classes of glycoproteins and KDEL sequence-containing proteins.[42-44] Loss of ERGIC53 from cells can result in the loss of the transport to the cell surface of specific classes of glycoproteins that regulate blood clotting.[45,46]

The medial-Golgi comprises the three to seven stacked cisternae situated between the tubular-vesicular elements of the cis- and trans-Golgi. It is here where monosaccharides are incorporated into glycoproteins and glycolipids.[13,14,47] An estimated 100-200 different glycosyltransferases are found within this region of the Golgi apparatus. These enzymes represent the bulk of resident membrane proteins in the Golgi. Though diverse in their amino acid sequence, the glycosyltransferases all have a short amino-terminal cytoplasmic domain, a single hydrophobic membrane-spanning domain (14-25 amino acids) and a large carboxy-terminal catalytic domain facing the Golgi lumen.[13,48,49] Also residing in the medial Golgi are nucleoside sugar transporters responsible for transferring nucleotide sugars (which are substrates for the glycotransferases) from the cytosol to the Golgi lumen, and nucleoside diphosphatases that act as antiports to exchange nucleotide sugars for nucleosides.[14,50]

The most common post-translational sugar modification occurring within the medial Golgi is the remodeling of N-linked glycoproteins. High mannose N-linked glycoproteins are initially generated in the ER.[13] Upon delivery to the medial Golgi these glycoproteins are remodeled to complex structures through removal of sugars by specific glycosidases.[48] These reactions occur primarily in the lumen of the medial Golgi and are catalyzed by the sequential enzymatic activity of mannosidase I, mannosidase II and galactosyltransferase. Also occurring in the medial-Golgi stacks is the initiation and extension of O-linked glycan chains of glycosaminoglycans.[51,52] In this process a tetrasaccharide of xylose is added to specific serine and threonine residues on the protein.

Phosphorylation of selected N-glycan chains on proteins and their modification to mannose-6-phosphate units also takes place in the medial Golgi stacks.[53,54] The latter modification enables the terminal glycan unit to interact with mannose-6-phosphate receptors, which are concentrated in the trans-Golgi network and are crucial for targeting acid hydrolases to lysosomes.[13] Failure to phosphorylate results in mistargeting of lysosomal hydrolases to the extracellular medium which can lead to the inability of lysosomes to function normally in degrading cellular debris.

Another modification that occurs in the Golgi is the noncovalent addition of lipids (including cholesterol and phospholipids) to secretory lipoproteins.[47,52,55] Golgi stacks are the primary site of sphingomyelin synthesis whose precursor, ceramide, is produced in the ER.[56-58] Sphingomyelin and ceramide concentrations have been reported to increase in the Golgi in the cis-to-trans direction.[28,59] This has led to the idea that sorting within the Golgi may be occurring through the preferential partitioning of membrane proteins into domains rich in sphingomyelin or ceramide.[59]

The trans region of the Golgi, known as the trans-Golgi network (TGN), mediates sorting and final exit of membrane and protein from the Golgi apparatus.[60] The TGN can be readily identified using the vital dye C6-NBD-ceramide, with the lectin WGA or with antibodies to TGN resident proteins such as TGN 38.[61,62] It appears as a sacculo-tubular network that varies in size and shape in different cell types.[63] Membranes bud out from the TGN in large transport intermediates that track out on microtubules to the plasma membrane and to endosomal membrane compartments (Fig. 5).[25,33,64] The sorting and vesicle budding events at the TGN are regulated by Arf1, the GGAs, adaptor proteins, clathrin, as well as protein kinase D.[63,65-69] These molecules coordinate sorting of secretory cargo with changes in membrane morphology so that budding and fission of post-Golgi carriers is properly regulated.

Many important functions are served by recycling of plasma membrane components back to the TGN. These include the remodeling of surface markers, processing of components internalized from the extracellular space, transfer of toxins to the ER, and replenishment of Golgi membranes with plasma membrane-like lipid necessary for driving export out of the Golgi apparatus.[70-76] Recent work has revealed that plasma membrane to Golgi transport is followed by membranes that are primarily enriched in glycosphingo lipids or rafts that are endocytosed by a clathrin-independent mechanism.[76]

Finally, a number of post-translational modifications of proteins occur in the TGN, including galactose α2,6-sialylation, tyrosine sulfation and proteolytic cleavage of dibasic residues on prohormones.[77-79] Also occurring in this compartment is the process of condensation of macromolecular lumenal content characteristic of cells producing secretion granules.[80,81] This condensation involves charge neutralization, protein aggregation and ion extrusion.[52,82]

Transport within the Golgi Complex

Traditional models describing intra-Golgi transport have assumed that Golgi cisternae are stable units that have a unique enzymatic identity.[2,83,84] In these models maintenance of discrete Golgi cisternae occurs amidst continuous vesicle budding and fusion events between cisternae. Vesicles laden with secretory cargo bud off from one cisterna and fuse with another, moving in cis-to-trans direction across the Golgi stack.[2,85] Vesicle fusion between cisternae is though to involve the activity of SNARE complexes,[86] which have been shown to be required for membrane fusion throughout the cell.[86,87] A typical SNARE complex is comprised of four stable helical bundles, two of which are in the vesicle membrane (so called v-SNAREs) and two of which are in the target membrane (so called t-SNAREs) to which the vesicle fuses.[88,89] It has been proposed that specific SNARE complexes not only regulate membrane fusion but determine what pairs of membranes undergo fusion at a particular intracellular site.[87,90,91]

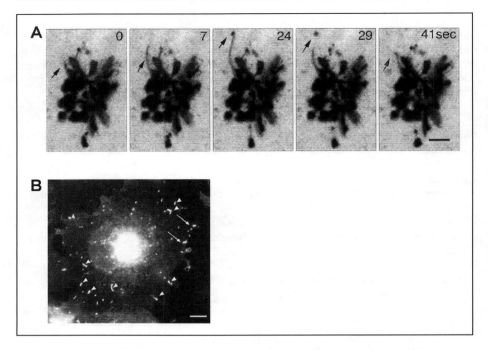

Figure 5. Post-Golgi trafficking. A) VSVG-GFP-containing membranes are shown emerging out of the TGN in tubules that pull off and eventually detach (indicated by arrow). Scale bar represents 5 microns. B) Post-Golgi transport intermediates carrying VSVG-GFP are shown docking and fusing with the plasma membrane (arrows). Scale bar represents 5 microns. Reproduced with permission from refs. 6 and 25.

Other models of intra-Golgi transport have been proposed in which secretory cargo does not move across the Golgi in transport vesicles. In one model secretory transport is proposed to occur by cisternal progression or maturation.[92-96] This model requires that resident enzymes undergo retrograde transport in order to maintain a constant distribution across the stack. In a different model cargo and Golgi enzymes are freely diffusible across the Golgi stack. Here the differential distribution of Golgi enzymes in cis versus trans cisternae would arise by a dynamic self-organizing process based on the directional flux of substrate (i.e., secretory cargo) through the stack. The high diffusional mobility of green fluorescent protein (GFP)-tagged Golgi enzymes measured in photobleaching experiments is consistent with this model.[34]

Intra-Golgi transport may be occurring through a combination of these proposed models and may also depend on the state of secretory activity in the cell.[8] More advanced imaging techniques will be needed to resolve these issues. Indeed thick section (200-400nm) high voltage[4] or thin section 3-dimensional reconstructions of electron micrographs in flash frozen secretory cells[97] has provided evidence for both tubular connections and vesicular transport taking place between cisternae.

Golgi Dynamics: Interphase

Despite its characteristic morphology and structure, the Golgi exists only as a result of the continued process of membrane transport out of the ER.[6] The size and distribution of the Golgi apparatus thus reflect the level of protein and lipid sorting/transport activities within a cell. When membrane flux out of the ER is blocked (for example, through using secretory mutants[98] or by drug treatments such as adding the fungal metabolite brefeldin A [BFA][99])

Golgi structure disassembles and often disappears within cells. How Golgi membranes disperse under these conditions is not clear, but is likely to be related to the membrane recycling pathways operating between the Golgi and ER.[6] The transport pathways operating between the ER and Golgi play an indispensable role in Golgi maintenance and biogenesis. For example, Golgi resident enzymes undergo constitutive cycling between the Golgi and ER compartments.[20,34,100] The first evidence for this came from observing the effects of BFA treatment.[99] BFA inhibits the activation of the Golgi associated small GTPase Arf1, whose activation is necessary to recruit coat proteins to the Golgi membranes.[101-103] Coat proteins are required for sorting and recycling of membrane components within preGolgi and Golgi intermediates.[22,24] When Arf1 is inactive, coat proteins are not recruited to membranes. This inhibits anterograde transport out of the ER and accelerates retrograde transport back to the ER.[29,99,104] The net result is redistribution of Golgi membranes into the ER.[32] When BFA is washed out of cells, Golgi membranes reappear within a few minutes and reassemble into stacks. This de novo formation of the Golgi apparatus can be visualized in real time with time-lapse confocal imaging of GFP-tagged Golgi resident proteins. Reformation of the Golgi apparatus after BFA-washout has been shown to require both Sar1/COPII and Arf1/COPI activities based on results from expression of dominant negative Sar1 and Arf1 proteins.[20,36,100]

Constitutive cycling of Golgi membrane proteins to and from the ER has been demonstrated in the absence of perturbants of membrane trafficking by photobleaching either the ER or Golgi pools of GFP-tagged Golgi proteins and observing their exchange with nonbleached ER or Golgi pools (Fig. 6).[100] Kinetic analysis of this type of data has suggested that the Golgi resident enzyme galactosyltransferase tagged with GFP (GalTase-GFP) cycles between the ER and Golgi every 85 minutes, spending approximately 57 minutes of its lifetime in the Golgi and 28 minutes of its lifetime in the ER.[100]

Because the Golgi is not a preexisting station through which protein and lipids pass, but instead undergoes growth and remodeling through constitutive cycling of its components through the ER, the intracellular distribution of the Golgi can easily change between cell types. This is readily observed in mammalian cells in which Golgi stacks are clustered together in a juxtanuclear arrangement[30,105,106] due to their association with microtubules.[8] Microtubule motors, in particular the microtubule minus end-directed motor protein called dynein is known to associate with Golgi and preGolgi membranes in mammalian cells resulting in their movement toward the minus ends of microtubules.[108-110] The translocation and fusion of preGolgi membranes leads to the juxtanuclear localization of the Golgi apparatus under normal conditions.[108,111]

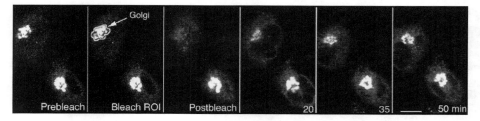

Figure 6. The Golgi complex (outlined and noted by arrow in second frame, and noted as the region of interest (ROI)) was photobleached with high intensity laser light in a cell expressing Galtase-GFP in the presence of cycloheximide to inhibit any new protein synthesis. The recovery of fluorescence in the Golgi region postbleach was monitored over time by acquiring images at low laser light intensity. The recovery observed indicated that the Galtase-GFP resident enzyme underwent continuous exchange with nonGolgi pools (i.e., an ER pool) during its lifetime. Scale bar represents 10 microns. Reproduced with permission from ref. 100.

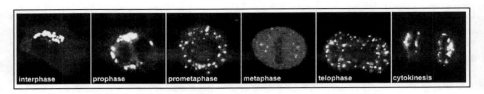

Figure 7. Golgi apparatus dynamics during mitosis in a mammalian cell. NRK cells expressing GalTase-YFP, a Golgi marker protein, were followed by time-lapse confocal microscopy as they underwent mitosis.

Golgi size and distribution are also affected by the rate of membrane flux through the secretory pathway. For example, in the yeast *Saccharomyces cerevisae*, the Golgi membranes exist as single cisternae that often have a basket-like appearance.[112,113] These structures are scattered through the cell and are in close association with the ER.[114] This simple Golgi organization in *S. cerevisae* is thought to be due to the fact that secretory cargo moves through the secretory pathway of yeast extremely fast with minimal processing by Golgi enzymes. When transport is slowed in these cells by expression of transport mutants, Golgi membranes quickly proliferate into a stack-like organization reminiscent of mammalian cells.[115,116]

Golgi Dynamics: Mitosis

The Golgi apparatus undergoes reversible disassembly during mitosis (Fig. 7).[117] The changes in Golgi morphology begin in prophase when the Golgi ribbon is extended around the nuclear envelope with the segregating centrosomes.[118,119] During prometaphase when cytoplasmic microtubules are disassembled,[120] the Golgi enzymes are found in scattered fragments across the cytoplasm. There is a further dispersal of these enzymes during metaphase. Currently there is disagreement on the fate of the Golgi complex during mitosis. The traditional model for disassembly proposes that the Golgi stacks progressively fragment into vesicles that are segregated between the two daughter cells.[121-123] At the end of mitosis these vesicles coalesce and homotypically fuse to reform the Golgi complex in each newly formed daughter cell. An alternative view is based on the finding that many Golgi resident proteins colocalize with ER proteins during metaphase.[100] This model proposes that the Golgi is progressively absorbed into the ER and reemerges from the ER in each daughter cell during mitosis. In this model mitotic Golgi disassembly is a result of perturbing existing (i.e., interphase) Golgi/ER transport pathways. In support of this model, an ER exit block early in mitosis has been reported.[124-127] This ER exit block is relieved during telophase and if the ER exit block becomes permanent by expressing an inactive Sar1 protein then the Golgi apparatus is not formed in each daughter cell.[100,127]

In many simple eukaryotes such as the protozoan *Toxiplasma gondii* and yeast *S. cerevisiae*, the Golgi does not disassemble in mitosis. Instead, a new Golgi is formed in the daughter cell.[128] Unlike in animal cells, secretion is not blocked in these simpler cells during mitosis and thus Golgi/ER cycling pathways are not perturbed. Hence, it is possible that the new Golgi in the daughter cell is created de novo from ER exit sites. Indeed in yeast it has been reported that the newly formed Golgi is localized to the ER exit sites.[128] In general, the manner in which cells duplicate their Golgi apparatus may depend on whether or not secretion is blocked in mitosis.

Golgi As a Scaffold for Signaling Molecules

In addition to its roles in processing and sorting, recent evidence suggests that the Golgi complex also serves as a platform for diversely functioning signaling and scaffolding molecules.[129] Many features of the Golgi complex make it an attractive location for signaling molecules. First, it is located juxta-nuclearly and hence access to the nucleus where gene expression takes place will be rapid for many signaling molecules. Second the Golgi exchanges membrane with the plasma membrane and ER compartments and thus functions at the interface of several membrane transport pathways. This results in the Golgi having an intermediate lipid composition, between the glycerolipid-rich ER and sterol/sphingolipid-rich plasma membrane and makes the Golgi lipid composition dynamic and responsive to changes in the rates of secretory transport.[127,129] Changes in lipid composition are known to effect the activity of a variety of signaling proteins that are associated with the Golgi membranes including heterotrimeric G proteins, small G protein Ras, PKA, PI(3) kinase, IQGAP, eNOS, PI4Kβ and Cdc42.[127,129-137] The Golgi membranes are also associated with cytoskeletal proteins. Ankyrin and spectrin form a mesh on Golgi membranes which in turn recruit a range of cytoskeletal proteins such as actin, tubulin, vimentin, dynein, dynamin, myosin as well as the kinases PKC and CaM kinase.[135] Other cytoplasmic proteins with roles in the nucleus and cytoplasm are also localized on the surface of the Golgi, including casein kinase, cyclin B2, tankyrase and Cullin family members.[138-141] Localizing to Golgi membranes could play a role in spatially and temporally restricting the activity of these proteins inside cells.[142,143]

Conclusions

The Golgi apparatus has intrigued cell biologists since its first description by Camillo Golgi over a century ago.[10] Understanding the complex structure of the Golgi apparatus and its remarkable dynamics remain challenging questions, whose answers are key for explaining the diverse functions of this organelle. Several characteristics of the Golgi distinguish it from other organelles. These include its unique stack-like architecture, its maintenance in the face of massive flux of membrane through the secretory pathway; and its capacity for rapid disassembly and de novo reassembly. While much headway has been made mechanistically in analyzing these features of the Golgi apparatus, the challenge remains in relating them to the evolutionarily conserved role of the Golgi apparatus in membrane transport and processing in all eukaryotic cells.

References

1. Palade G. Intracellular aspects of the process of protein synthesis. Science 1975; 189(4200):347-358.
2. Rothman JE. Mechanisms of intracellular protein transport. Nature 1994; 372(6501):55-63.
3. Farquhar MG, Palade GE. The Golgi apparatus: 100 years of progress and controversy. Trends Cell Biol 1998; 8(1):2-10.
4. Rambourg A, Clermont Y. Three-dimensional electron microscopy: Structure of the Golgi apparatus. Eur J Cell Biol 1990; 51(2):189-200.
5. Mellman I, Simons K. The Golgi complex: in vitro veritas? Cell 1992; 68(5):829-840.
6. Lippincott-Schwartz J, Roberts TH, Hirschberg K. Secretory protein trafficking and organelle dynamics in living cells. Annu Rev Cell Dev Biol 2000; 16:557-589.
7. Pelham HR. Traffic through the Golgi apparatus. J Cell Biol 2001; 155(7):1099-1101.
8. Marsh BJ, Howell KE. The mammalian Golgi-complex debates. Nat Rev Mol Cell Biol 2002; 3(10):789-795.
9. Dean N, Pelham HR. Recycling of proteins from the Golgi compartment to the ER in yeast. J Cell Biol 1990; 111(2):369-377.
10. Golgi C. On the structure of nerve cells. J Microsc 1989; 155(Pt 1):3-7.
11. Rambourg A, Clermont Y, Hermo L et al. Tridimensional structure of the Golgi apparatus of nonciliated epithelial cells of the ductuli efferentes in rat: An electron microscope stereoscopic study. Biol Cell 1987; 60(2):103-115.
12. Ladinsky MS, Mastronarde DN, McIntosh JR et al. Golgi structure in three dimensions: functional insights from the normal rat kidney cell. J Cell Biol 1999; 144(6):1135-1149.
13. Kornfeld R, Kornfeld S. Assembly of asparagine-linked oligosaccharides. Annu Rev Biochem 1985; 54:631-664.
14. Hirschberg CB, Snider MD. Topography of glycosylation in the rough endoplasmic reticulum and Golgi apparatus. Annu Rev Biochem 1987; 56:63-87.

15. Tartakoff AM, Vassalli P. Lectin-binding sites as markers of Golgi subcompartments: Proximal-to-distal maturation of oligosaccharides. J Cell Biol 1983; 97(4):1243-1248.

16. Farquhar MG. Protein Traffic through the Golgi complex. In: Steer CJ, Hanover JA, eds. Intracellular trafficking of proteins. Cambridge: Cambridge University Press, 1991:431-471

17. Slusarewicz P, Nilsson T, Hui N et al. Isolation of a matrix that binds medial Golgi enzymes. J Cell Biol 1994; 124(4):405-413.

18. Seemann J, Jokitalo E, Pypaert M et al. Matrix proteins can generate the higher order architecture of the Golgi apparatus. Nature 2000; 407(6807):1022-1026.

19. Shorter J, Warren G. Golgi architecture and inheritance. Annu Rev Cell Dev Biol 2002; 18:379-420.

20. Ward TH, Polishchuk RS, Caplan S et al. Maintenance of Golgi structure and function depends on the integrity of ER export. J Cell Biol 2001; 155(4):557-570.

21. Rothman JE, Wieland FT. Protein sorting by transport vesicles. Science 1996; 272(5259):227-234.

22. Schekman R, Orci L. Coat proteins and vesicle budding. Science 1996; 271(5255):1526-1533.

23. Presley JF, Ward TH, Pfeifer AC et al. Dissection of COPI and Arf1 dynamics in vivo and role in Golgi membrane transport. Nature 2002; 417(6885):187-193.

24. Bonifacino JS, Lippincott-Schwartz J. Coat proteins: Shaping membrane transport. Nat Rev Mol Cell Biol 2003; 4(5):409-414.

25. Hirschberg K, Miller CM, Ellenberg J et al. Kinetic analysis of secretory protein traffic and characterization of golgi to plasma membrane transport intermediates in living cells. J Cell Biol 1998; 143(6):1485-1503.

26. Kreitzer G, Marmorstein A, Okamoto P et al. Kinesin and dynamin are required for post-Golgi transport of a plasma-membrane protein. Nat Cell Biol 2000; 2(2):125-127.

27. Holthuis JC, Pomorski T, Raggers RJ et al. The organizing potential of sphingolipids in intracellular membrane transport. Physiol Rev 2001; 81(4):1689-1723.

28. Bretscher MS, Munro S. Cholesterol and the Golgi apparatus. Science 1993; 261(5126):1280-1281.

29. Cole NB, Ellenberg J, Song J et al. Retrograde transport of Golgi-localized proteins to the ER. J Cell Biol 1998; 140(1):1-15.

30. Thyberg J, Moskalewski S. Role of microtubules in the organization of the Golgi complex. Exp Cell Res 1999; 246(2):263-279.

31. Rios RM, Bornens M. The Golgi apparatus at the cell centre. Curr Opin Cell Biol 2003; 15(1):60-66.

32. Sciaky N, Presley J, Smith C et al. Golgi tubule traffic and the effects of brefeldin A visualized in living cells. J Cell Biol 1997; 139(5):1137-1155.

33. Polishchuk RS, Polishchuk EV, Marra P et al. Correlative light-electron microscopy reveals the tubular-saccular ultrastructure of carriers operating between Golgi apparatus and plasma membrane. J Cell Biol 2000; 148(1):45-58.

34. Cole NB, Sciaky N, Marotta A et al. Golgi dispersal during microtubule disruption: Regeneration of Golgi stacks at peripheral endoplasmic reticulum exit sites. Mol Biol Cell 1996; 7(4):631-650.

35. Storrie B, White J, Rottger S et al. Recycling of golgi-resident glycosyltransferases through the ER reveals a novel pathway and provides an explanation for nocodazole-induced Golgi scattering. J Cell Biol 1998; 143(6):1505-1521.

36. Miles S, McManus H, Forsten KE et al. Evidence that the entire Golgi apparatus cycles in interphase HeLa cells: Sensitivity of Golgi matrix proteins to an ER exit block. J Cell Biol 2001; 155(4):543-555.

37. Rothman JE. The Golgi apparatus: Roles for distinct 'cis' and 'trans' compartments. Ciba Found Symp 1982; (92):120-137.

38. Hsu VW, Yuan LC, Nuchtern JG et al. A recycling pathway between the endoplasmic reticulum and the Golgi apparatus for retention of unassembled MHC class I molecules. Nature 1991; 352(6334):441-444.

39. Hammond C, Helenius A. Quality control in the secretory pathway. Curr Opin Cell Biol 1995; 7(4):523-529.

40. Schweizer A, Fransen JA, Matter K et al. Identification of an intermediate compartment involved in protein transport from endoplasmic reticulum to Golgi apparatus. Eur J Cell Biol 1990; 53(2):185-196.

41. Chavrier P, Parton RG, Hauri HP et al. Localization of low molecular weight GTP binding proteins to exocytic and endocytic compartments. Cell 1990; 62(2):317-329.

42. Pelham HR. Recycling of proteins between the endoplasmic reticulum and Golgi complex. Curr Opin Cell Biol 1991; 3(4):585-591.

43. Appenzeller C, Andersson H, Kappeler F et al. The lectin ERGIC-53 is a cargo transport receptor for glycoproteins. Nat Cell Biol 1999; 1(6):330-334.

44. Hauri HP, Kappeler F, Andersson H et al. ERGIC-53 and traffic in the secretory pathway. J Cell Sci 2000; 113(Pt 4):587-596.

45. Nichols WC, Seligsohn U, Zivelin A et al. Mutations in the ER-Golgi intermediate compartment protein ERGIC-53 cause combined deficiency of coagulation factors V and VIII. Cell 1998; 93(1):61-70.

46. Zhang B, Cunningham MA, Nichols WC et al. Bleeding due to disruption of a cargo-specific ER-to-Golgi transport complex. Nat Genet 2003; 34(2):220-225.

47. Maccioni HJ, Giraudo CG, Daniotti JL. Understanding the stepwise synthesis of glycolipids. Neurochem Res 2002; 27(7-8):629-636.

48. Moremen KW. Golgi alpha-mannosidase II deficiency in vertebrate systems: Implications for asparagine-linked oligosaccharide processing in mammals. Biochim Biophys Acta 2002; 1573(3):225-235.

49. Giraudo CG, Daniotti JL, Maccioni HJ. Physical and functional association of glycolipid N-acetyl-galactosaminyl and galactosyl transferases in the Golgi apparatus. Proc Natl Acad Sci USA 2001; 98(4):1625-1630.

50. Martinez-Duncker I, Mollicone R, Codogno P et al. The nucleotide-sugar transporter family: A phylogenetic approach. Biochimie 2003; 85(3-4):245-260.

51. Ernst JF, Prill SK. O-glycosylation. Med Mycol 2001; 39(Suppl 1):67-74.

52. Turner JR, Tartakoff AM, Greenspan NS. Cytologic assessment of nuclear and cytoplasmic O-linked N-acetylglucosamine distribution by using anti-streptococcal monoclonal antibodies. Proc Natl Acad Sci USA 1990; 87(15):5608-5612.

53. Kornfeld S. Trafficking of lysosomal enzymes in normal and disease states. J Clin Invest 1986; 77(1):1-6.

54. Ghosh P, Dahms NM, Kornfeld S. Mannose 6-phosphate receptors: New twists in the tale. Nat Rev Mol Cell Biol 2003; 4(3):202-212.

55. Sandhoff K, Kolter T. Biosynthesis and degradation of mammalian glycosphingolipids. Philos Trans R Soc Lond B Biol Sci 2003; 358(1433):847-861.

56. Jeckel D, Karrenbauer A, Birk R et al. Sphingomyelin is synthesized in the cis Golgi. FEBS Lett 1990; 261(1):155-157.

57. Fang M, Rivas MP, Bankaitis VA. The contribution of lipids and lipid metabolism to cellular functions of the Golgi complex. Biochim Biophys Acta 1998; 1404(1-2):85-100.

58. van Meer G, Holthuis JC. Sphingolipid transport in eukaryotic cells. Biochim Biophys Acta 2000; 1486(1):145-170.

59. Simons K, Ikonen E. Functional rafts in cell membranes. Nature 1997; 387(6633):569-572.

60. Griffiths G, Simons K. The trans Golgi network: Sorting at the exit site of the Golgi complex. Science 1986; 234(4775):438-443.

61. Pagano RE, Sepanski MA, Martin OC. Molecular trapping of a fluorescent ceramide analogue at the Golgi apparatus of fixed cells: Interaction with endogenous lipids provides a trans-Golgi marker for both light and electron microscopy. J Cell Biol 1989; 109(5):2067-2079.

62. Humphrey JS, Peters PJ, Yuan LC et al. Localization of TGN38 to the trans-Golgi network: Involvement of a cytoplasmic tyrosine-containing sequence. J Cell Biol 1993; 120(5):1123-1135.

63. Ladinsky MS, Kremer JR, Furcinitti PS et al. HVEM tomography of the trans-Golgi network: Structural insights and identification of a lace-like vesicle coat. J Cell Biol 1994; 127(1):29-38.

64. Keller P, Simons K. Post-Golgi biosynthetic trafficking. J Cell Sci 1997; 110(Pt 24):3001-3009.

65. Sabatini DD, Adesnik M, Ivanov IE et al. Mechanism of formation of post Golgi vesicles from TGN membranes: Arf-dependent coat assembly and PKC-regulated vesicle scission. Biocell 1996; 20(3):287-300.

66. Puertollano R, Aguilar RC, Gorshkova I et al. Sorting of mannose 6-phosphate receptors mediated by the GGAs. Science 2001; 292(5522):1712-1716.

67. Robinson MS, Bonifacino JS. Adaptor-related proteins. Curr Opin Cell Biol 2001; 13(4):444-453.
68. Baron CL, Malhotra V. Role of diacylglycerol in PKD recruitment to the TGN and protein transport to the plasma membrane. Science 2002; 295(5553):325-328.
69. Liljedahl M, Maeda Y, Colanzi A et al. Protein kinase D regulates the fission of cell surface destined transport carriers from the trans-Golgi network. Cell 2001; 104(3):409-420.
70. Farquhar MG, Palade GE. The Golgi apparatus (complex)-(1954-1981)-from artifact to center stage. J Cell Biol 1981; 91(3 Pt 2):77s-103s.
71. Kornfeld S, Mellman I. The biogenesis of lysosomes. Annu Rev Cell Biol 1989; 5:483-525.
72. Sandvig K, van Deurs B. Membrane traffic exploited by protein toxins. Annu Rev Cell Dev Biol 2002; 18:1-24.
73. Nelson WJ, Yeaman C. Protein trafficking in the exocytic pathway of polarized epithelial cells.Trends Cell Biol 2001; 11(12):483-486
74. Le Borgne R, Hoflack B. Protein transport from the secretory to the endocytic pathway in mammalian cells.Biochim Biophys Acta 1998; 1404(1-2):195-209
75. Nichols BJ, Lippincott-Schwartz J. Endocytosis without clathrin coats. Trends Cell Biol 2001; 11(10):406-412.
76. Nichols BJ, Kenworthy AK, Polishchuk RS et al. Rapid cycling of lipid raft markers between the cell surface and Golgi complex. J Cell Biol 2001; 153(3):529-541.
77. Duncan JR, Kornfeld S. Intracellular movement of two mannose 6-phosphate receptors: Return to the Golgi apparatus. J Cell Biol 1988; 106(3):617-628.
78. Aeuerle PA, Huttner WB. Tyrosine sulfation is a trans-Golgi-specific protein modification. J Cell Biol 1987; 105(6 Pt 1):2655-2664.
79. Sossin WS, Fisher JM, Scheller RH. Sorting within the regulated secretory pathway occurs in the trans-Golgi network. J Cell Biol 1990; 110(1):1-12.
80. Molinete M, Irminger JC, Tooze SA et al. Trafficking/sorting and granule biogenesis in the beta-cell. Semin Cell Dev Biol 2000; 11(4):243-251.
81. Tooze SA, Martens GJ, Huttner WB. Secretory granule biogenesis: Rafting to the SNARE. Trends Cell Biol 2001; 11(3):116-122.
82. De Lisle RC. Role of sulfated O-linked glycoproteins in zymogen granule formation. J Cell Sci 2002; 115(Pt 14):2941-2952.
83. Jamieson JD, Palade GE. Role of the Golgi complex in the intracellular transport of secretory proteins. Proc Natl Acad Sci USA 1966; 55(2):424-431.
84. Palade G. Intracellular aspects of the process of protein synthesis. Science 1975; 189(4200):347-358.
85. Orci L, Amherdt M, Ravazzola M et al. Exclusion of golgi residents from transport vesicles budding from Golgi cisternae in intact cells. J Cell Biol 2000; 150(6):1263-1270.
86. Parlati F, Varlamov O, Paz K et al. Distinct SNARE complexes mediating membrane fusion in Golgi transport based on combinatorial specificity. Proc Natl Acad Sci USA 2002; 99(8):5424-5429
87. McNew JA, Parlati F, Fukuda R et al. Compartmental specificity of cellular membrane fusion encoded in SNARE proteins. Nature 2000; 407(6801):153-159.
88. Sutton RB, Fasshauer D, Jahn R et al. Crystal structure of a SNARE complex involved in synaptic exocytosis at 2.4 A resolution. Nature 1998; 395(6700):347-353.
89. Nickel W, Weber T, McNew JA et al. Content mixing and membrane integrity during membrane fusion driven by pairing of isolated v-SNAREs and t-SNAREs. Proc Natl Acad Sci USA 1999; 96(22):12571-12576.
90. Sollner T, Whiteheart SW, Brunner M et al. SNAP receptors implicated in vesicle targeting and fusion. Nature 1993; 362(6418):318-324.
91. Rothman JE, Warren G. Implications of the SNARE hypothesis for intracellular membrane topology and dynamics. Curr Biol 1994; 4(3):220-233.
92. Grasse PP. Ultrastructure polarite reproduction de l'appareil de Golgi. C. R. Acad Sci 1957; 245:1278-1281.
93. Melkonian M, Becker B, Becker D. Scale formation in Algae. J. Electron Microsc Tech 1991; 17(2):165-178.
94. Glick BS, Elston T, Oster G. A cisternal maturation mechanism can explain the asymmetry of the Golgi stack. FEBS Lett 1997; 414(2):177-181.

95. Mollenhauer HH, Morre DJ. The tubular network of the Golgi apparatus. Histochem Cell Biol 1998; 109(5-6):533-543.

96. Bonfanti L, Mironov Jr AA, Martinez-Menarguez JA et al. Procollagen traverses the Golgi stack without leaving the lumen of cisternae: Evidence for cisternal maturation. Cell 1998; 95(7):993-1003.

97. Marsh BJ, Mastronarde DN, Buttle KF et al. Organellar relationships in the Golgi region of the pancreatic beta cell line, HIT-T15, visualized by high resolution electron tomography. Proc Natl Acad Sci USA 2001; 98(5):2399-2406.

98. Dascher C, Balch WE. Dominant inhibitory mutants of ARF1 block endoplasmic reticulum to Golgi transport and trigger disassembly of the Golgi apparatus. J Biol Chem 1994; 269(2):1437-48.

99. Lippincott-Schwartz J, Yuan LC, Bonifacino JS et al. Rapid redistribution of Golgi proteins into the ER in cells treated with brefeldin A: Evidence for membrane cycling from Golgi to ER. Cell 1989; 56(5):801-813.

100. Zaal KJ, Smith CL, Polishchuk RS et al. Golgi membranes are absorbed into and reemerge from the ER during mitosis. Cell 1999; 99(6):589-601.

101. Donaldson JG, Finazzi D, Klausner RD. Brefeldin A inhibits Golgi membrane-catalysed exchange of guanine nucleotide onto ARF protein. Nature 1992; 360(6402):350-352.

102. Helms JB, Rothman JE. Inhibition by brefeldin A of a Golgi membrane enzyme that catalyses exchange of guanine nucleotide bound to ARF. Nature 1992; 360(6402):352-354.

103. Peyroche A, Antonny B, Robineau S et al. Brefeldin A acts to stabilize an abortive ARF-GDP-Sec7 domain protein complex: Involvement of specific residuesof the Sec7 domain. Mol Cell 1999; 3(3):275-285.

104. Presley JF, Ward TH, Pfeifer AC et al. Dissection of COPI and Arf1 dynamics in vivo and role in Golgi membrane transport. Nature 2002; 417(6885):187-193

105. Boevink P, Oparka K, Santa Cruz S et al. Stacks on tracks: The plant Golgi apparatus traffics on an actin/ER network. Plant J 1998; 15(3):441-447.

106. Nebenfuhr A, Frohlick JA, Staehelin LA. Redistribution of Golgi stacks and other organelles during mitosis and cytokinesis in plant cells. Plant Physiol 2000; 124(1):135-151.

107. Chabin-Brion K, Marceiller J, Perez F et al. The Golgi complex is a microtubule-organizing organelle. Mol Biol Cell 2001; 12(7):2047-2060.

108. Presley JF, Cole NB, Schroer TA et al. ER-to-Golgi transport visualized in living cells. Nature 1997; 389(6646):81-85.

109. Quintyne NJ, Gill SR, Eckley DM et al. Dynactin is required for microtubule anchoring at centrosomes. J Cell Biol 1999; 147(2):321-334.

110. Allan VJ, Thompson HM, McNiven MA. Motoring around the Golgi. Nat Cell Biol 2002; 4(10):E236-E242.

111. Scales SJ, Pepperkok R, Kreis TE. Visualization of ER-to-Golgi transport in living cells reveals a sequential mode of action for COPII and COPI. Cell 1997; 90(6):1137-1148.

112. Rambourg A, Clermont Y, Ovtracht L et al. Three-dimensional structure of tubular networks, presumably Golgi in nature, in various yeast strains: A comparative study. Anat Rec 1995; 243(3):283-923.

113. Rambourg A, Jackson CL, Clermont Y. Three dimensional configuration of the secretory pathway and segregation of secretion granules in the yeast Saccharomyces cerevisiae. J Cell Sci 2001; 114(Pt 12):2231-2239.

114. Rossanese OW, Soderholm J, Bevis BJ et al. Golgi structure correlates with transitional endoplasmic reticulum organization in Pichia pastoris and Saccharomyces cerevisiae. J Cell Biol 1999; 145(1):69-81.

115. Rambourg A, Clermont Y, Jackson CL et al. Ultrastructural modifications of vesicular and Golgi elements in the Saccharomyces cerevisiae sec21 mutant at permissive and nonpermissive temperatures. Anat Rec 1994; 240(1):32-41.

116. Rambourg A, Clermont Y, Nicaud JM et al. Transformations of membrane-bound organelles in sec 14 mutants of the yeast Saccharomyces cerevisiae and Yarrowia lipolytica. Anat Rec 1996; 245(3):447-458.

117. Warren G. Membrane partitioning during cell division. Annu Rev Biochem 1993; 62:323-348.

118. Misteli T, Warren G. Mitotic disassembly of the Golgi apparatus in vivo. J Cell Sci 1995; 108(Pt 7):2715-2727.

119. Thyberg J, Moskalewski S. Partitioning of cytoplasmic organelles during mitosis with special reference to the Golgi complex. Microsc Res Tech 1998; 40(5):354-368.
120. Zhai Y, Kronebusch PJ, Simon PM et al. Microtubule dynamics at the G2/M transition: abrupt breakdown of cytoplasmic microtubules at nuclear envelope breakdown and implications for spindle morphogenesis. J Cell Biol 1996; 135(1):201-214.
121. Shima DT, Haldar K, Pepperkok R et al. Partitioning of the Golgi apparatus during mitosis in living HeLa cells. J Cell Biol 1997; 137(6):1211-1228
122. Shorter J, Warren G. Golgi architecture and inheritance. Annu Rev Cell Dev Biol 2002; 18:379-420.
123. Colanzi A, Deerinck TJ, Ellisman MH et al. A specific activation of the mitogen-activated protein kinase kinase 1 (MEK1) is required for Golgi fragmentation during mitosis. J Cell Biol 2000; 149(2):331-339.
124. Warren G, Featherstone C, Griffiths G et al. Newly synthesized G protein of vesicular stomatitis virus is not transported to the cell surface during mitosis. J Cell Biol 1983; 97(5 Pt 1):1623-1628.
125. Farmaki T, Ponnambalam S, Prescott AR et al. Forward and retrograde trafficking in mitotic animal cells. ER-Golgi transport arrest restricts protein export from the ER into COPII-coated structures. J Cell Sci 1999; 112(Pt 5):589-600.
126. Prescott AR, Farmaki T, Thomson C et al. Evidence for prebudding arrest of ER export in animal cell mitosis and its role in generating Golgi partitioning intermediates. Traffic 2001; 2(5):321-335.
127. Hammond AT, Glick BS. Dynamics of transitional endoplasmic reticulum sites in vertebrate cells. Mol Biol Cell 2000; 11(9):3013-3030.
128. Rossanese OW, Glick BS. Deconstructing Golgi inheritance. Traffic 2001; 2(9):589-596.
129. Donaldson JG, Lippincott-Schwartz J. Sorting and signaling at the Golgi complex. Cell 2000; 101(7):693-696.
130. Bomsel M, Mostov K. Role of heterotrimeric G proteins in membrane traffic. Mol Biol Cell 1992; 3(12):1317-1328.
131. Denker SP, McCaffery JM, Palade GE et al. Differential distribution of alpha subunits and beta gamma subunits of heterotrimeric G proteins on Golgi membranes of the exocrine pancreas. J Cell Biol 1996; 133(5):1027-1040.
132. Erickson JW, Zhang C, Kahn RA et al. Mammalian Cdc42 is a brefeldin A-sensitive component of the Golgi apparatus. J Biol Chem 1996; 271(43):26850-26854.
133. McCallum SJ, Erickson JW, Cerione RA. Characterization of the association of the actin-binding protein, IQGAP, and activated Cdc42 with Golgi membranes. J Biol Chem 1998; 273(35):22537-22544.
134. Stow JL, Heimann K. Vesicle budding on Golgi membranes: Regulation by G proteins and myosin motors. Biochim Biophys Acta 1998; 1404(1-2):161-171.
135. De Matteis MA, Morrow JS. Spectrin tethers and mesh in the biosynthetic pathway. J Cell Sci 2000; 113 (Pt 13):2331-2343.
136. Cockcroft S, De Matteis MA. Inositol lipids as spatial regulators of membrane traffic. J Membr Biol 2001; 180(3):187-194.
137. Bivona TG, Perez De Castro I, Ahearn IM et al. Phospholipase Cgamma activates Ras on the Golgi apparatus by means of RasGRP1. Nature 2003; 424(6949):694-698.
138. Jackman M, Firth M, Pines J. Human cyclins B1 and B2 are localized to strikingly different structures: B1 to microtubules, B2 primarily to the Golgi apparatus. EMBO J 1995; 14(8):1646-1654.
139. Singer JD, Gurian-West M, Clurman B et al. Cullin-3 targets cyclin E for ubiquitination and controls S phase in mammalian cells. Genes Dev 1999; 13(18):2375-2387.
140. Smith S, de Lange T. Cell cycle dependent localization of the telomeric PARP, tankyrase, to nuclear pore complexes and centrosomes. J Cell Sci 1999; 112(Pt 21):3649-3656.
141. Milne DM, Looby P, Meek DW. Catalytic activity of protein kinase CK1 delta (casein kinase 1delta) is essential for its normal subcellular localization. Exp Cell Res 2001; 263(1):43-54.
142. Lippincott-Schwartz J. The endoplasmic reticulum and Golgi complex in secretory membrane transport. In: Arias IM, Boyer JL, Chiasari FV et al, eds. The Liver: Biology and Pathobiology. Lippincott: Williams & Wilkins, 2001:119-131.
143. Altan-Bonnet N, Phair RD, Polishchok RS et al. A role for Arf1 in mitotic Golgi disassembling chromosome secrecation and cytokenesis. Proc Natl Acad Sci USA 2003; 100:13314-13319.

CHAPTER 6

Lysosome Biogenesis and Dynamics

Diane McVey Ward, Shelly L. Shiflett and Jerry Kaplan

Abstract

Lysosomes are membrane-bound organelles that serve as the site for delivery of molecules destined for degradation. These molecules, along with lysosomal hydrolases, are delivered to lysosomes by a series of heterotypic vesicle fusion events. Lysosomes are also capable of homotypic fusion and yet cells are able to maintain a relatively constant size and number of lysosomes. To maintain lysosome size and number, highly regulated sorting and vesicle fission events must occur. The specificity of these processes is determined largely by targeting molecules that traffic vesicles to and away from lysosomes. Misregulated trafficking can result in alterations in the "normal" number and size of lysosomes within a cell. Such critical changes in lysosomes are often associated with human disease. The identification and characterization of the molecules involved in lysosome biogenesis and maintenance continues to advance our understanding of intracellular trafficking and endocytosis, as well as other basic cell biological processes.

Introduction

Lysosomes, or vacuoles as they are referred to in fungi and plants, are membrane-bound organelles that function as the major degradative compartment within eukaryotic cells.[1,2] Lysosomes are typified by having an acid pH and contain a wide variety of hydrolases capable of degrading most biological macromolecules. They are the terminal organelle in the endocytic pathway and are the repository for internalized material, most of which is degraded. Lysosomes can fuse with intracellular organelles and effect their digestion, a process referred to as autophagy.[3-7] Morphologically, lysosomes appear as dense membrane bound bodies containing whirls of membranous material.[8] Lysosomes are frequently localized near the nucleus adjacent to the microtubule organizing centers.[9] Lysosomes usually appear as spherical structures but can also be found as long tubules in cell types such as fibroblasts and macrophages (Fig. 1).[10,11] Currently, a lysosome is defined by the presence of lysosomal acid hydrolases and lysosomal integral membrane glycoproteins.[12-14] The absence of mannose 6-phosphate receptors (M6PRs) and recycling cell surface receptors from lysosomes distinguish lysosomes from late endosomes, which also contain degradative enzymes.

Lysosomes are constantly undergoing fusion with endocytic vesicles that are delivering internalized molecules destined for degradation. Lysosomes also show a remarkable capacity for homotypic fusion, which permits an extensive redistribution of lysosomal contents through the complement of cellular lysosomes.[10,15-19] Even though lysosomes are continually fusing with vesicles, the cellular complement of lysosomes is relatively constant with respect to volume,

The Biogenesis of Cellular Organelles, edited by Chris Mullins. ©2005 Eurekah.com and Kluwer Academic/Plenum Publishers.

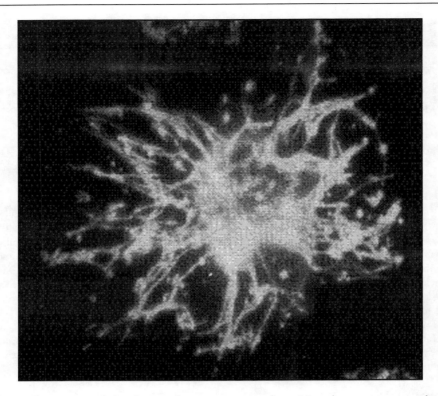

Figure 1. Lysosome morphology in mouse bone marrow macrophages. Mouse bone marrow macrophages were incubated with 1 mg/ml of the fluid-phase marker Lucifer Yellow-CH. This marker is endocytosed and localized to lysosomes. The image shown is presented as an example of the dynamic tubular structure of lysosomes.

size and number. This constancy suggests that fusion, which adds both membrane and volume, must be balanced by fission events.[20]

The importance of lysosomes in cellular homeostasis, as shown by human diseases caused by lysosome dysfunction,[21,22] has led to extensive research on the biogenesis of these organelles. In this chapter we will review theories of lysosome formation. We will discuss the molecular and biochemical data supporting these theories and describe the recent identification of molecules involved in lysosome biogenesis and maintenance through heterotypic and homotypic fusion.

Models for Lysosome Biogenesis

Lysosomes were initially postulated to form de novo by budding from the Golgi because of their proximity to the Golgi apparatus.[23,24] It became clear, however, that these membrane systems are quite dissimilar. Studies on endocytosis and on the delivery of soluble hydrolases to lysosomes suggested two models for lysosome biogenesis (Fig. 2).[25-28] The first model, termed the maturation model, suggests that endosomes, formed by plasma membrane internalization, are transformed into lysosomes by the addition and removal of molecules. Thus, endosomes "mature" into lysosomes and without endocytosis lysosomes would not be formed. A second model, the vesicular transport model, suggests that endosomes, late endosomes and lysosomes are pre-existing structures that communicate by continuous rounds of fusion and fission.

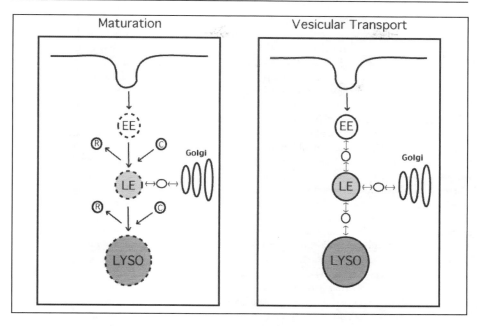

Figure 2. Models of lysosome formation. Two models of lysosome formation have been postulated. The maturation model hypothesizes that early (EE) and late (LE) endosomes, formed by plasma membrane internalization, gain (C) and lose molecules (R) as they develope into lysosomes (LYSO). The vesicular transport model suggests that endosomes (EE and LE) and lysosomes (LYSO) are pre-existing organelles that exchange contents by continuous rounds of fusion and fission.

Early endosomes are steady-state organelles. Most early endosomal membrane is not retained within cells but is recycled back to the plasma membrane.[29-31] In the absence of continued membrane internalization, the early endocytic apparatus virtually disappears.[32,33] The lysosome, however, retains its identity in the absence of continued membrane internalization. The fact that lysosomes exist in the absence of endocytosis rules out formation strictly by maturation. It is unclear whether late endosomes are solely derived from endocytosis or if they are pre-existing structures. It is apparent that late endosomes play a critical role in lysosomal biogenesis and in the sorting of lysosomal hydrolases.[12,14,34-38] It is clear that either hypothesis in its purest form can not describe lysosome formation and that a final model will have elements from both hypotheses.

Synthesis and Delivery of Lysosomal Hydrolases

Lysosomal hydrolases are synthesized in the lumen of the endoplasmic reticulum (ER), as are molecules destined for secretion.[39-42] Due to the presence of a leader sequence, these molecules enter the lumen of the endoplasmic reticulum where they become N-glycosylated. A high mannose carbohydrate is transferred from a dolichol phosphate intermediate to both secreted and lysosomal hydrolases. The high mannose containing proteins are transferred to the Golgi apparatus where further modification of the carbohydrate chains occurs. In the case of lysosomal hydrolases, however, a specific GlcNAc phosphotransferase recognizes determinates in the polypeptide chain and catalyzes the addition of a diphospho-N-acetyl glucosamine to a mannose residue. A second enzyme cleaves off phospho-N-acetyl glucosamine, leaving a phospho mannose. The absence of either enzyme results in the lack of retention of lysosomal hydrolases, resulting in their secretion. In humans the loss of either of these two enzymes results in a severe disease referred to as I-cell disease. It was through analysis of the molecular basis of I-cell disease that the mannose-phosphate marking system was discovered.[43-47]

Within the trans-Golgi network (TGN) mannose-phosphate containing proteins are recognized by the mannose 6-phosphate receptors (M6PRs).[12,48-50] There are two different receptors encoded by separate genes: a cation-independent receptor (CI-M6PR), which can also bind insulin-like growth factor, and a second much smaller cation-dependent receptor (CD-M6PR). These receptors have overlapping specificity in terms of mannose-6 phosphate recognition.[51] The role of these receptors in the trafficking of lysosomal hydrolases has been confirmed by study of animals in which one or both of the receptors have been deleted by gene targeting. The absence of either receptor leads to decreased hydrolase retention.[41,52-54] Cells with a deletion in both receptor genes show an enhanced secretion of lysosomal enzymes. These ligand-receptor complexes are localized at the TGN where they are then pinched off into vesicles that fuse with late endosomes. Late endosomes are acidic organelles and the low pH dissociates the mannose-phosphate hydrolase from the M6PR. Unoccupied receptors are then recycled back to the Golgi and can enter into further rounds of ligand capture and delivery.[36] The mannose-phosphate containing hydrolases, present as soluble proteins within the lumen of the late endosome, are delivered to the lysosome. M6PRs that cannot recycle back to the Golgi are also delivered to the lysosome where they are degraded.

It has been thought that M6PRs interact with the adaptor protein complex–1 (AP-1).[55] AP complexes are key constituents of protein coats mediating selective protein sorting in the late-secretory and endocytic pathways. AP-1 is specifically associated with Golgi membranes and was thought to transport lysosomal hydrolases to the late endosome.[56] In vitro studies have shown that the M6PR tail can bind to elements of the AP-1 complex.[57,58] Generation of a targeted deletion of the μ1A subunit of AP-1 in mice has revealed a novel finding. It might be expected that an AP-1 deletion would trap M6PRs in the Golgi. However, AP-1 deficient mice show clustering of M6PRs in an early endosome.[59,60] This suggests that another coat molecule may be responsible for M6PR trafficking from the Golgi, and that AP-1 might be required for trafficking from the endosome to the Golgi.

More recent studies have suggested that a class of protein coat components termed the GGAs (for Golgi-localized, γ-ear-containing, ARF binding) might function as adaptors between the scaffolding protein clathrin and M6PRs.[61-64] GGAs are a novel family of proteins characterized by an amino-terminal Vps27/Hrs/STAM (VHS) homology domain, an ADP-ribosylation factor (ARF) binding domain, a "hinge" region, and a carboxyl-terminal domain with homology to the "ear" domain of the AP-1 subunit.[42,65] Several groups[66-69] have demonstrated that the VHS domain of GGA proteins recognizes the dileucine signals from CI-M6PR and CD-M6PR. Expression of truncated versions of GGAs result in the specific missorting of M6PRs while other TGN sorted proteins are unaffected. These data suggest that the GGA proteins may be responsible for appropriate lysosomal hydrolase sorting.

Synthesis and Trafficking of Lysosomal Membrane Proteins

While soluble lysosomal hydrolases are sorted to the lysosome by the mannose-phosphate recognition system, lysosomal membrane proteins take a different route.[40,70,71] This difference in trafficking was first recognized through analysis of I-cell disease.[72] In the absence of the mannose-phosphate system, lysosomal membrane proteins show a normal distribution. Similarly, deletion of M6PRs affects the proper trafficking of hydrolases but has no affect on the trafficking of lysosomal proteins.[73] Our current understanding of the trafficking of lysosomal membrane proteins comes from analysis of targeting signal motifs on membrane proteins[74-76] using site specific mutagenesis, analysis of pigmentation mutants in eukaryotes and analysis of vacuolar mutants in yeast.[77-79]

Motifs in the cytoplasmic tail of lysosomal membrane proteins define their targeting to the lysosome. Two motifs, GYXXΦ and dileucine, have been identified for lysosomal targeting. The current data suggest that these motifs are recognized by the adaptor protein-3 complex, AP-3.[80-85] This complex consists of four polypeptide subunits and appears to assemble into protein coats localized to medial and trans regions of the Golgi. AP-3 recognition of targeting motifs on lysosomal membrane proteins may lead to their capture as cargo in vesicles that then transport the lysosomal proteins to a late endosomal compartment. Researchers have shown that the absence of any one of the subunits of the AP-3 complex results in the missorting of lysosomal membrane proteins.[86-90] In the absence of AP-3, proteins still traffic to the lysosome but they take a circuitous route. Instead of being targeted to the late endosome, they are first sorted to the cell surface. From the cell surface they are internalized into an early endosome and trafficked to late endosomes. The hallmark of this missorting is the presence of large amounts of lysosomal membrane proteins on the cell surface.[84,86,90] The lysosomal membrane protein motifs that interact with the AP-3 complex can also interact with AP-2 at the plasma membrane, resulting in their internalization into clathrin coated pits and delivery to the endocytic pathway.[41,86]

Disruption of the AP-3 trafficking route is seen most dramatically in mutants of the AP-3 complex, which lead to alterations in pigment distribution in melanosomes of mice and humans or pigment granules in *Drosophila melanogaster*. There are over 20 different mouse mutants with alterations in coat color[91] and 10-15 Drosophila mutants with altered eye color due to changes in pigment granules.[77] Many of these mutations are within genes required for transfer of lysosomal membrane proteins e.g., AP-3 or in proteins that regulate vesicular trafficking.

Lysosomes and Endosomes Undergo Fusion and Fission

Dynamics of Fusion and Fission

The endocytic apparatus traffics molecules by vesicular fusion and fission, yet the organelles of this apparatus remain fairly discreet.[92] This implies a high degree of regulation in fusion and fission events in the endocytic pathway.[37] While early endosomes can fuse with each other,[93,94] they cannot fuse with lysosomes. The specificity of fusion among endocytic organelles can be reproduced in vitro. Using a system in which endocytic vesicle fusion can be synchronized and then isolated, Ward et al[19,95] demonstrated that endosomes isolated four minutes after internalization could readily fuse with endosomes isolated eight minutes after internalization but not with endosomes isolated 12 minutes after internalization. Endosomes isolated 12 minutes after internalization could fuse with lysosomes but not with either four or eight minute endosomes. Lysosomes could fuse with each other and with 12 minute endosomes but not with four or eight minute endosomes. This specificity implies that there are unique recognition molecules gained by vesicles in the endocytic pathway that regulate homotypic and heterotypic fusion.

A heterotypic fusion event is required for the transfer of lysosomal hydrolases from the lumen of the late endosome to the lumen of the lysosome. Another heterotypic fusion event in the late endocytic pathway is the transfer of endocytosed material from an endosome to the lysosome.[11,92] Data from both in vitro and in vivo studies demonstrate that lysosomes can fuse with late endosomes.[35,38,95-108] This fusion event has been proposed to lead to the formation of a hybrid-organelle with a density intermediate to that of a late endosome and a lysosome.[109-111] This hybrid organelle is both lgp120 (a lysosomal membrane protein) and M6PR positive suggestive of a fusion between late endosomes and lysosomes. In vitro analysis of these hybrid organelles has shown an ATP-dependent change in the density of the hybrid organelle, ostensibly reforming late endosomes and lysosomes.[112]

There is little debate regarding the fact that late endosomes and lysosomes fuse. There is, however, no consensus on how late endosomal membrane is retrieved. Two mechanisms have been suggested. The first is that late endosomal membrane proteins are recycled through a process that involves budding.[113] The budding process would require the formation of a coat. While there is evidence for coat formation on lysosomes, most of the evidence utilizes in vitro systems.[114] A second hypothesis is that a fission event separates late endosomes and lysosomes. Storrie et al suggested that lysosomes repeatedly fuse with endosomes in a series of transient fusion and fission events.[20,115,116] During these events, small amounts of material are exchanged and recycled between the two organelles. A "kiss and run" sampling, as the hypothesis is called, may allow for microdomains of sorting prior to content mixing.

The ability of lysosomes to engage in heterotypic fusion is readily understandable; both for lysosomes to obtain newly synthesized components and to effect the degradation of internalized material. The reasons for homotypic lysosome fusion are less clear. Lysosome-lysosome fusion may guarantee that the amount of substrate in a given lysosome does not overwhelm the amount of enzymes available for degradation. Thus, lysosomal fusion may ensure that substrates are always exposed to conditions in which there is an excess of degradative enzymes. Several laboratories have demonstrated lysosome-lysosome fusion.[10] UV-Sendai virus cell fusions have shown that the lysosomal contents from one set of cells mix with the lysosomal contents of the fusion partner cells in a time and temperature dependent fashion.[117,118] Lysosome-lysosome fusion has also been reconstituted in vitro.[19,95,119]

The Molecular Machinery Mediating Fusion and Fission

Fusion of endocytic vesicles requires energy, specific addressing molecules, and other regulatory molecules. All fusion events examined to date require the cytosolic ATPase N-ethylmaleimide-sensitive factor (NSF) and an energy source, ATP. Fusion also requires targeting molecules that address which vesicles fuse together. These targeting molecules/proteins are hypothesized to be the NSF attachment protein (SNAP) receptors, or SNAREs.[120] They can be found in both the donor and acceptor membranes and it is hypothesized that the appropriate pairing will mediate fusion of donor and acceptor membranes. Recent studies have shown that the SNAREs Syntaxin 7, vesicle associated membrane protein-7 (VAMP-7) and VAMP-8 are involved in heterotypic and homotypic lysosome fusion.[95,106-108] In the case of Syntaxin 7, it has been localized throughout the endocytic apparatus but appears to be concentrated on late endosomes and lysosomes. Furthermore, expression of mammalian Syntaxin 7 in Saccharomyces cerevisiae permitted vacuolar trafficking in yeast mutants defective in the yeast SNARE Pep12p.[107] VAMP-7 has been localized primarily to late endosomes.[106] Coimmunoprecipitation experiments utilizing a cultured melanoma cell line showed Syntaxin 7 in a complex with VAMP-8, Syntaxin 6, mouse Vps10p tail interactor 1b (mVti1b), α-synaptosome-associated protein (α-SNAP), VAMP-7 and the protein phosphatase 1M regulatory subunit.[121] These data suggest that a complex may be required for mediating heterotypic and homotypic lysosome fusion. Caplan and colleagues[119] have also shown a role for Vam6p in homotypic lysosome fusion. Overexpression of Vam6p results in a specific clustering and fusion of lysosomes and late endosomes, whereas early endocytic and secretory organelles were unaffected. They further demonstrated that specific citron homology and clathrin homology repeat domains present in Vam6p are required for lysosome/late endosome clustering and fusion.

Biochemical dissection of lysosome fusion has shown a requirement for a heterotrimeric G proteins and Rabs.[19,110] Exactly what role these molecules play is less clear. Small GTP binding molecules, Rabs, have been shown to regulate vesicle fusion events and yet no Rab has been identified in lysosome fusion. Both Rab7 and Rab9 have been found on late endosomes.[122] Rab9 plays a demonstrable role in regulating M6PR recycling from late endosomes to the Golgi.[123] Rab7 appears to be required for transport to the late endosome/lysosome.[122,124-126]

Expression of a dominant negative Rab7 prevents the transfer of soluble molecules from the late endosome to the lysosome and[119,127] results in dispersion of perinuclear lysosomes. Studies by Cantalupo et al showed that Rab7, in its GTP bound state, recruits the cytosolic protein Rab-interacting lysosomal protein (RILP) onto late endosomes and lysosomes. RILP contains a domain comprising two coiled-coil regions typical of myosin-like proteins. Overexpression of RILP prevents the dispersion of perinuclear lysosomes due to the effects of Rab7 dominant-negative mutants. In addition, a dominant negative construct of RILP inhibited degradation of ligands destined for the lysosome. These data suggest that RILP may act as a downstream effector of Rab7 in late endosome-lysosome trafficking. The overexpression phenotype of dominant-negative Rab7 was examined in the context of Vam6p overexpression, another molecule implicated in lysosome fusion events.[119] The lysosomal clustering and fusion mediated by overexpression of Vam6p was unchanged in the context of a dominant-negative Rab7. These studies suggest that Vam6p works downstream of Rab7 or in a parallel pathway in mediating lysosome fusion.

Studies on the endocytic pathway have also indicated an important role for phosphoinositides in membrane trafficking.[128-130] Phosphoinositides are clearly important throughout the endocytic apparatus specifically in endocytosis and sorting in the early endocytic apparatus. A role in the late endocytic apparatus is less well defined. Analysis in mammalian systems has shown that addition of the fungal chemical wortmannin, which inhibits mammalian phosphoinositide-3 kinases, decreases sorting of the lysosomal hydrolase Cathepsin D and results in late endosomal swelling.[131,132] The importance of phosphoinositides in the late endocytic pathway has been analyzed extensively in *S. cerevisiae*. Mutants with defects in phosphoinositide synthesis and metabolism show defects in vesicular trafficking to the vacuole and in vacuolar morphology.[133-140] The high degree of conservation in eukaryotes suggests that phosphoinositide metabolism must also alter trafficking in the late endocytic pathway of mammalian cells and studies support this view.[132,135,141,142] The specificity of fusion in the late endocytic pathway probably arises from the combination of appropriate tethering, docking factors, SNAREs, Rabs and lipid components.

Lysosomes Are Capable of Fusion with the Plasma Membrane

Recent studies have provided evidence that lysosomes are capable of fusing with the plasma membrane. The first reports of lysosome-plasma membrane fusion were observed in *Trypanosoma cruzi* invasion in mammalian cells.[143-145] During *T. cruzi* invasion, lysosomes are recruited to the parasite entry site and fuse with the plasma membrane. Other studies have shown that lysosomal contents could be released upon stimulation of polymorphonuclear leukocytes with a wide variety of agents, including activated complement,[146,147] phorbol esters,[148] calcium ionophores and the chemotactic agent Formyl-Met-Leu-Phe.[149] These treatments resulted in a release of intracellular calcium, thereby promoting lysosomal secretion.

More recently it was discovered that fusion of lysosomes with the plasma membrane is a physiological mechanism of wound repair.[150,151] Cells that are subject to motility, stretching and/or mechanical manipulations are known to have their plasma membrane disrupted. These disruptions are resealed by fusion of lysosomes with the cell surface. Resealing requires the regulated movement of lysosomes to the cell periphery, docking of the lysosomes with the plasma membrane and finally fusion with the plasma membrane. The fusion event is dependent upon Ca^{2+}, temperature and ATP.[152] This resealing process has been used to introduce exogenous proteins or nucleic acids into cells.[153-159] To examine this, cells are deliberately abraded by either scraping (i.e. scrape-loading) or by interaction with glass beads. During the abrasion process, tears in the plasma membrane permit the entry of exogenous molecules. The presence of calcium then promotes lysosome-cell surface fusion resulting in the resealing of the plasma membrane and thus entrapping the molecules within cells.

Movement of Lysosomes

Several studies have shown that targeting of internalized material to lysosomes requires an intact cytoskeleton and actin based motor system.[160-162] In many cell types, microtubule inhibitors prevent degradation of internalized material by inhibiting the movement of endosomes.[101,163-165] Addition of microtubule inhibitors also leads to disruption of tubular lysosomes,[166,167] suggesting that microtubules are involved in tethering lysosomes and defining lysosome morphology. A particularly notable example of lysosome-microtubule based movement was shown by Swanson and co-workers.[166] Treatment of macrophages with acid-containing solutions decreases cytosolic pH and results in the fragmentation of lysosomes. The fragmented lysosomes are transported to the periphery of the cell by microtubule-based motors. Introduction of a kinesin antibody by scrape loading demonstrated that the outward movement of lysosomes was due to the microtubule motor kinesin. When cytosolic pH was returned to normal, by removal of cells from acid-containing buffers, lysosomes moved from the periphery back to a perinuclear region in a microtubule-dependent manner. Because kinesin is a plus-directed motor, a different microtubule motor must be involved in this retrograde movement.

In addition to microtubules, data indicate that actin based cytoskeletal elements are required for lysosome-endosome movement.[151,168,169] Inhibitors of actin affect the movement of endosomes preventing endosome-lysosome fusion. In addition, the movement of lysosomes on actin may also involve myosin-like motors.[127,161,170] There are a number of unconventional myosins that have been shown to mediate organelle movement.[171-178] Myosin-based organelle movement has been studied most extensively in pigment containing cells of vertebrates, particularly mammals. The pigmentation defects in the mouse mutants *dilute* and *viral* have been shown to result from mutations in a gene encoding an unconventional myosin, myosin 5a.[179-183] In humans, a mutation in myosin 5a results in Type 2 Griscelli syndrome, which affects both melanocytes and immune cells.[184] In order for melanocytes to produce and deposit melanin they must transport melanosomes to the cell periphery. The defect in these cell types results from an inability to move granules in either pigment cells or immune effector cells. A related disorder, Griscelli Type 1 in humans and *ashen* in mice, is due to a mutation in Rab27a, a gene required for association of myosin 5a with granules.[185,186] These results clearly show a role for unconventional myosins in pigment granule movement.[187-189] While melanosomes are considered lysosome-related organelles, defects in rab27a or myosin 5a do not result in alterations in lysosome movement.

A recent study has suggested that myosin 1a may be involved in endosome-lysosome fusion. Myosin1a was shown to be bound to endosomes and lysosomes by both subcellular fractionation and immunofluorescence.[190] Transfection of mammalian cells with a truncated form of myosin 1a affected the delivery of fluid phase markers to lysosomes. There was, however, no evidence that the number of lysosomes or their distribution was altered in the cells transfected with the truncated myosin 1a.

One gene product has been identified that affects lysosome size, movement, and distribution. Mutations in the human Chediak-Higashi gene (CHS1), or in orthologous genes in other mammals (e.g., *Beige* in mice, *Aleution blue* in mink), result in dramatic changes in lysosome size, number and distribution.[191-193] Large granule size is also seen in melanosomes, platelet dense granules and cytolytic granules. In the absence of the CHS1/*Beige* gene product, cells show a reduction in lysosome number, the remaining lysosomes are giant, and these large lysosomes are clustered in a perinuclear region as opposed to a dispersed distribution normally. In humans, Chediak-Higashi syndrome is a life threatening disorder, in part because the large size of lysosomes reduces their ability to fuse with phagosomes containing internalized bacteria. Similarly, the abnormal size of the other granules affects their movement and function. Patients with CHS have coagulation defects, pigmentation defects and recurrent bacterial infections. In the case of cytolytic granules, such defects reduce immune-surveillance by NK cells and T-effector cells. The Chediak/Beige protein is an enormous protein that appears to be soluble.[194] However, the function of this protein in regulating lysosome and lysosome-related organelle size is still unknown. Cells that overexpress the protein show a novel phenotype characterized by smaller than normal lysosomes, which tend to be found in the cell periphery.[194] One extrapolation from this observation is the Chediak/Beige protein regulates association of a motor system with lysosomes. In the absence of the motor system, lysosomes can fuse but cannot undergo fission, as fission may require a mechanical force to generate fragmented lysosomes. The absence of the protein would result in giant lysosomes, clustered near the nucleus. Conversely, an excess of Chediak/Beige protein might lead to increased association of lysosomes with motor proteins, increased occupancy on the cytoskeletal system and thus, smaller than normal lysosomes in the periphery of cells. Where and how the Chediak/Beige protein functions in lysosome formation/morphology remains unknown.

Conclusions

The importance of understanding lysosome biogenesis and maintenance is underscored by the fact that several human diseases result from defects in the lysosomal pathway. Determining the biochemical function of each of the molecules involved in the biogenesis and maintenance of the lysosome will be the primary challenge of future studies. The fact that so much of the required machinery has been identified yet we still do not truly understand lysosome formation reflects the sophistication of the biochemical pathways involved. Defining the biochemical functions of required factors may resolve some of the controversies surrounding lysosome formation and function and could possibly translate to therapies for patients suffering from lysosomal storage diseases as well as other conditions resulting from aberrant protein trafficking.

References

1. DeDuve C, Wattiaux R. Functions of lysosomes. Annu Rev Physiol 1966; 28:435-92.
2. DeDuve C. General properties of lysosomes: The lysosome concept. Lysosomes 1963; 1-31.
3. Glaumann H, Ericsson JL, Marzella L. Mechanisms of intralysosomal degradation with special reference to autophagocytosis and heterophagocytosis of cell organelles. Int Rev Cytol 1981; 73:149-82.
4. Lawrence BP, Brown WJ. Autophagic vacuoles rapidly fuse with pre-existing lysosomes in cultured hepatocytes. J Cell Sci 1992; 102(Pt 3):515-26.
5. Sakai M, Araki N, Ogawa K. Lysosomal movements during heterophagy and autophagy: With special reference to nematolysosome and wrapping lysosome. J Electron Microsc Tech 1989; 12(2):101-31.
6. Klionsky DJ, Emr SD. Autophagy as a regulated pathway of cellular degradation. Science 2000; 290(5497):1717-21.
7. Stromhaug PE, Klionsky DJ. Approaching the molecular mechanism of autophagy. Traffic 2001; 2(8):524-31.
8. Holtzmann E. Lysosomes. Plenum Press, 1989:439.
9. Matteoni R, Kreis TE. Translocation and clustering of endosomes and lysosomes depends on microtubules. J Cell Biol 1987; 105(3):1253-65.
10. Heuser J. Changes in lysosome shape and distribution correlated with changes in cytoplasmic pH. J Cell Biol 1989; 108(3):855-64.
11. Racoosin EL, Swanson JA. Macropinosome maturation and fusion with tubular lysosomes in macrophages. J Cell Biol 1993; 121(5):1011-20.
12. Griffiths G, Hoflack B, Simons K et al. The mannose 6-phosphate receptor and the biogenesis of lysosomes. Cell 1988; 52(3):329-41.
13. Kornfeld S, Mellman I. The biogenesis of lysosomes. Annu Rev Cell Biol 1989; 5:483-525.
14. Luzio JP. Lysosomes. The Encyclopaedia of Molecular Biology 1994; 597-600.

15. Deng YP, Storrie B. Animal cell lysosomes rapidly exchange membrane proteins. Proc Natl Acad Sci USA 1988; 85(11):3860-4.

16. Deng YP, Griffiths G, Storrie B. Comparative behavior of lysosomes and the pre-lysosome compartment (PLC) in in vivo cell fusion experiments. J Cell Sci 1991; 99(Pt 3):571-82.

17. Perou CM, Kaplan J. Chediak-Higashi syndrome is not due to a defect in microtubule-based lysosomal mobility. J Cell Sci 1993; 106(Pt 1):99-107.

18. Bakker AC, Webster P, Jacob WA et al. Homotypic fusion between aggregated lysosomes triggered by elevated [Ca2+]i in fibroblasts. J Cell Sci 1997; 110(Pt 18):2227-38.

19. Ward DM, Leslie JD, Kaplan J. Homotypic lysosome fusion in macrophages: Analysis using an in vitro assay. J Cell Biol 1997; 139(3):665-73.

20. Jahraus A, Storrie B, Griffiths G et al. Evidence for retrograde traffic between terminal lysosomes and the prelysosomal/late endosome compartment. J Cell Sci 1994; 107(Pt 1):145-57.

21. Kornfeld S. Trafficking of lysosomal enzymes in normal and disease states. J Clin Invest 1986; 77(1):1-6.

22. Karageorgos LE, Isaac EL, Brooks DA et al. Lysosomal biogenesis in lysosomal storage disorders. Exp Cell Res 1997; 234(1):85-97.

23. Bainton DF. The discovery of lysosomes. J Cell Biol 1981; 91(3 Pt 2):66s-76s.

24. Farquhar MG, Palade GE. The Golgi apparatus (complex)-(1954-1981)-from artifact to center stage. J Cell Biol 1981; 91(3 Pt 2):77s-103s.

25. Helenius A, Mellman I, Wall D et al. Endosomes. Trends Biochem Sci 1983; 8:245-9.

26. Murphy RF. Maturation models for endosome and lysosome biogenesis. Trends Cell Biol 1991; 1:77-82.

27. Stoorvogel W, Strous GJ, Geuze HJ et al. Late endosomes derive from early endosomes by maturation. Cell 1991; 65(3):417-27.

28. Gruenberg J, Maxfield FR. Membrane transport in the endocytic pathway. Curr Opin Cell Biol 1995; 7(4):552-63.

29. Steinman RM, Mellman IS, Muller WA et al. Endocytosis and the recycling of plasma membrane. J Cell Biol 1983; 96(1):1-27.

30. van Deurs B, Christensen EI. Endocytosis in kidney proximal tubule cells and cultured fibroblasts: A review of the structural aspects of membrane recycling between the plasma membrane and endocytic vacuoles. Eur J Cell Biol 1984; 33(1):163-73.

31. Thilo L. Quantification of endocytosis-derived membrane traffic. Biochim Biophys Acta 1985; 822(2):243-66.

32. Tsuruhara T, Koenig JH, Ikeda K. Synchronized endocytosis studied in the oocyte of a temperature- sensitive mutant of Drosophila melanogaster. Cell Tissue Res 1990; 259(2):199-207.

33. Ward DM, Perou CM, Lloyd M et al. "Synchronized" endocytosis and intracellular sorting in alveolar macrophages: The early sorting endosome is a transient organelle. J Cell Biol 1995; 129(5):1229-40.

34. Ludwig T, Griffiths G, Hoflack B. Distribution of newly synthesized lysosomal enzymes in the endocytic pathway of normal rat kidney cells. J Cell Biol 1991; 115(6):1561-72.

35. Futter CE, Pearse A, Hewlett LJ et al. Multivesicular endosomes containing internalized EGF-EGF receptor complexes mature and then fuse directly with lysosomes. J Cell Biol 1996; 132(6):1011-23.

36. Mellman I. Endocytosis and molecular sorting. Annu Rev Cell Dev Biol 1996; 12:575-625.

37. Luzio JP, Mullock BM, Pryor PR et al. Relationship between endosomes and lysosomes. Biochem Soc Trans 2001; 29(Pt 4):476-80.

38. Piper RC, Luzio JP. Late endosomes: Sorting and partitioning in multivesicular bodies. Traffic 2001; 2(9):612-21.

39. Hasilik A. The early and late processing of lysosomal enzymes: proteolysis and compartmentation. Experientia 1992; 48(2):130-51.

40. Hunziker W, Geuze HJ. Intracellular trafficking of lysosomal membrane proteins. Bioessays 1996; 18(5):379-89.

41. Rouille Y, Rohn W, Hoflack B. Targeting of lysosomal proteins. Semin Cell Dev Biol 2000; 11(3):165-71.

42. Dell'Angelica EC, Payne GS. Intracellular cycling of lysosomal enzyme receptors: Cytoplasmic tails' tales. Cell 2001; 106(4):395-8.

43. von Figura K, Hasilik A, Pohlmann R et al. Mutations affecting transport and stability of lysosomal enzymes. Enzyme 1987; 38(1-4):144-53.
44. Leroy JG. I-cell disease: Elucidation of the enzyme defect and its molecular biology significance. Verh K Acad Geneeskd Belg 1989; 51(3):231-67.
45. Suzuki Y. Lysosomal enzymes, sphingolipid activator proteins, and protective protein. Nippon Rinsho 1995; 53(12):2887-91.
46. McDowell G, Gahl WA. Inherited disorders of glycoprotein synthesis: Cell biological insights. Proc Soc Exp Biol Med 1997; 215(2):145-57.
47. Himeno M, Tanaka Y. Lysosomal hydrolases have specific conformational domains for acquisition of mannose-6-phosphate. Nippon Rinsho 1995; 53(12):2892-7.
48. von Figura K, Hasilik A. Lysosomal enzymes and their receptors. Annu Rev Biochem 1986; 55:167-93.
49. Kornfeld S. Trafficking of lysosomal enzymes. Faseb J 1987; 1(6):462-8.
50. Kornfeld S. Structure and function of the mannose 6-phosphate/insulinlike growth factor II receptors. Annu Rev Biochem 1992; 61:307-30.
51. Ludwig T, Le Borgne R, Hoflack B. Roles for mannose 6-phosphate receptors in lysosomal enzyme sorting, IGF-II binding and clathrin-coat assembly. Trends Cell Biol 1995; 5:202-6.
52. Le Borgne R, Hoflack B. Mannose 6-phosphate receptors regulate the formation of clathrin-coated vesicles in the TGN. J Cell Biol 1997; 137(2):335-45.
53. Zhu Y, Traub LM, Kornfeld S. High-affinity binding of the AP-1 adaptor complex to trans-golgi network membranes devoid of mannose 6-phosphate receptors. Mol Biol Cell 1999; 10(3):537-49.
54. Rohn WM, Rouille Y, Waguri S et al. Bi-directional trafficking between the trans-Golgi network and the endosomal/lysosomal system. J Cell Sci 2000; 113(Pt 12):2093-101.
55. Pearse BM, Robinson MS. Clathrin, adaptors, and sorting. Annu Rev Cell Biol 1990; 6:151-71.
56. Ohno H, Stewart J, Fournier MC et al. Interaction of tyrosine-based sorting signals with clathrin-associated proteins. Science 1995; 269(5232):1872-5.
57. Ohno H, Aguilar RC, Yeh D et al. The medium subunits of adaptor complexes recognize distinct but overlapping sets of tyrosine-based sorting signals. J Biol Chem 1998; 273(40):25915-21.
58. Honing S, Sosa M, Hille-Rehfeld A et al. The 46-kDa mannose 6-phosphate receptor contains multiple binding sites for clathrin adaptors. J Biol Chem 1997; 272(32):19884-90.
59. Meyer C, Eskelinen EL, Guruprasad MR et al. Mu 1A deficiency induces a profound increase in MPR300/IGF-II receptor internalization rate. J Cell Sci 2001; 114(Pt 24):4469-76.
60. Meyer C, Zizioli D, Lausmann S et al. mu1A-adaptin-deficient mice: Lethality, loss of AP-1 binding and rerouting of mannose 6-phosphate receptors. Embo J 2000; 19(10):2193-203.
61. Boman AL, Zhang C, Zhu X et al. A family of ADP-ribosylation factor effectors that can alter membrane transport through the trans-Golgi. Mol Biol Cell 2000; 11(4):1241-55.
62. Dell'Angelica EC, Puertollano R, Mullins C et al. GGAs: A family of ADP ribosylation factor-binding proteins related to adaptors and associated with the Golgi complex. J Cell Biol 2000; 149(1):81-94.
63. Hirst J, Lui WW, Bright NA et al. A family of proteins with gamma-adaptin and VHS domains that facilitate trafficking between the trans-Golgi network and the vacuole/lysosome. J Cell Biol 2000; 149(1):67-80.
64. Poussu A, Lohi O, Lehto VP. Vear, a novel Golgi-associated protein with VHS and gamma-adaptin "ear" domains. J Biol Chem 2000; 275(10):7176-83.
65. Lohi O, Poussu A, Mao Y et al. VHS domain — a longshoreman of vesicle lines. FEBS Lett 2002; 513(1):19-23.
66. Nielsen MS, Madsen P, Christensen EI et al. The sortilin cytoplasmic tail conveys Golgi-endosome transport and binds the VHS domain of the GGA2 sorting protein. Embo J 2001; 20(9):2180-90.
67. Puertollano R, Aguilar RC, Gorshkova I et al. Sorting of mannose 6-phosphate receptors mediated by the GGAs. Science 2001; 292(5522):1712-6.
68. Takatsu H, Katoh Y, Shiba Y et al. Golgi-localizing, gamma-adaptin ear homology domain, ADP-ribosylation factor-binding (GGA) proteins interact with acidic dileucine sequences within the cytoplasmic domains of sorting receptors through their Vps27p/Hrs/STAM (VHS) domains. J Biol Chem 2001; 276(30):28541-5.

69. Zhu Y, Doray B, Poussu A et al. Binding of GGA2 to the lysosomal enzyme sorting motif of the mannose 6- phosphate receptor. Science 2001; 292(5522):1716-8.
70. Peters C, von Figura K. Biogenesis of lysosomal membranes. FEBS Lett 1994; 346(1):108-14.
71. Sandoval IV, Bakke O. Targeting of membrane proteins to endosomes and lysosomes. Trends Cell Biol. 1994; 4:292-7.
72. Kornfeld S, Sly WS. I-cell disease and pseudo-Hurler polydystropy: Disorders of lysosomal enzyme phosphorylation and localization. New York, NY: McGraw-Hill, 1995.
73. Ludwig T, Munier-Lehmann H, Bauer U et al. Differential sorting of lysosomal enzymes in mannose 6-phosphate receptor-deficient fibroblasts. Embo J 1994; 13(15):3430-7.
74. Le Borgne R, Hoflack B. Protein transport from the secretory to the endocytic pathway in mammalian cells. Biochim Biophys Acta 1998; 1404(1-2):195-209.
75. Bonifacino JS, Dell'Angelica EC. Molecular bases for the recognition of tyrosine-based sorting signals. J Cell Biol 1999; 145(5):923-6.
76. Kirchhausen T. Adaptors for clathrin-mediated traffic. Annu Rev Cell Dev Biol 1999; 15:705-32.
77. Lloyd V, Ramaswami M, Kramer H. Not just pretty eyes: Drosophila eye-colour mutations and lysosomal delivery. Trends Cell Biol 1998; 8(7):257-9.
78. Spritz RA. Multi-organellar disorders of pigmentation: Tied up in traffic. Clin Genet 1999; 55(5):309-17.
79. Odorizzi G, Cowles CR, Emr SD. The AP-3 complex: A coat of many colours. Trends Cell Biol 1998; 8(7):282-8.
80. Cowles CR, Odorizzi G, Payne GS et al. The AP-3 adaptor complex is essential for cargo-selective transport to the yeast vacuole. Cell 1997; 91(1):109-18.
81. Dell'Angelica EC, Ohno H, Ooi CE et al. AP-3: An adaptor-like protein complex with ubiquitous expression. Embo J 1997; 16(5):917-28.
82. Darsow T, Burd CG, Emr SD. Acidic di-leucine motif essential for AP-3-dependent sorting and restriction of the functional specificity of the Vam3p vacuolar t-SNARE. J Cell Biol 1998; 142(4):913-22.
83. Honing S, Sandoval IV, von Figura K. A di-leucine-based motif in the cytoplasmic tail of LIMP-II and tyrosinase mediates selective binding of AP-3. Embo J 1998; 17(5):1304-14.
84. Le Borgne R, Alconada A, Bauer U et al. The mammalian AP-3 adaptor-like complex mediates the intracellular transport of lysosomal membrane glycoproteins. J Biol Chem 1998; 273(45):29451-61.
85. Tabuchi N, Akasaki K, Tsuji H. Two acidic amino acid residues, Asp(470) and Glu(471), contained in the carboxyl cytoplasmic tail of a major lysosomal membrane protein, LGP85/LIMP II, are important for its accumulation in secondary lysosomes. Biochem Biophys Res Commun 2000; 270(2):557-63.
86. Dell'Angelica EC, Shotelersuk V, Aguilar RC et al. Altered trafficking of lysosomal proteins in Hermansky-Pudlak syndrome due to mutations in the beta 3A subunit of the AP-3 adaptor. Mol Cell 1999; 3(1):11-21.
87. Simpson F, Peden AA, Christopoulou L et al. Characterization of the adaptor-related protein complex, AP-3. J Cell Biol 1997; 137(4):835-45.
88. Hirst J, Robinson MS. Clathrin and adaptors. Biochim Biophys Acta 1998; 1404(1-2):173-93.
89. Zhen L, Jiang S, Feng L et al. Abnormal expression and subcellular distribution of subunit proteins of the AP-3 adaptor complex lead to platelet storage pool deficiency in the pearl mouse. Blood 1999; 94(1):146-55.
90. Yang W, Li C, Ward DM et al. Defective organellar membrane protein trafficking in Ap3b1-deficient cells. J Cell Sci 2000; 113(Pt 22):4077-86.
91. Robinson MS, Bonifacino JS. Adaptor-related proteins. Curr Opin Cell Biol 2001; 13(4):444-53.
92. Clague MJ. Molecular aspects of the endocytic pathway. Biochem J 1998; 336(Pt 2):271-82.
93. Mills IG, Jones AT, Clague MJ. Regulation of endosome fusion. Mol Membr Biol 1999; 16(1):73-9.
94. Clague MJ. Membrane transport: Take your fusion partners. Curr Biol 1999; 9(7):R258-60.
95. Ward DM, Pevsner J, Scullion MA et al. Syntaxin 7 and VAMP-7 are soluble N-ethylmaleimide-sensitive factor attachment protein receptors required for late endosome-lysosome and homotypic lysosome fusion in alveolar macrophages. Mol Biol Cell 2000; 11(7):2327-33.
96. Mullock BM, Branch WJ, van Schaik M et al. Reconstitution of an endosome-lysosome interaction in a cell-free system. J Cell Biol 1989; 108(6):2093-9.

97. Salzman NH, Maxfield FR. Fusion accessibility of endocytic compartments along the recycling and lysosomal endocytic pathways in intact cells. J Cell Biol 1989; 109(5):2097-104.

98. Ward DM, Hackenyos DP, Davis-Kaplan S et al. Inhibition of late endosome-lysosome fusion: Studies on the mechanism by which isotonic-K+ buffers alter intracellular ligand movement. J Cell Physiol 1990; 145(3):522-30.

99. Mullock BM, Luzio JP. Reconstitution of rat liver endosome-lysosome fusion in vitro. Methods Enzymol 1992; 219:52-60.

100. Mullock BM, Perez JH, Kuwana T et al. Lysosomes can fuse with a late endosomal compartment in a cell-free system from rat liver. J Cell Biol 1994; 126(5):1173-82.

101. van Deurs B, Holm PK, Kayser L et al. Delivery to lysosomes in the human carcinoma cell line HEp-2 involves an actin filament-facilitated fusion between mature endosomes and preexisting lysosomes. Eur J Cell Biol 1995; 66(4):309-23.

102. Kuwana T, Mullock BM, Luzio JP. Identification of a lysosomal protein causing lipid transfer, using a fluorescence assay designed to monitor membrane fusion between rat liver endosomes and lysosomes. Biochem J 1995; 308(Pt 3):937-46.

103. van Deurs B, Holm PK, Sandvig K. Inhibition of the vacuolar H(+)-ATPase with bafilomycin reduces delivery of internalized molecules from mature multivesicular endosomes to lysosomes in HEp-2 cells. Eur J Cell Biol 1996; 69(4):343-50.

104. Schmid JA, Ellinger I, Kosma P. In vitro fusion of tissue-derived endosomes and lysosomes. Eur J Cell Biol 1998; 77(3):166-74.

105. Ohashi M, Miwako I, Nakamura K et al. An arrested late endosome-lysosome intermediate aggregate observed in a Chinese hamster ovary cell mutant isolated by novel three-step screening. J Cell Sci 1999; 112(Pt 8):1125-38.

106. Advani RJ, Yang B, Prekeris R et al. VAMP-7 mediates vesicular transport from endosomes to lysosomes. J Cell Biol 1999; 146(4):765-76.

107. Nakamura N, Yamamoto A, Wada Y et al. Syntaxin 7 mediates endocytic trafficking to late endosomes. J Biol Chem 2000; 275(9):6523-9.

108. Mullock BM, Smith CW, Ihrke G et al. Syntaxin 7 is localized to late endosome compartments, associates with Vamp 8, and Is required for late endosome-lysosome fusion. Mol Biol Cell 2000; 11(9):3137-53.

109. Bright NA, Reaves BJ, Mullock BM et al. Dense core lysosomes can fuse with late endosomes and are re-formed from the resultant hybrid organelles. J Cell Sci 1997; 110(Pt 17):2027-40.

110. Mullock BM, Bright NA, Fearon CW et al. Fusion of lysosomes with late endosomes produces a hybrid organelle of intermediate density and is NSF dependent. J Cell Biol 1998; 140(3):591-601.

111. Luzio JP, Rous BA, Bright NA et al. Lysosome-endosome fusion and lysosome biogenesis. J Cell Sci 2000; 113(Pt 9):1515-24.

112. Pryor PR, Mullock BM, Bright NA et al. The role of intraorganellar Ca(2+) in late endosome-lysosome heterotypic fusion and in the reformation of lysosomes from hybrid organelles. J Cell Biol 2000; 149(5):1053-62.

113. Higgins ME, Davies JP, Chen FW et al. Niemann-Pick C1 is a late endosome-resident protein that transiently associates with lysosomes and the trans-Golgi network. Mol Genet Metab 1999; 68(1):1-13.

114. Traub LM, Bannykh SI, Rodel JE et al. AP-2-containing clathrin coats assemble on mature lysosomes. J Cell Biol 1996; 135(6 Pt 2):1801-14.

115. Storrie B, Desjardins M. The biogenesis of lysosomes: Is it a kiss and run, continuous fusion and fission process? Bioessays 1996; 18(11):895-903.

116. Duclos S, Diez R, Garin J et al. Rab5 regulates the kiss and run fusion between phagosomes and endosomes and the acquisition of phagosome leishmanicidal properties in RAW 264.7 macrophages. J Cell Sci 2000; 113 Pt 19:3531-41.

117. Ferris AL, Brown JC, Park RD et al. Chinese hamster ovary cell lysosomes rapidly exchange contents. J Cell Biol 1987; 105(6 Pt 1):2703-12.

118. Perou CM, Kaplan J. Complementation analysis of Chediak-Higashi syndrome: The same gene may be responsible for the defect in all patients and species. Somat Cell Mol Genet 1993; 19(5):459-68.

119. Caplan S, Hartnell LM, Aguilar RC et al. Human Vam6p promotes lysosome clustering and fusion in vivo. J Cell Biol 2001; 154(1):109-22.
120. Rothman JE, Warren G. Implications of the SNARE hypothesis for intracellular membrane topology and dynamics. Curr Biol 1994; 4(3):220-33.
121. Wade N, Bryant NJ, Connolly LM et al. Syntaxin 7 complexes with mouse Vps10p tail interactor 1b, syntaxin 6, vesicle-associated membrane protein (VAMP)8, and VAMP7 in b16 melanoma cells. J Biol Chem 2001; 276(23):19820-7.
122. Soldati T, Rancano C, Geissler H et al. Rab7 and Rab9 are recruited onto late endosomes by biochemically distinguishable processes. J Biol Chem 1995; 270(43):25541-8.
123. Riederer MA, Soldati T, Shapiro AD et al. Lysosome biogenesis requires Rab9 function and receptor recycling from endosomes to the trans-Golgi network. J Cell Biol 1994; 125(3):573-82.
124. Meresse S, Gorvel JP, Chavrier P. The rab7 GTPase resides on a vesicular compartment connected to lysosomes. J Cell Sci 1995; 108(Pt 11):3349-58.
125. Feng Y, Press B, Wandinger-Ness A. Rab 7: An important regulator of late endocytic membrane traffic. J Cell Biol 1995; 131(6 Pt 1):1435-52.
126. Bottger G, Nagelkerken B, van der Sluijs P. Rab4 and Rab7 define distinct nonoverlapping endosomal compartments. J Biol Chem 1996; 271(46):29191-7.
127. Cantalupo G, Alifano P, Roberti V et al. Rab-interacting lysosomal protein (RILP): The Rab7 effector required for transport to lysosomes. Embo J 2001; 20(4):683-93.
128. De Camilli P, Emr SD, McPherson PS et al. Phosphoinositides as regulators in membrane traffic. Science 1996; 271(5255):1533-9.
129. Roth MG. Lipid regulators of membrane traffic through the Golgi complex. Trends Cell Biol 1999; 9(5):174-9. _00001535.
130. Corvera S, D'Arrigo A, Stenmark H. Phosphoinositides in membrane traffic. Curr Opin Cell Biol 1999; 11(4):460-5.
131. Reaves BJ, Bright NA, Mullock BM et al. The effect of wortmannin on the localisation of lysosomal type I integral membrane glycoproteins suggests a role for phosphoinositide 3- kinase activity in regulating membrane traffic late in the endocytic pathway. J Cell Sci 1996; 109(Pt 4):749-62.
132. Bright NA, Lindsay MR, Stewart A et al. The relationship between lumenal and limiting membranes in swollen late endocytic compartments formed after wortmannin treatment or sucrose accumulation. Traffic 2001; 2(9):631-42.
133. Foti M, Audhya A, Emr SD. Sac1 lipid phosphatase and Stt4 phosphatidylinositol 4-kinase regulate a pool of phosphatidylinositol 4-phosphate that functions in the control of the actin cytoskeleton and vacuole morphology. Mol Biol Cell 2001; 12(8):2396-411.
134. Burd CG, Babst M, Emr SD. Novel pathways, membrane coats and PI kinase regulation in yeast lysosomal trafficking. Semin Cell Dev Biol 1998; 9(5):527-33.
135. Row PE, Reaves BJ, Domin J et al. Overexpression of a rat kinase-deficient phosphoinositide 3-kinase, Vps34p, inhibits cathepsin D maturation. Biochem J 2001; 353(Pt 3):655-61.
136. Stack JH, Emr SD. Vps34p required for yeast vacuolar protein sorting is a multiple specificity kinase that exhibits both protein kinase and phosphatidylinositol-specific PI 3-kinase activities. J Biol Chem 1994; 269(50):31552-62.
137. Wurmser AE, Emr SD. Phosphoinositide signaling and turnover: PtdIns(3)P, a regulator of membrane traffic, is transported to the vacuole and degraded by a process that requires lumenal vacuolar hydrolase activities. Embo J 1998; 17(17):4930-42.
138. Gary JD, Wurmser AE, Bonangelino CJ et al. Fab1p is essential for PtdIns(3)P 5-kinase activity and the maintenance of vacuolar size and membrane homeostasis. J Cell Biol 1998; 143(1):65-79.
139. Mayer A, Scheglmann D, Dove S et al. Phosphatidylinositol 4,5-bisphosphate regulates two steps of homotypic vacuole fusion. Mol Biol Cell 2000; 11(3):807-17.
140. Cheever ML, Sato TK, de Beer T et al. Phox domain interaction with PtdIns(3)P targets the Vam7 t-SNARE to vacuole membranes. Nat Cell Biol 2001; 3(7):613-8.
141. Fernandez-Borja M, Wubbolts R, Calafat J et al. Multivesicular body morphogenesis requires phosphatidyl-inositol 3- kinase activity. Curr Biol 1999; 9(1):55-8.
142. Sachse M, Urbe S, Oorschot V et al. Bilayered Clathrin Coats on Endosomal Vacuoles Are Involved in Protein Sorting toward Lysosomes. Mol Biol Cell 2002; 13(4):1313-28.

143. Andrews NW. From lysosomes into the cytosol: The intracellular pathway of Trypanosoma cruzi. Braz J Med Biol Res 1994; 27(2):471-5.

144. Andrews NW. Living dangerously: How Trypanosoma cruzi uses lysosomes to get inside host cells, and then escapes into the cytoplasm. Biol Res 1993; 26(1-2):65-7.

145. Tardieux I, Webster P, Ravesloot J et al. Lysosome recruitment and fusion are early events required for trypanosome invasion of mammalian cells. Cell 1992; 71(7):1117-30.

146. Goldstein IM, Kaplan HB, Radin A et al. Independent effects of IgG and complement upon human polymorphonuclear leukocyte function. J Immunol 1976; 117(4):1282-7.

147. Hatherill JR, Stephens KE, Nagao K et al. Effects of anti-C5a antibodies on human polymorphonuclear leukocyte function: Chemotaxis, chemiluminescence, and lysosomal enzyme release. J Biol Response Mod 1989; 8(6):614-24.

148. Goldstein IM, Hoffstein ST, Weissmann G. Mechanisms of lysosomal enzyme release from human polymorphonuclear leukocytes. Effects of phorbol myristate acetate. J Cell Biol 1975; 66(3):647-52.

149. Naccache PH, Showell HJ, Becker EL et al. Changes in ionic movements across rabbit polymorphonuclear leukocyte membranes during lysosomal enzyme release. Possible ionic basis for lysosomal enzyme release. J Cell Biol 1977; 75(3):635-49.

150. Reddy A, Caler EV, Andrews NW. Plasma membrane repair is mediated by Ca(2+)-regulated exocytosis of lysosomes. Cell 2001; 106(2):157-69.

151. McNeil PL. Repairing a torn cell surface: Make way, lysosomes to the rescue. J Cell Sci 2002; 115(Pt 5):873-9.

152. Rodriguez A, Webster P, Ortego J et al. Lysosomes behave as Ca2+-regulated exocytic vesicles in fibroblasts and epithelial cells. J Cell Biol 1997; 137(1):93-104.

153. Fechheimer M, Boylan JF, Parker S et al. Transfection of mammalian cells with plasmid DNA by scrape loading and sonication loading. Proc Natl Acad Sci USA 1987; 84(23):8463-7.

154. Morris JD, Price B, Lloyd AC et al. Scrape-loading of Swiss 3T3 cells with ras protein rapidly activates protein kinase C in the absence of phosphoinositide hydrolysis. Oncogene 1989; 4(1):27-31.

155. Swanson JA, Lee M, Knapp PE. Cellular dimensions affecting the nucleocytoplasmic volume ratio. J Cell Biol 1991; 115(4):941-8.

156. Daum T, Engels JW, Mag M et al. Antisense oligodeoxynucleotide: Inhibitor of splicing of mRNA of human immunodeficiency virus. Intervirology 1992; 33(2):65-75.

157. Boes R, Obe G. Scrape-loading: A simple method to induce chromosomal aberrations with restriction enzymes in CHO cells. Mutat Res 1993; 292(3):225-30.

158. Kumar S, O'Dowd C, Dunckley MG et al. A comparative evaluation of three transfection procedures as assessed by resistance to G418 conferred to HEPG2 cells. Biochem Mol Biol Int 1994; 32(6):1059-66.

159. Partridge M, Vincent A, Matthews P et al. A simple method for delivering morpholino antisense oligos into the cytoplasm of cells. Antisense Nucleic Acid Drug Dev 1996; 6(3):169-75.

160. Taunton J. Actin filament nucleation by endosomes, lysosomes and secretory vesicles. Curr Opin Cell Biol 2001; 13(1):85-91.

161. DePina AS, Langford GM. Vesicle transport: The role of actin filaments and myosin motors. Microsc Res Tech 1999; 47(2):93-106.

162. Andrews NW. Regulated secretion of conventional lysosomes. Trends Cell Biol 2000; 10(8):316-21.

163. Sakai T, Yamashina S, Ohnishi S. Microtubule-disrupting drugs blocked delivery of endocytosed transferrin to the cytocenter, but did not affect return of transferrin to plasma membrane. J Biochem (Tokyo) 1991; 109(4):528-33.

164. Aniento F, Emans N, Griffiths G et al. Cytoplasmic dynein-dependent vesicular transport from early to late endosomes. J Cell Biol 1993; 123(6 Pt 1):1373-87.

165. Sonee M, Barron E, Yarber FA et al. Taxol inhibits endosomal-lysosomal membrane trafficking at two distinct steps in CV-1 cells. Am J Physiol 1998; 275(6 Pt 1):C1630-9.

166. Swanson J, Bushnell A, Silverstein SC. Tubular lysosome morphology and distribution within macrophages depend on the integrity of cytoplasmic microtubules. Proc Natl Acad Sci USA 1987; 84(7):1921-5.

167. Swanson JA, Locke A, Ansel P et al. Radial movement of lysosomes along microtubules in permeabilized macrophages. J Cell Sci 1992; 103(Pt 1):201-9.

168. Brown SS. Cooperation between microtubule- and actin-based motor proteins. Annu Rev Cell Dev Biol 1999; 15:63-80.

169. Apodaca G. Endocytic traffic in polarized epithelial cells: Role of the actin and microtubule cytoskeleton. Traffic 2001; 2(3):149-59.
170. Cordonnier MN, Dauzonne D, Louvard D et al. Actin filaments and Myosin I alpha cooperate with microtubules for the movement of lysosomes. Mol Biol Cell 2001; 12(12):4013-29.
171. Zhu Q, Clarke M. Association of calmodulin and an unconventional myosin with the contractile vacuole complex of Dictyostelium discoideum. J Cell Biol 1992; 118(2):347-58.
172. D'Andrea L, Danon MA, Sgourdas GP et al. Identification of coelomocyte unconventional myosin and its association with in vivo particle/vesicle motility. J Cell Sci 1994; 107(Pt 8):2081-94.
173. Hill KL, Catlett NL, Weisman LS. Actin and myosin function in directed vacuole movement during cell division in Saccharomyces cerevisiae. J Cell Biol 1996; 135(6 Pt 1):1535-49.
174. Sturmer K, Baumann O. Immunolocalization of a putative unconventional myosin on the surface of motile mitochondria in locust photoreceptors. Cell Tissue Res 1998; 292(2):219-27.
175. Krendel M, Sgourdas G, Bonder EM. Disassembly of actin filaments leads to increased rate and frequency of mitochondrial movement along microtubules. Cell Motil Cytoskeleton 1998; 40(4):368-78.
176. Wu X, Hammer 3rd JA. Making sense of melanosome dynamics in mouse melanocytes. Pigment Cell Res 2000; 13(4):241-7.
177. Titus MA. A class VII unconventional myosin is required for phagocytosis. Curr Biol 1999; 9(22):1297-303.
178. Ong LL, Lim AP, Er CP et al. Kinectin-kinesin binding domains and their effects on organelle motility. J Biol Chem 2000; 275(42):32854-60.
179. Mercer JA, Seperack PK, Strobel MC et al. Novel myosin heavy chain encoded by murine dilute coat colour locus. Nature 1991; 349(6311):709-13.
180. Provance Jr DW, Wei M, Ipe V et al. Cultured melanocytes from dilute mutant mice exhibit dendritic morphology and altered melanosome distribution. Proc Natl Acad Sci USA 1996; 93(25):14554-8.
181. Zhao LP, Koslovsky JS, Reinhard J et al. Cloning and characterization of myr 6, an unconventional myosin of the dilute/myosin-V family. Proc Natl Acad Sci USA 1996; 93(20):10826-31.
182. Wu X, Bowers B, Wei 3rd Q et al. Myosin V associates with melanosomes in mouse melanocytes: Evidence that myosin V is an organelle motor. J Cell Sci 1997; 110(Pt 7):847-59.
183. Wei Q, Wu X, Hammer 3rd JA. The predominant defect in dilute melanocytes is in melanosome distribution and not cell shape, supporting a role for myosin V in melanosome transport. J Muscle Res Cell Motil 1997; 18(5):517-27.
184. Westbroek W, Lambert J, Naeyaert JM. The dilute locus and Griscelli syndrome: Gateways towards a better understanding of melanosome transport. Pigment Cell Res 2001; 14(5):320-7.
185. Seabra MC, Mules EH, Hume AN. Rab GTPases, intracellular traffic and disease. Trends Mol Med 2002; 8(1):23-30.
186. Wilson SM, Yip R, Swing DA et al. A mutation in Rab27a causes the vesicle transport defects observed in ashen mice. Proc Natl Acad Sci USA 2000; 97(14):7933-8.
187. Haddad EK, Wu X, Hammer 3rd JA. Defective granule exocytosis in Rab27a-deficient lymphocytes from Ashen mice. J Cell Biol 2001; 152(4):835-42.
188. Stinchcombe JC, Barral DC, Mules EH et al. Rab27a is required for regulated secretion in cytotoxic T lymphocytes. J Cell Biol 2001; 152(4):825-34.
189. Hume AN, Collinson LM, Rapak A et al. Rab27a regulates the peripheral distribution of melanosomes in melanocytes. J Cell Biol 2001; 152(4):795-808.
190. Raposo G, Cordonnier MN, Tenza D et al. Association of myosin I alpha with endosomes and lysosomes in mammalian cells. Mol Biol Cell 1999; 10(5):1477-94.
191. Introne W, Boissy RE, Gahl WA. Clinical, molecular, and cell biological aspects of Chediak-Higashi syndrome. Mol Genet Metab 1999; 68(2):283-303.
192. Ward DM, Griffiths GM, Stinchcombe JC et al. Analysis of the lysosomal storage disease Chediak-Higashi syndrome. Traffic 2000; 1(11):816-22.
193. Huizing M, Anikster Y, Gahl WA. Hermansky-Pudlak syndrome and Chediak-Higashi syndrome: Disorders of vesicle formation and trafficking. Thromb Haemost 2001; 86(1):233-45.
194. Perou CM, Leslie JD, Green W et al. The Beige/Chediak-Higashi syndrome gene encodes a widely expressed cytosolic protein. J Biol Chem 1997; 272(47):29790-4.

Nucleogenesis

Sui Huang

Abstract

The vertebrate cell nucleus undergoes disassembly and reassembly at each cell division. Elaborate and well-regulated mechanisms ensure faithful and precise cellular duplication throughout this process. This chapter is intended to summarize our current understanding of nuclear biogenesis, or nucleogenesis, with a specific focus on nuclear envelope assembly and nucleolar reformation following mitosis.

Introduction

Eukaryotic cells are divided by a nuclear envelope into the nucleus and the cytoplasm. The nucleus contains chromosomal DNA that carries genetic information from one generation to the next and encodes the majority of products required for cell viability. In addition, the nucleus facilitates and regulates DNA replication, transcription, processing of RNA precursors, and transport of macromolecules across the nuclear envelope, which consists of lipid membranes and associated proteins. In addition to the nuclear envelope, the nucleus contains many nonmembrane bound structural domains that spatially and temporally organize various nuclear functions (for a review see ref. 1). For example, nucleoli, the most morphologically distinct of nuclear organelles, are involved in the synthesis of preribosomal particles.

Nuclei and their enclosed genetic material are highly dynamic in cycling cells. Chromosomes undergo replication and nuclei enlarge as cells transition from G1 to the G2 phase of the cell cycle (Fig. 1). Following G2 and upon entering mitosis, chromosomal DNA condenses followed by the disintegration of the nuclear envelope. During metaphase mitotic chromosomes are aligned on the metaphase plate and are segragated during anaphase on a microtubule-based spindle that pulls replicated chromosomes (i.e., sister chromatids) in opposite directions. At this point daughter cells, which are still attached to each other, reassemble their nuclear envelopes around their respective diploid sets of chromosomes. Daughter cells are subsequently separated from one another through a processes termed cytokenisis. The disassembly and reformation of nuclei during eukaryotic cell division are highly regulated process critical to ensuring faithful and precise cellular duplication.

The following review will describe recent findings and models for the post-mitotic biogenesis of the nucleus, with special emphasis on the nuclear envelope and nucleoli.

The Biogenesis of Cellular Organelles, edited by Chris Mullins. ©2005 Eurekah.com and Kluwer Academic/Plenum Publishers.

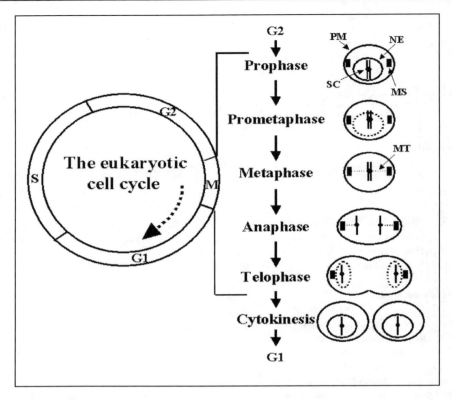

Figure 1. A schematic diagram of the eukaryotic cell cycle is presented. The respective phases of the eukaryotic cell cycle are indicated: mitosis (M), gap 1 (G1), synthesis (S) and gap 2 (G2). The relative amount of time spent by a typical eukaryotic cell in each phase is roughly equal to the depicted lengths of the respective phases. The hatched arrow represents the direction of the cycle. The individual stages of mitosis are listed to the right in temporal order. Respective cellular events of each mitotic stage and cytokinesis are depicted in the highly schematic model of a dividing cell. Only select events relevant to this discussion are shown and events/structures depicted may span more stages than indicated. See text for relevant references and discussion. PM= plasma membrane; NE= nuclear envelope; MS= mitotic spindle; SC= sister chromatids (separated chromosomes are also indicated); MT= microtubules. Disassembling (prometaphase) and reassembling (telophase) NEs are indicated by hatch marks

The Nuclear Envelope in Mitosis

Nuclear Envelope Disassembly and Assembly

The nuclear envelope is composed of a double membrane (outer and inner) riveted by nuclear pore complexes (NPCs). The outer membrane is the extension of endoplasmic reticulum (ER) membrane while the inner membrane is supported by an underlying nuclear lamina that consists of nuclear lamins, an intermediate filament network, and associated proteins. The proteinous lamina intimately associates with intranuclear components including chromosomes and the nuclear matrix, and may play important roles in DNA replication, transcription, and chromatin structure (for reviews see refs. 2-5).

When cells enter mitosis, cell cycle specific phosphorylation mediates the depolymerization of lamins and fragmentation of nuclear membrane structures, leading to the breakdown of the nuclear envelope at the end of prophase. There are two models for the disassembly of the nuclear envelope during mitosis (for a review see ref. 6). One, primarily based on electron microscopic observations, suggests that the nuclear membrane fragments and vesiculates at prophase forming vesicles that are distinct from ER networks. More recently, accumulating evidence from live cell and immunolocalization studies supports another model in which the fragmented nuclear membranes are absorbed into the network of ER membranes.[7,8] Although the physical forces behind nuclear envelope breakdown are not clear, two new studies suggest that microtubules, dynein and dynactin are involved in the tearing of the nuclear envelope.[9,10]

Nuclear envelope assembly has been extensively investigated using reconstitutions of nuclei in cell free extracts and observations from mammalian somatic cells. Studies using a cell free system with Xenopus egg extracts identified vesicles on the surface of sperm DNA around which nuclear envelopes form. Two types of membrane vesicles are classified by their ability to fuse in such a system, the nonfusogenic and fusogenic vesicles. These vesicles can be separated by differential centrifugation.[11,12] Nuclear reconstitution assays demonstrate that the nonfusogenic vesicles dock first onto condensed chromosomes followed by the fusogenic vesicles that associate with docked vesicles or the chromosome and facilate fusion with the nonfusogenic vesicles to form a complete nuclear membrane (Fig. 2).[11,13-16] Upon the formation of the nuclear membrane, nuclear pore complexes are then assembled in a stepwise manner.[17]

In mammalian cells, there is no clear evidence of vesicle docking and fusion during nuclear envelope assembly. Instead, immunolabeling and more recent live cell studies show that protein components of the nuclear envelope begin to dock onto condensed chromosomes at late anaphase and that the formation of a complete envelope is a sequential event extending into

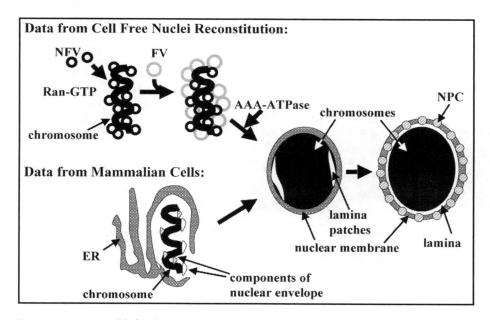

Figure 2. A current model of nuclear envelope assembly. Events of nuclear envelope assembly as derived from nuclear reconstitution and mammalian cellular studies are depicted in highly schematic model. See text for relevant references and discussion. NFV= nonfusogenic vesicles; FV= fusogenic vesicles; NPC= nuclear pore complex; ER= endoplasmic reticulum.

early G1 (Fig. 2) (for reviews see refs. 2,5,18,19). The earliest proteins associated with anaphase chromosomes prior to obvious chromosome decondensation are lamin B receptor (LBR), lamin associated protein 2B, emerin (a nuclear lamina protein), and NUP153 and p62 (NPC proteins).[8,20-23] While LBR and lamin associated protein 2B begin their association with the lateral sides of early telophase chromosomes, probably due to their inability to penetrate the spindles, NUP153 covers the entire chromosome surface. In comparison, emerin associates with the center portions of chromosomes on both sides (those facing the spindle and those facing the midbody). Subsequently, lamin B associates with the spindle side of the dividing chromosome, forming discontinuous patches.[22] During transit to G1, these polarized localizations to the chromosome surface eventually extend into a continuous encircling of the chromosome in parallel with the recruitment of nuclear membranes, NPC components, and other envelope proteins.

In contrast to the vesicle docking and fusion observed in cell free systems, the formation of a complete nuclear envelope membrane in cycling cells is thought to be the result of the extension of ER membranes that become associated with some of the nuclear envelope components already anchored onto chromosome.[7,8] Upon formation of the nuclear membrane, NPCs begin to assemble onto the membrane, in a stepwise manner that involves the recruitment of numerous proteins.[17,19,21,23,24] In vertebrates, the pore complex contains two known integral membrane proteins, POM 121 and gp210. POM121 associates with the developing envelope earlier than gp210 and thus may facilitate the membrane fusion step required for NPC formation.[23] A complete assembly of the nuclear lamina occurs in early G1 when lamin A becomes associated with the nuclear envelope.[22]

The Machinery Mediating Nuclear Envelope Dynamics

The mechanisms that initiate and facilitate nuclear envelope formation have been an active area of research. Recent studies have identified some of the key players involved in these processes using cell free nuclei reconstitution assays or genetic systems. This section will summarize the roles of three of these factors in nuclear envelope assembly: Ran, importin B, and lamin β.

The emerging picture of the biogenesis of the nucleus, a process referred to as nucleogenesis, suggests that Ran, a small GTPase protein, is essential for nuclear import and export, spindle formation during mitosis and the initiation of nuclear envelope assembly (for reviews see refs. 25-28). Similar to other related small GTPases, Ran has a low intrinsic GTPase activity and a slow nucleotide exchange rate. These activities are greatly enhanced in vivo by a nucleotide exchange factor (RCC1) and a GTPase activating factor (RanGAP).

In interphase (i.e., nondividing) cells, the nuclear Ran is predominantly in a GTP bound form and cytoplasmic Ran is in a GDP bound form. This differential distribution of Ran forms plays an important role in nuclear import and export processes (for reviews see refs. 29,30). Importins, which transport cargo into the nucleus through NPCs (see below), interact with Ran-GTP (converted from Ran-GDP by RCC1) in the nucleus. This interaction dislodges cargo from the importins (e.g., importin β). Subsequently, the Ran-GTP-importin β complex is exported out of the nucleus into the cytoplasm. Importin β then dissociates after RanGAP stimulates Ran to hydrolyze GTP to GDP, thus completing the cycle of nuclear import and export of the importins. The concentration gradient of Ran-GTP in the nucleus and Ran-GDP in the cytoplasm has been shown to be essential for nucleocytoplasmic trafficking. More recently, several groups have found that Ran-GTP is also required for mitotic spindle formation in a cell free system using Xenopus egg extracts.[31-35] Similar to nucleo-cytoplasmic trafficking, the Ran-GTP/Ran-GDP gradient appears to regulate nucleation of spindle microtubules and their association with chromosomes.[36-38]

In addition to its role in nucleo-cytoplasmic trafficking and spindle formation, a potential role for Ran in nuclear envelope assembly has been revealed in both cell free systems as well as in in vivo studies using genetic models.[38-41] Using Xenopus egg extracts, Zhang and Clarke[40] reconstituted a pseudonuclear envelope on Ran-GTP coated beads. This envelope contains many hallmark components of the nuclear envelope, including NPC proteins and a lipid bilayer, and is capable of facilitating the import and export of macromolecules. The depletion of Ran or RCC1, or the addition of Ran mutants that fail to undergo nucleotide exchange or GTP hydrolysis, block the nuclear envelope assembly, thus suggesting that active Ran-GTP ↔ Ran-GDP cycling is essential for nuclear envelope assembly.[31] More recently Zhang and Clarke[41] have demonstrated that the conversion of Ran-GDP to Ran-GTP by RCC1 in human mitotic cell extracts is necessary to recruit precursor vesicles while Ran-GTP hydrolysis is crucial for the vesicle fusions required to generate a complete envelope. Furthermore, RNA interference (RNAi) experiments in *Caenorhabditis elegans* demonstrate that depletion of Ran prevents nuclear envelope assembly in addition to inducing abnormalities in chromosome segregation during mitosis.[38] These findings demonstrate an essential requirement for Ran in nuclear envelope assembly in vivo.

To explore the potential mechanistic link between Ran and vesicle docking and fusion, Zhang et al[42] evaluated the role of importin β, a Ran effector protein,[28] in nuclear envelope assembly in Xenopus egg extracts. Importin β alone proved sufficient to restore nuclear envelope assembly in RanBP (Ran binding protein) depleted egg extracts. Furthermore, importin β coated beads are capable of inducing formation of a psudeonuclear envelope similar to those formed around the Ran coated beads. A mutant importin β, with decreased binding affinity for FxFG repeat-containing nucleoporins but not for other types of nucleoporins, fails to induce nuclear envelope formation. These findings suggest that the Ran-GTP generated by RCC1 on the chromatin surface may recruit importin β bound to FxFG nucleoporins and release the nucleoporins locally.[42] Ran-GTP may also directly interact with some nucleoporins.[43] Since importin β coated beads could recruit Ran-GTP, it remains to be clarified whether other components, probably in a small amounts, in addition to importin β could also be involved in Ran-GTP dependent nuclear envelope assembly. These findings indicate that importin β may act to recruit essential elements involved in nuclear envelope development when cells exit mitosis. Although investigations using cell free systems have significantly increased our understanding of the apparent roles that Ran plays in nuclear envelope assembly in vitro, much less is known regarding its involvement in post-mitotic nuclear assembly in mammalian cells, where the assembly does not appear to involve vesicle fusions.

Nuclear lamins, including lamins A/C and B, form a filamentous network on the inner surface of the nuclear envelope.[44] Lamins have been shown to be important for nuclear shape in mammalian cells. In addition to being localized to the nuclear envelope, lamins are also observed in the nucleoplasm as a veil or sometimes in foci.[22,45] Lamin B has been implicated in other nuclear functions, including DNA replication, transcription, and chromatin structure.[22,45-47] When cells exit mitosis, lamin B appears to associate with telophase chromosomes in patches early during nuclear envelope assembly, whereas lamin A/C does not become associated with the envelope until G1.[22]

A longstanding question in the field of nucleogenesis is whether lamins are necessary for nuclear envelope assembly. Several groups have addressed this question using cell free nuclear reconstitution assays. In some studies, immunodepletion of lamins prevents chromosome decondensation and nuclear envelope assembly,[48-52] while in other studies, the depletion results in smaller nuclei with fragile envelopes that do not have a lamina.[53,54] These studies, although controversial in regard to the need for lamins in the process of nuclear envelope assembly, do suggest that formation of the lamina layer is not required for envelope assembly.

More recent studies suggest that lamins, as functional intra-nuclear proteins rather than constituents of the lamina network, are important for nuclear envelope assembly. Lopez-Soler et al[55] evaluated nuclear envelope assembly in the presence of the carboxy-terminus of Xenopus lamin B3 (LB3T), a fragment that blocks the in vitro polymerization of lamin B3 beyond dimer formation. Here, the addition of LB3T to the Xenopus egg extracts inhibits sperm chromosome decondensation and the assembly of the nuclear envelope and NPCs. LB3T demonstrates such blocking activity only in the presence of the wild type LB3. Electron microscopic analyses show some association of membrane vesicles to the condensed chromosome surface but these vesicles fail to fuse. LB3T appears to block the fusogenic vesicles from associating with chromatin or the nonfusogenic vesicles by blocking lamin-lamin interactions, leading to inhibition of nuclear envelope assembly. These findings suggest that lamin-lamin interactions may be involved in facilitating the association of membrane vesicles to chromatin surfaces as lamins are present on both chromatin and in these vesicles.[55] The role of lamins in nuclear envelope assembly has also been addressed in vivo in genetic models. A mutation that significally reduces expression of Drosophila lamin DM0, the homologue of vertebrate lamin B, inhibits nuclear membrane assembly in flies.[56] Similarly, suppression of lamin expression in *C. elegans* using RNAi results in defects in DNA segregation and nuclear envelope assembly. However, in genetic studies it is difficult to interpret the specific roles of lamins in nuclear envelope assembly since the mutations affect other lamin functions as well.

The discoveries described above raise new questions and provide new approaches regarding nuclear envelope assembly. In addition to Ran, importin β, and lamins, recently Hetzer et al[57] found that an AAA-ATPase involved in Golgi and ER fusions plays important roles in mediating two types of nuclear membrane fusion, the enclosure of nuclear membrane around the chromosomes and subsequent nuclear envelope growth (Fig. 2). It is clear that nuclear envelope biogenesis is a rapidly evolving area of cell biology investigation.

Post-Mitotic Biogenesis of the Nucleolus

Nucleoli are characterized as nonmembrane bound, highly dense nuclear structures that function as sites of ribosome biosynthesis. Each cell contains hundreds of copies of ribosomal DNA (rDNA) in tandem repeats. Approximately 400 of these rDNA repeats are localized to five chromosome pairs in human cells. Clusters of such rDNA repeats are termed nucleolar organization regions (NORs) and active NORs are found within nucleoli. High-resolution electron microscopic studies demonstrate that an individual nucleolus contains three distinct and highly conserved substructural features, the fibrillar centers (FCs), dense fibrillar components (DFCs), and the granular components (GCs) (for reviews see refs. 58,59). FCs are pale fibrillar regions that are enriched in factors mediating RNA polymerase I (Pol I) specific transcription including Pol I itself, DNA topoisomerase I, and UBF (upstream binding factor). DFCs are highly electron dense fibrillar regions that partially or completely surround FCs. Each nucleolus can contain multiple FCs surrounded by DFCs. DFCs intensely label with antibodies that recognize select Pol I transcription factors and pre-rRNA processing factors, including fibrillarin, a component of all box C/D snoRNPs, complexes involved in preribosomal RNA processing, modification, and/or assembly. GCs represent granular regions outside of FCs and DFCs and constitute the rest of the nucleolus. GCs are enriched with assembly factors, including B23, and ribosomal proteins. Studies using pulse-chase labeling, in situ hybridization to prerRNAs, and immunolabeling of trans-acting factors involved in ribosome biogenesis suggest a vectorial process by which pre-rRNAs migrate from fibrillar regions to granular regions and subsequently into the nucleoplasm during maturation into preribosomal particles (for reviews see refs. 60, 61). More recently, nucleoli have been implicated in numerous other functions, including transcriptional silencing, cellular aging, cell cycle control, and intranuclear trafficking.[62-65]

Nucleoli are distorted and disassembled at prophase and prometaphase and reassemble in daughter cell nuclei at early G1. Although structurally disassembled, some of the nucleolar components, particularly the RNA polymerase I transcription apparatus, remain associated with the NORs that are transcriptionally active in interphase cells. This association is maintained throughout mitosis in spite of the transcriptional silencing of the rDNA during this period.[66-69]

In late telophase, the NORs recruit nucleolar components to reassemble nucleoli. The reformation of nucleoli following mitosis (i.e., in G1) is so precisely regulated that daughter cell nucleoli are often mirror images of each other with regards to their position, shape, size, and numbers.[70] At least two mechanisms are involved in biogenesis of nucleoli (i.e., nucleologenesis). Fusions of NORs probably take place during nucleolar assembly, as the number of nucleoli per cell (one to four) is often less than the number of NORs (10 for a diploid human cell). However, the mechanism and participants involved in NOR fusion are entirely unknown. Secondarily, there is a growth in the size of nucleoli during early G1 through a continuous recruitment of nucleolar components (for reviews see refs. 63,71).

Early studies attribute the growth of nucleoli during early G1 to the fusion of structures termed prenucleolar bodies (PNBs) with NORs.[72-75] PNBs are electron dense fibril-granular structures found in the nucleoplasm and contain pre-rRNA processing factors and preribosome assembly factors.[72,73] Pol I specific transcription factors are not detectable in the PNBs. There are two types of PNBs, fibrillarin-containing (early appearing) and B23-containing (late appearing).[76-78] Since they gradually disappear in parallel with the growth of nucleoli, it was once speculated that PNBs might fuse with the early nucleoli to form typical nucleoli in late G1. However, recent live-cell studies demonstrate that PNBs do not directly fuse with growing nucleoli. Instead, prerRNA processing factors appear to be delivered to nascent nucleoli by directional funneling from PNBs.[78] The formation of PNBs is controlled by the cell cycle specific CDK1 (cyclin-dependent kinase 1) activities while the flow of pre-rRNA processing factors towards the growing nucleoli is controlled by an unidentified CDK.[79] Together, these results demonstrate that PNB formation plays an important role in nucleologenesis at early G1.

A fascinating question in nucleologenesis is whether transcriptional activation of Pol I at the end of mitosis contributes to the assembly and growth of nucleoli. Several studies have attempted to address this question. Using a yeast rDNA deletion mutant, Oakes et al[80] has shown that the transcription of rDNA by Pol I from a plasmid induces multiple small dense structures (termed "mininucleoli") while transcription of rDNA by Pol II forms a larger, aggregated structure. In addition, insertion of actively transcribing rDNA repeats into Drosophila polytene chromosomes results in dense mininucleoli around the sites of transcription.[81] However, these dense structures do not resemble the typical nucleoli with their three distinct substructures. More recently, Verheggen et al[82] showed that during Xenopus embryogenesis maternal pre-rRNAs are present in nucleolin (a pre-rRNA processing and preribosomal particle assembly factor)-enriched structures with features of nucleoli prior to detectable Pol I transcription. This suggests that active Pol I transcription is not required for nucleolar formation. Furthermore, nucleoli can form even upon selective inhibition of Pol I transcription, although the nucleoli are smaller and exhibit a distorted structure similar to that found in interphase cells treated with pol I transcription inhibitors.[73,83-85] These findings suggest that atypical nucleoli can assemble in the absence of rDNA transcription. However, normal architecture and growth of nucleoli requires transcription activation of pol I.

Concluding Remarks

During exit from mitosis a highly precise and regulated organization and assembly of daughter cell nuclei ensures that parental nuclear morphologies are maintained in the new daughter cells.[70] Our current understanding of this process, although growing rapidly, is still very limited. There are many questions concerning nuclear biogenesis that remain to be addressed. For example, what is involved in ensuring the fidelity of sister chromatin segregation? What signals the initiation of nuclear envelope assembly? What triggers the cell cycle related events upon exiting mitosis, such as chromosome decondesation? How does chromosome decondensation relate to nuclear envelope assembly? What determines the morphological similarity between the daughter cell nuclei? What triggers the cell cycle specific regulation and controls? These and many other questions represent exciting and intriguing areas of cell biology that await further investigation.

Acknowledgements

My thanks go to Drs. Steve Adam, Robert Moir, Tim Spann, Rajesh Kamath, Daniel Leary, and Barry Feldman for their helpful discussion and critical reading during the manuscript preparation.

References

1. Spector DL. Nuclear domains. J Cell Sci 2001; 114(Pt 16):2891-3.
2. Goldman RD, Gruenbaum Y, Moir RD et al. Nuclear lamins: Building blocks of nuclear architecture. Genes Dev 2002; 16(5):533-47.
3. Moir RD, Spann TP. The structure and function of nuclear lamins: Implications for disease. Cell Mol Life Sci 2001; 58(12-13):1748-57.
4. Gant TM, Wilson KL. Nuclear assembly. Annu Rev Cell Dev Biol 1997; 13:669-95.
5. Holaska JM, Wilson KL, Mansharamani M. The nuclear envelope, lamins and nuclear assembly. Curr Opin Cell Biol 2002; 14(3):357-64.
6. Collas I, Courvalin JC. Sorting nuclear membrane proteins at mitosis. Trends Cell Biol 2000; 10(1):5-8.
7. Ellenberg J, Siggia ED, Moreira JE et al. Nuclear membrane dynamics and reassembly in living cells: Targeting of an inner nuclear membrane protein in interphase and mitosis. J Cell Biol 1997; 138(6):1193-206.
8. Yang L, Guan T, Gerace L. Integral membrane proteins of the nuclear envelope are dispersed throughout the endoplasmic reticulum during mitosis. J Cell Biol 1997; 137(6):1199-210.
9. Salina D, Bodoor K, Eckley DM et al. Cytoplasmic dynein as a facilitator of nuclear envelope breakdown. Cell 2002; 108(1):97-107.
10. Beaudouin J, Gerlich D, Daigle N et al. Nuclear envelope breakdown proceeds by microtubule-induced tearing of the lamina. Cell 2002; 108(1):83-96.
11. Vigers GP, Lohka MJ. A distinct vesicle population targets membranes and pore complexes to the nuclear envelope in Xenopus eggs. J Cell Biol 1991; 112(4):545-56.
12. Lourim D, Krohne G. Membrane-associated lamins in Xenopus egg extracts: Identification of two vesicle populations. J Cell Biol 1993; 123(3):501-12.
13. Sullivan KM, Busa WB, Wilson KL. Calcium mobilization is required for nuclear vesicle fusion in vitro: Implications for membrane traffic and IP3 receptor function. Cell 1993; 73(7):1411-22.
14. Newport J, Dunphy W. Characterization of the membrane binding and fusion events during nuclear envelope assembly using purified components. J Cell Biol 1992; 116(2):295-306.
15. Boman AL, Delannoy MR, Wilson KL. GTP hydrolysis is required for vesicle fusion during nuclear envelope assembly in vitro. J Cell Biol 1992; 116(2):281-94.
16. Drummond S, Ferrigno P, Lyon C et al. Temporal differences in the appearance of NEP-B78 and an LBR-like protein during Xenopus nuclear envelope reassembly reflect the ordered recruitment of functionally discrete vesicle types. J Cell Biol 1999; 144(2):225-40.

17. Macaulay C, Forbes DJ. Assembly of the nuclear pore: Biochemically distinct steps revealed with NEM, GTP gamma S, and BAPTA. J Cell Biol 1996; 132(1-2):5-20.
18. Buendia B, Courvalin JC, Collas P. Dynamics of the nuclear envelope at mitosis and during apoptosis. Cell Mol Life Sci 2001; 58(12-13):1781-9.
19. Vasu SK, Forbes DJ. Nuclear pores and nuclear assembly. Curr Opin Cell Biol 2001; 13(3):363-75.
20. Chaudhary N, Courvalin JC. Stepwise reassembly of the nuclear envelope at the end of mitosis. J Cell Biol 1993; 122(2):295-306.
21. Haraguchi T, Koujin T, Hayakawa T et al. Live fluorescence imaging reveals early recruitment of emerin, LBR, RanBP2, and Nup153 to reforming functional nuclear envelopes. J Cell Sci 2000; 113(Pt 5):779-94.
22. Moir RD, Yoon M, Khuon S et al. Nuclear lamins A and B1: Different pathways ofassembly during nuclear envelope formation in living cells. J Cell Biol 2000; 151(6):1155-68.
23. Bodoor K, Shaikh S, Salina D et al. Sequential recruitment of NPC proteins to the nuclear periphery at the end of mitosis. J Cell Sci 1999; 112(Pt 13):2253-64.
24. Goldberg MW, Wiese C, Allen TD et al. Dimples, pores, star-rings, and thin rings on growing nuclear envelopes: Evidence for structural intermediates in nuclear pore complex assembly. J Cell Sci 1997; 110(Pt 4):409-20.
25. Kuersten S, Ohno M, Mattaj IW. Nucleocytoplasmic transport: Ran, beta and beyond. Trends Cell Biol 2001; 11(12):497-503.
26. Macara IG. Transport into and out of the nucleus. Microbiol Mol Biol Rev 2001; 65(4):570-94.
27. Macara IG. Why FRET about Ran? Dev Cell 2002; 2(4):379-80.
28. Dasso M. Running on Ran: Nuclear transport and the mitotic spindle. Cell 2001; 104(3):321-4.
29. Gorlich D, Kutay U. Transport between the cell nucleus and the cytoplasm. Annu Rev Cell Dev Biol 1999; 15:607-60.
30. Mattaj IW, Englmeier L. Nucleocytoplasmic transport: The soluble phase. Annu Rev Biochem 1998; 67:265-306.
31. Kalab P, Pu RT, Dasso M. The ran GTPase regulates mitotic spindle assembly. Curr Biol 1999; 9(9):481-4.
32. Ohba T, Nakamura M, Nishitani H et al. Self-organization of microtubule astersinduced in Xenopus egg extracts by GTP-bound Ran. Science 1999; 284(5418):1356-8.
33. Wilde A, Zheng Y. Stimulation of microtubule aster formation and spindle assembly by the small GTPase Ran. Science 1999; 284(5418):1359-62.
34. Zhang C, Hughes M, Clarke PR. Ran-GTP stabilises microtubule asters and inhibits nuclear assembly in Xenopus egg extracts. J Cell Sci 1999; 112(Pt 14):2453-61.
35. Carazo-Salas RE, Guarguaglini G, Gruss OJ et al. Generation of GTP-bound Ran by RCC1 is required for chromatin-induced mitotic spindle formation. Nature 1999; 400(6740):178-81.
36. Carazo-Salas RE, Gruss OJ, Mattaj IW et al. Ran-GTP coordinates regulation of microtubule nucleation and dynamics during mitotic-spindle assembly. Nat Cell Biol 2001; 3(3):228-34.
37. Wilde A, Lizarraga SB, Zhang L et al. Ran stimulates spindle assembly by altering microtubule dynamics and the balance of motor activities. Nat Cell Biol 2001; 3(3):221-7.
38. Bamba C, Bobinnec Y, Fukuda M et al. The GTPase Ran Regulates Chromosome Positioning and Nuclear Envelope Assembly In Vivo. Curr Biol 2002; 12(6):503-7.
39. Hetzer M, Bilbao-Cortes D, Walther TC et al. GTP hydrolysis by Ran is required for nuclear envelope assembly. Mol Cell 2000; 5(6):1013-24.
40. Zhang C, Clarke PR. Chromatin-independent nuclear envelope assembly induced by Ran GTPase in Xenopus egg extracts. Science 2000; 288(5470):1429-32.
41. Zhang C, Clarke PR. Roles of Ran-GTP and Ran-GDP in precursor vesicle recruitment and fusion during nuclear envelope assembly in a human cell-free system. Curr Biol 2001; 11(3):208-12.
42. Zhang C, Hutchins JR, Muhlhausser P et al. Role of Importin-beta in the Control of Nuclear Envelope Assembly by Ran. Curr Biol 2002; 12(6):498-502.
43. Yokoyama N, Hayashi N, Seki T et al. A giant nucleopore protein that binds Ran/TC4. Nature 1995; 376(6536):184-8.
44. Aebi U, Cohn J, Buhle L et al. The nuclear lamina is a meshwork of intermediate-type filaments. Nature 1986; 323(6088):560-4.

45. Spann TP, Moir RD, Goldman AE et al. Disruption of nuclear lamin organization alters the distribution of replication factors and inhibits DNA synthesis. J Cell Biol 1997; 136(6):1201-12.
46. Moir RD, Spann TP, Herrmann H et al. Disruption of nuclear lamin organization blocks the elongation phase of DNA replication. J Cell Biol 2000; 149(6):1179-92.
47. Spann TP, Goldman AE, Wang C et al. Alteration of nuclear lamin organization inhibits RNA polymerase II- dependent transcription. J Cell Biol 2002; 156(4):603-8.
48. Dabauvalle MC, Loos K, Merkert H et al. Spontaneous assembly of pore complex-containing membranes ("annulate lamellae") in Xenopus egg extract in the absence of chromatin. J Cell Biol 1991; 112(6):1073-82.
49. Burke B, Gerace L. A cell free system to study reassembly of the nuclear envelope at the end of mitosis. Cell 1986; 44(4):639-52.
50. Ulitzur N, Gruenbaum Y. Nuclear envelope assembly around sperm chromatin in cell-free preparations from Drosophila embryos. FEBS Lett 1989; 259(1):113-6.
51. Ulitzur N, Harel A, Feinstein N et al. Lamin activity is essential for nuclear envelope assembly in a Drosophila embryo cell-free extract. J Cell Biol 1992; 119(1):17-25.
52. Ulitzur N, Harel A, Goldberg M et al. Nuclear membrane vesicle targeting to chromatin in a Drosophila embryo cell-free system. Mol Biol Cell 1997; 8(8):1439-48.
53. Newport JW, Wilson KL, Dunphy WG. A lamin-independent pathway for nuclear envelope assembly. J Cell Biol 1990; 111(6 Pt 1):2247-59.
54. Meier J, Campbell KH, Ford CC et al. The role of lamin LIII in nuclear assembly and DNA replication, in cell- free extracts of Xenopus eggs. J Cell Sci 1991; 98(Pt 3):271-9.
55. Lopez-Soler RI, Moir RD, Spann TP et al. A role for nuclear lamins in nuclear envelope assembly. J Cell Biol 2001; 154(1):61-70.
56. Lenz-Bohme B, Wismar J, Fuchs S et al. Insertional mutation of the Drosophila nuclear lamin Dm0 gene results in defective nuclear envelopes, clustering of nuclear pore complexes, and accumulation of annulate lamellae. J Cell Biol 1997; 137(5):1001-16.
57. Hetzer M, Meyer HH, Walther TC et al. Distinct AAA-ATPase p97 complexes function in discrete steps of nuclear assembly. Nat Cell Biol 2001; 3(12):1086-91.
58. Busch H, Smetana K. The nucleolus New York: Academic Press, 1970.
59. Hadjiolov AA. The nucleolus and ribosome biogenesis. Cell Biology Monographs New York: Springer-Verlag, 1985:1-263.
60. Scheer U, Hock R. Structure and function of the nucleolus. Curr Opin Cell Biol 1999; 11(3):385-90.
61. Shaw PJ, Jordan EG. The nucleolus. Annu Rev Cell Dev Biol 1995; 11:93-121.
62. Carmo-Fonseca M, Mendes-Soares L, Campos I. To be or not to be in the nucleolus. Nat Cell Biol 2000; 2(6):E107-12.
63. Garcia SN, Pillus L. Net results of nucleolar dynamics. Cell 1999; 97(7):825-8.
64. Pederson T. The plurifunctional nucleolus. Nucleic Acids Research 1998; 26(17):3871-6.
65. Johnson FB, Marciniak RA, Guarente L. Telomeres, the nucleolus and aging. Curr Opin Cell Biol 1998; 10(3):332-8.
66. Scheer U, Rose KM. Localization of RNA polymerase I in interphase cells and mitotic chromosomes by light and electron microscopic immuncytochemistry. Proc Natl Acad Sci USA 1984; 81:1431-35.
67. Roussel P, Andre C, Masson C et al. Localization of the RNA polymerase I transcription factor hUBF during the cell cycle. J Cell Sci 1993; 104(Pt 2):327-37.
68. Gebrane-Younes J, Fomproix N, Hernandez-Verdun D. When rDNA transcription is arrested during mitosis, UBF is still associated with noncondensed rDNA. Journal of Cell Science 1997; 110(Pt 19):2429-40.
69. Grummt I. Regulation of mammalian ribosomal gene transcription by RNA polymerase I. Prog Nucleic Acid Res Mol Biol 1999; 62:109-54.
70. Locke M, Leung H. The pairing of nucleolar patterns in an epithelium as evidence for a conserved nuclear skeleton. Tissue & Cell 1985; 17:573-88.
71. Hernandez-Verdun D, Roussel P, Gebrane-Younes J. Emerging concepts of nucleolar assembly. J Cell Sci 2002; 115(Pt 11):2265-70.

72. Jimenez-Garcia LF, Segura-Valdez ML, Ochs RL et al. Nucleologenesis: U3 snRNA-containing prenucleolar bodies move to sites of active prerRNA transcription after mitosis. Mol Biol Cell 1994; 5(9):955-66.

73. Ochs RL, Lischwe MA, Shen E et al. Nucleologenesis: Composition and fate of prenucleolar bodies. Chromosoma 1985; 92(5):330-6.

74. Benavente R. Postmitotic nuclear reorganization events analyzed in living cells. Chromosoma 1991; 100(4):215-20.

75. Bell P, Dabauvalle MC, Scheer U. In vitro assembly of prenucleolar bodies in Xenopus egg extract. J Cell Biol 1992; 118(6):1297-304.

76. Verheggen C, Almouzni G, Hernandez-Verdun D. The ribosomal RNA processing machinery is recruited to the nucleolar domain before RNA polymerase I during Xenopus laevis development. J Cell Biol 2000; 149(2):293-306.

77. Fomproix N, Gebrane-Younes J, Hernandez-Verdun D. Effects of anti-fibrillarin antibodies on building of functional nucleoli at the end of mitosis. J Cell Sci 1998; 111(Pt 3):359-72.

78. Savino TM, Gebrane-Younes J, De Mey J et al. Nucleolar assembly of the rRNA processing machinery in living cells. J Cell Biol 2001; 153(5):1097-110.

79. Sirri V, Hernandez-Verdun D, Roussel P. Cyclin-dependent kinases govern formation and maintenance of the nucleolus. J Cell Biol 2002; 156(6):969-81.

80. Oakes M, Aris JP, Brockenbrough JS et al. Nomura M. Mutational analysis of the structure and localization of the nucleolus in the yeast Saccharomyces cerevisiae. J Cell Biol 1998; 143(1):23-34.

81. Karpen GH, Schaefer JE, Laird CD. A Drosophila rRNA gene located in euchromatin is active in transcription and nucleolus formation. Genes & Dev 1988; 2(12B):1745-63.

82. Verheggen C, Le Panse S, Almouzni G et al. Presence of prerRNAs before activation of polymerase I transcription in the building process of nucleoli during early development of Xenopus laevis. J Cell Biol 1998; 142(5):1167-80.

83. Dousset T, Wang C, Verheggen C et al. Initiation of nucleolar assembly is independent of RNA polymerase I transcription. Mol Biol Cell 2000; 11(8):2705-17.

84. Benavente R, Rose KM, Reimer G et al. Inhibition of nucleolar reformation after microinjection of antibodies to RNA polymerase I into mitotic cells. J Cell Biol 1987; 105(4):1483-91.

85. Weisenberger D, Scheer U, Benavente R. The DNA topoisomerase I inhibitor camptothecin blocks postmitotic reformation of nucleoli in mammalian cells. Euro J Cell Biol 1993; 61(1):189-92.

86. Wiese C, Goldberg MW, Allen TD et al. Nuclear envelope assembly in Xenopus extracts visualized by scanning EM reveals a transport-dependent 'envelope smoothing' event. J Cell Sci 1997; 110(Pt 13):1489-502.

CHAPTER 8

Mitochondrial Biogenesis

Danielle Leuenberger, Sean P. Curran and Carla M. Koehler

Abstract

The mitochondrion is especially complex and interesting because of its prokaryotic origins and subsequent integration into the eukaryotic cell and establishment as an essential organelle. As a result of this evolutionary history, the mitochondrion is a mix of "old and new" biology. For example, this organelle has maintained its own small genome that codes for a handful of inner membrane proteins and utilizes a prokaryotic-like system for transcription and translation. In addition, novel pathways for mitochondrial biogenesis and movement within the cell have evolved concurrently with its endosymbiosis. The importance of this unique organelle to cellular physiology is obvious from the broad spectrum of human diseases arising from defects in mitochondrial energy production, ion homeostasis, and morphology. The molecular mechanisms of mitochondrial biogenesis and protein import and export, as well as metal ion transport, are being dissected at a rapid pace and are the subjects of the following review.

Introduction

In cytological studies performed over 100 years ago, Altman first described mitochondria and noted that they were similar in size and shape to bacteria.[1] These early observations proved insightful as the resolving power of the electron microscope later revealed the mitochondrion is a two-membrane organelle that contains its own small genome, thus resembling a bacterium. In the first half the 19th century, the role of the mitochondrion in energy production was characterized. Additional details on the origin and function of mitochondria and the history of mitochondrial research can be found in the various reviews cited throughout this chapter, as well as in several books.[2-4]

Critical questions of recent interest in mitochondrial biology focus on the biogenesis and maintenance of the organelle. For example, in the past twenty years, the basic mechanisms of mitochondrial fission, fusion, and division and mitochondrial protein import and export have and continue to be subjects of key interest. Investigations into topics of mitochondrial biogenesis and maintenance have been aided by studies of the mitochondrial system of the budding yeast *Saccharomyces cerevisiae*. These molecular and genetic studies have also yielded greater insights into the relationship between mitochondrial dysfunction and disease in humans. It is now clear that the processes by which mitochondria are formed are highly conserved between eukaryotic cells. Indeed, most of the differences found so far are not fundamental but variations on a common theme.

The Biogenesis of Cellular Organelles, edited by Chris Mullins. ©2005 Eurekah.com and Kluwer Academic/Plenum Publishers.

Because it maintains its own small genome and has two functionally distinct membranes, the mitochondrion is one of the most complex and unique organelles in nonphotosynthetic cells. Mitochondria biogenesis occurs through growth and division of preexisting organelles. Processes mediating mitochondrial import and export, fission, and fusion are thus requisite for the biogenesis and maintenance of this organelle. In *S. cerevisiae*, which is able to grow anaerobically, the genes required for mitochondrial respiration and the mitochondrial genome itself are not essential for viability. However, genes coding for protein import and iron-sulfur cluster assembly components are essential,[5-7] thus confirming that biogenesis of the mitochondrion can not be achieved de novo.

The mitochondrial outer and inner membranes are functionally distinct and, as a result, the membranes differ in their lipid and protein complements. The outer membrane contains metabolic enzymes, particularly those for phospholipid biosynthesis, and the protein porin, which forms a pore that allows passage of proteins less than 6 kDa and small molecules between the cytosol and mitochondrial intermembrane space. The outer membrane also contains components involved in mitochondrial movement and the TOM (translocase of the outer membrane) complex, through which imported proteins and RNAs pass from the cytosol. The lipids of the outer membrane are predominantly phospholipids, and have a content similar to that of microsomes. The inner membrane is the "industrial site" of the mitochondrion and is comprised of 50% protein. In density gradients, the heavier inner membrane can be separated from the more buoyant outer membrane. The protein complexes in the inner membrane are involved in oxidative phosphorylation, transport, protein translocation and assembly, and protein turnover. The lipid content of the membrane is comprised of phospholipids and cardiolipin, which may play an integral role in the stability of the inner membrane protein complexes.[8]

Mitochondrial Dynamics

Current topics in mitochondrial biogenesis being characterized at the molecular level include mitochondrial division and movement within the cell.[9-11] When mitochondria are observed using electron microscopy they appear as "sausage-shaped" organelles with several copies per cell. In vivo, however, mitochondria form a highly mobile tubular network that spans the entire cell. The shape of this reticulum is characterized by a series of fusion and fission events. This network has to maintain a high motility to relocalize within the cell to meet the current energy requirements. Examples occur during spermatogenesis in insects where the mitochondria fuse to form two separate organelles that wrap around the base of the flagellum and during division in *S. cerevisiae* where the mitochondrial network fragments and a subset of the organelles travel through the mother-bud neck and into the daughter cell. The combination of yeast genetics and visual observation with green fluorescent protein and confocal microscopy in *Caenorhabditis elegans*, *Drosophila melanogaster*, *S. cerevisiae*, and *Schizosaccharomyces pombe* have advanced this field rapidly in the past five years. Our current knowledge of mitochondrial fusion, fission, and movement during inheritance are summarized in the following sections.

Mitochondrial Fusion

The first molecular regulator of mitochondrial fusion, *fuzzy onions* or Fzo1p, was identified in *D. melanogaster*, where it regulated mitochondrial fusion during spermatogenesis (Fig. 1).[12] Fzo1p is a GTPase with one transmembrane domain that localizes to the mitochondrial outer membrane and faces into the cytosol.[12] From studies with yeast mutants, loss of Fzo1p results in rapid fragmentation of mitochondrial tubules and in failure of mitochondria to fuse when two haploid yeast cells are mated.[13] A novel outer mitochondrial membrane protein,

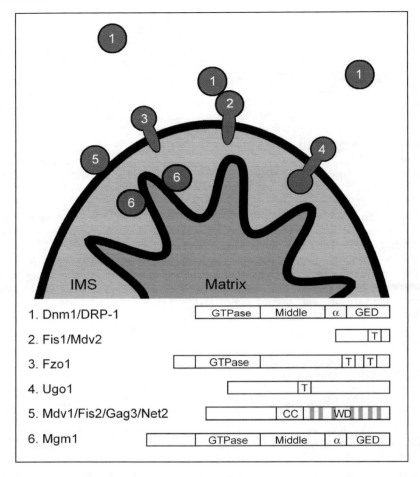

Figure 1. Location of components mediating mitochondrial dynamics. The cytosolic Dnm1 protein (role in mitochondrial fission) may bind to the outer membrane protein Fis1, which is a potential nucleation point for fission components. Mdv1 is associated with the mitochondrial outer membrane and most likely is a fission component. Mdv1 colocalizes with Dnm1 but partner proteins have not been identified by biochemical methods. Fzo1 and Ugo1 are involved in mitochondrial fusion but biochemical methods have not shown that these proteins are partners. Mgm1 is associated with the mitochondrial inner membrane, most likely in the intermembrane space, and mediates fission. Conserved domains among the components have been marked: GTPase= GTPase domain; Middle= domain shared by Dnm1 and Mgm1; α= alpha-helical region; GED= GTPase effector domain; T= transmembrane domain; CC= coiled coil motif; WD= WD-40 repeats.

Ugo1p, has recently been identified as a regulator of mitochondrial fusion.[14] The 58-kDa Ugo1p resides in the outer membrane and contains one membrane spanning domain near the middle of the protein that localizes the amino-terminus to the cytosol and the carboxy-terminus to the intermembrane space. Fzo1p and Ugo1p do not partner in a larger complex,[14] but further studies are clearly needed to determine their role in mitochondrial fusion and if they are part of a fusion machinery.

Mitochondrial Fission

There has been more progress towards understanding the mechanism of mitochondrial division than for fusion. Much of this progress has been seen since the discovery that mutations in the dynamin-related protein, Dnm1p/DRP-1 (in yeast and *C. elegans* respectively), block mitochondrial fission and result in the formation of elaborate "net-like" structures.[15,16] The dynamin protein family has a well-established role in membrane fission and vesicle release during endocytosis.[17] However, Dnm1p/DRP-1 is a cytosolic protein with no membrane-spanning domains, so it is not initially apparent how it could associate with the mitochondria (Fig. 1). This suggests additional components of the fission machinery must exist. Several such factors recently identified are discussed below.

The dynamin GTPase Mgm1p is a second fission machinery component and contains a mitochondrial targeting signal.[18] Though its sub-mitochondrial localization is under debate, Mgm1p appears to be localized largely to the intermembrane space.[19-21] Alternatively, it might associate with different compartments during different stages of fission. When Mgm1p function in yeast is impaired, mitochondrial tubules rapidly fragment and the mitochondrial DNA is subsequently lost.[20,21] Genetic studies in yeast have also identified Fis1p/Mdv2p and Mdv1p/Fis2p/Gag3p/Net2p that assist the Dnm1p/DRP-1 GTPase with mitochondrial fission. Fis1p spans the mitochondrial outer membrane and might serve as a nucleation point for the fission complex.[22,23] Mdv1p has only been identified in *S. cerevisiae* and also is a soluble protein, but colocalizes with Dnm1p in punctate structures on the mitochondrial outer membrane.[22-25]

Based on molecular and cellular studies from many laboratories, a molecular model for mitochondrial division is developing that may involve processes similar to those seen in endocytosis at the cell surface. During endocytosis in mammalian cells, homotetramers of dynamin assemble into collars around the necks of clathrin-coated pits at the plasma membrane.[17] GTP hydrolysis catalyzed by dynamin is required for the efficient "pinching" or fission and release of clathrin-coated vesicles. The dynamin-related GTPases Mgm1p and Dnm1p/DRP-1 might operate on the mitochondrial inner and outer membranes, respectively, via a similar mechanism. Indeed, Dnm1p/DPR-1 assembles to form rings in vitro, suggesting that dynamin family members might form rings around mitochondrial membranes in vivo.[26] Fis1p might serve as a scaffold or nucleation site on the outer membrane and Mdv1p may assist Dnm1p/DRP-1.

Mitochondrial Movement During Inheritance

Mitochondria move through the cell with the help of the cytoskeleton.[10,27] In higher eukaryotes, mitochondria are transported along microtubules to synapses or growth cones in neurons.[28] In the dividing yeast cell, mitochondria must be transferred from the mother to the bud. This directional transport is obtained with motor proteins and mitochondrial-specific kinesin proteins in higher eukaryotes.[29,30] In contrast, mitochondria in budding yeast are tethered to the actin cytoskeleton.[31] Genetic screens for yeast mutants with abnormal mitochondrial distribution identified a series of cytoskeletal elements, mitochondrial attachment proteins, and regulatory proteins involved in mitochondrial movement.[10,27] Cytoskeletal elements important for maintaining mitochondrial movement include actin, tropomyosin, and the Arp2/3 complex, which plays a role in actin nucleation.[32,33] A cytosolic protein, Mdm20p, maintains the integrity of actin cables,[34] while Mdm1p is an intermediate filament-like protein that may act as a cytoskeletal scaffold.[35] On the mitochondrial outer membrane, the proteins Mmm1p, Mdm10p, and Mdm12p may coordinate attachment to the actin cytoskeleton.[36-38]

The temporal coordination of cell cycle events with the distribution of mitochondria into the bud in *S. cerevisiae* suggests tightly controlled regulation. While little is known about this aspect of mitochondrial inheritance, two mechanisms might be involved. Regulation may be mediated in part through phosphorylation because mitochondrial inheritance, but not morphology, is lost in a mutant carrying a deletion of the *PTC1* gene, which codes a serine/threonine phosphatase.[39] Ptc1p is a negative regulator of the high-osmolarity glycerol response pathway, a MAP kinase cascade. Rsp5p, an ubiquitin-protein ligase, suppresses a *mdm1* mutation, suggesting ubiquitination acts as a second regulatory mechanism.[40,41] Mutations in *RSP5* result in small, round mitochondria, and defects in mitochondrial distribution and transfer into the bud.[40] The ubiquitin degradation pathway thus may regulate mitochondrial inheritance. In support of this observation, cells with defective ubiquitin conjugating enzymes, Ubc4p and Ubc5p, also show specific mitochondrial aggregation.

Along with transmission of mitochondria, the mitochondrial genome must be inherited faithfully. The mitochondrial genome is tethered to the mitochondrial inner membrane via a DNA-protein complex termed the nucleoid, which is the segregating unit of the genome.[42] The fission protein Mmm1p may play a role in mitochondrial DNA segregation.[43] Although Mmm1p is an outer membrane protein, Mmm1p tagged with green fluorescent protein localizes to small, punctate structures, adjacent to a subset of matrix-localized nucleoids. In an *mmm1* mutant, nucleoid structure also collapse in concurrence with a defect in mitochondrial DNA transmission.

Mitochondrial Protein Import

Correct assembly of the mitochondrion is an essential process to insure that protein complexes, requisite for energy production and metabolism, function as expected. The mitochondria therefore has developed an elaborate apparatus to accommodate the import of nuclear-coded proteins and export/assembly of mitochondrial-coded proteins. The mitochondrion contains approximately 1000 proteins. Of these mitochondrial proteins, approximately 3 to 32,[44] depending on the organism, are encoded by the mitochondrial genome. The remainder are encoded by the nuclear genome and are translated in the cytosol and imported into mitochondria to one of four locations: the outer membrane, the intermembrane space, the inner membrane, or the matrix (Fig. 2). Precursor proteins destined for the mitochondrion thus contain targeting as well as fine sorting information, while the mitochondrion has developed an elaborate translocation machinery that mediates selective protein transport. The mitochondrial translocation machinery includes the TOM (translocase of the outer membrane) complex, which mediates protein translocation across the outer membrane and insertion of outer membrane proteins. The inner membrane contains the TIM23 (translocase of inner membrane) complex for the translocation of proteins residing predominantly in the matrix and intermembrane space and the TIM22 complex for translocation of many inner membrane proteins (the nomenclature of the mitochondrial protein transport systems has been unified such that proteins are named Tom or Tim corresponding to translocase of outer membrane and inner membrane, respectively, followed by the number indicating the component's molecular weight[45]). Assembly of protein translocation complexes is mediated by processing peptidases that remove targeting sequences and a battery of chaperones that guide protein folding. In addition, a protein surveillance system is present to regulate the assembly and degradation of mitochondrial protein complexes.

The vast majority of mitochondrial proteins are imported post-translationally from the cytosol. This requires that proteins are maintained in an import-competent state by chaperones during transport to their final destinations.[46-48] Most soluble proteins of the matrix and some proteins of the inner membrane and intermembrane space have an amino-terminal extension of 20-50 amino acid residues, with a range of 10-80 residues, which is generally cleaved after import. Other precursors do not contain an amino-terminal targeting sequence; rather the targeting information resides within the mature protein. This group includes outer membrane proteins, and some intermembrane space and inner membrane proteins.

Regardless of the targeting sequence, all precursors are recognized by receptors of the outer membrane TOM complex and then pass through the TOM channel. This translocation requires that the precursors must be at least partially unfolded. After crossing the outer membrane, precursors are directed to either the TIM23 or TIM22 machinery of the inner membrane (Fig. 2). Proteins containing an amino-terminal presequence are imported via the TIM23 complex,[49] which forms a tightly regulated channel across the inner membrane. The membrane potential ($\Delta\Psi$) across the inner membrane is requisite for translocation across the inner membrane,[50] while an ATP-dependent translocation motor drives import to completion.[51-53] Mitochondrial heat shock protein 70 (mHsp70) serves as such a molecular motor. The matrix contains a mitochondrial processing peptidase (MPP) that cleaves the presequence,[54] and the protein folds into its active form, possibly with the assistance of chaperones such as mHsp70, Hsp60, and Hsp10.[51,55] Proteins destined for the inner membrane such as the metabolic carriers and import components are directed through the aqueous intermembrane space by the small Tim proteins to the TIM22 complex.[56-58] The TIM22 complex mediates insertion of mitochondrial proteins typically lacking a cleavable targeting presequence into the inner membrane in a $\Delta\Psi$ dependent manner.

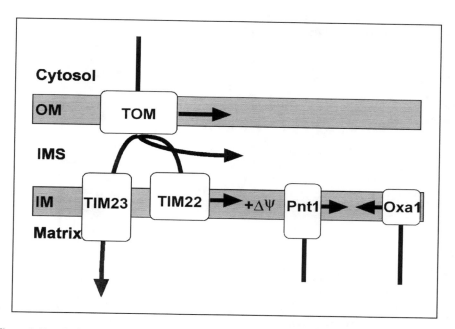

Figure 2. Protein import and export pathways in the mitochondrion. Cytosolic proteins are imported through the translocase of the outer membrane (TOM) and then, depending upon their destination, remain in the outer membrane (OM), remain in the intermembrane space (IMS), or engage the translocases of the inner membrane (TIM). Precursors with a typical amino-terminal targeting sequence generally utilize the TIM23 complex, whereas proteins that reside in the inner membrane (IM), often lacking a targeting sequence, utilize the TIM22 complex. Mitochondrial encoded proteins may be exported to the inner membrane from the matrix via Oxa1p and Pnt1p. Pathways are depicted schematically by arrows. The membrane potential is depicted by $\Delta\Psi$ symbols. See text for additional details and relevant references.

The TOM Translocase of the Outer Mitochondrial Membrane

Whether a precursor protein has been released from the ribosome, or remains in the process of translation, the precursor interacts with the receptors of the TOM complex to initiate translocation across the mitochondrial outer membrane (Fig. 3). There are eight subunits of the TOM complex in *S. cerevisiae* (Fig. 3).[59] Receptors include Tom20p and Tom22p, which are highly conserved in fungi and animals, and Tom70p and Tom37p.[60] The translocation channel consists of Tom40p and the small Tom proteins, Tom5p, Tom6p, and Tom7p.[61,62] The stable Tom core complex is approximately 400 kDa.[59] In yeast, the pore-forming Tom40p and multifunctional receptor Tom22p are essential for viability.

Tom20p preferentially binds to precursors with amino-terminal presequences and then passes the precursor to Tom22p. Tom20p consists of a soluble cytosolic domain that is anchored to the membrane by an amino-terminal transmembrane domain. The cytosolic domain contains a single tetratricopeptide repeat motif, a 34-residue motif implicated in protein-protein interactions,[63] and specifically binds to mitochondrial precursors.[64] Initial NMR structural studies have revealed the interaction between Tom20p and the presequence.[65] Tom20p con-

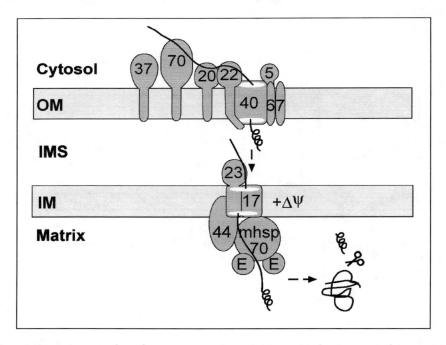

Figure 3. Protein import pathway for precursor proteins containing a typical amino-terminal presequence. This pathway is mediated by the Tim17p/Tim23p complex and an associated ATP-driven protein transport motor on the inner face of the inner membrane (IM). As a precursor with an amino-terminal basic matrix-targeting signal (depicted as helical line) emerges from the TOM complex (consisting of Tom5, 6, 7, 20, 22, 37, 40 and 70 proteins) in the outer membrane (OM), it binds to an acidic Tim23p domain in the intermembrane space (IMS) and thereby induces transient docking of the TOM and Tim17p/Tim23p systems. In the presence of a membrane potential $\Delta\Psi$, the presequence passes through the IM. The ATP-drive translocation motor consisting of mitochondrial Hsp70 (mHsp70p), the nucleotide exchange factor mitochondrial GrpE (E) and the membrane anchor Tim44p drives translocation to completion. In the matrix, the matrix processing protease (represented as scissors) removes the matrix-targeting sequence and a battery of matrix chaperones may aid in folding to generate the mature protein. See text for additional details and relevant references.

tains four α-helices that form a stable structure with a shallow hydrophobic groove flanked by hydrophilic residues at the periphery. The presequence peptide is bound to Tom20p in a α-helical structure, with the hydrophobic amino acids sitting in the groove and the hydrophilic residues oriented to the aqueous solvent.

In contrast, Tom70p preferentially binds to the β-subunit of the F_1-ATPase; precursors with internal targeting sequences, such as members of the mitochondrial carrier family, through hydrophobic interactions; and cytosolic chaperones.[66] Like Tom20p, Tom70p contains a large cytosolic domain with tetratricopeptide repeats, anchored to the membrane by an amino-terminal transmembrane domain.[66] Several Tom70p dimers bind simultaneously to one carrier protein, potentially preventing aggregation before subsequent passage to Tom22p.[67,68] Yeast mitochondria also have a related protein, Tom72p. Although its specific role has not been defined, Tom72p may mediate interactions between mitochondria and the cytoskeleton.[69,70]

Tom22p is a multifunctional organizer of the TOM complex. Tom22p is essential for viability. However, a yeast mutant lacking Tom22p exhibits slow growth,[61] thus helping to confirm Tom22p plays diverse functions in vivo. Tom22p contains domains on both sides of the outer membrane, with the amino-terminus forming a large cytosolic domain and the carboxy-terminus forming a small domain in the intermembrane space.[71] Both domains are negatively-charged and mediate the import of precursors through the TOM complex. In fact, Tom22p serves as a convergence point for precursors that initially bind to either Tom20p or Tom70p.[71,72] The Tom22p transmembrane domain maintains association between the individual Tom40 channels. Tom22p also seems to regulate the gating activity of the Tom 40p channels.[61]

Tom37p was originally identified in a screen for yeast mutants defective in phospholipid biosynthesis.[73] Subsequent biochemical and genetic studies indicate that Tom37p associates with Tom70p and deletion of *TOM37* results in decreased in vitro import of a set of precursors that are preferentially imported via Tom70p.[73] However, Tom37p was recently shown to exhibit characteristics of a peripheral membrane protein, thus its specific role in protein import remains to be defined.[72] The human Tom37p homolog metaxin has similar properties to the yeast protein. Metaxin was identified serendipitously because of its chromosomal location between thrombospondin 3 and glucocerebrosidase.[74] Overexpression of metaxin in mammalian cells decreased the import of preproteins, suggesting it may function as a receptor.[75] Metaxin however is not a central component of the Tom complex, but does form a complex with a related cytosolic protein metaxin 2.[76] The early embryonic lethal phenotype of mice lacking metaxin demonstrates that efficient import of proteins into mitochondria is critical for development and the identification of metaxin 2 indicates that the import pathway in mammalian systems may be more complex than fungi.

Functions of TOM Pore Proteins

Tom40p is the core component of the TOM complex and is essential for viability in yeast. Tom40p is a β-barrel protein containing eight membrane-spanning domains and probably forms a dimer. Recently, Tom40p was reconstituted in lipid vesicles and shown to be a cationic-specific channel.[77] In another major achievement, the TOM complex was purified from *Neurospora crassa* mitochondria using a hexahistidine-tagged Tom22p.[62] Electron microscopy and image reconstruction experiments reveals that the complex is 138 Å wide and contains up to two pores with an internal diameter of 20 Å. The purified TOM complex was reconstituted into lipid vesicles and shown to be both voltage-gated and cation-selective.[78] The current model of TOM structure proposes that a single channel is formed by two Tom40p molecules and that a complete TOM complex contains two to three such channels.[60,78] In addition to forming the pore, Tom40p contains binding sites for mitochondrial precursor proteins.

The TOM pore also contains three small Tom proteins, Tom5p, Tom6p, and Tom7p. Tom5p acts as a receptor for the small Tim proteins of the intermembrane space.[79] Tom6p and Tom7p are involved with TOM complex assembly and disassembly.[80] Tom6p also promotes assembly of Tom22p with Tom40p. In contrast, Tom7p mediates dissociation and thereby a lateral release of precursors into the outer membrane. Sorting of outer membrane proteins, such as porin, is strongly inhibited in mitochondria lacking Tom7p.[80,81]

All this begs a question as to how proteins pass through the TOM complex. Other than the release of precursors from cytosolic chaperones, an ATP requirement has not been shown. Instead, the "acid chain hypothesis" predicts that increased affinity for negatively-charged domains on the receptors on the outer membrane and then the inner membrane, followed by Tim23p in the intermembrane space, may serve as a driving force for import.[82,83] However, hydrophobic interactions are also important in precursor recognition,[84] suggesting that a combination of binding interactions facilitates transport across the outer membrane.

The TIM23 Import Pathway

The mitochondrial inner membrane has various translocons to mediate protein import. Precursors with an amino-terminal targeting presequence follow the "general import pathway" (Fig. 3); their import is mediated by the Tim17p/Tim23p complex (designated TIM23) and the translocation motor consisting of Tim44p, mitochondrial hsp70, and the nucleotide exchange factor mitochondrial GrpE.[46-48] This translocation is dependent upon the presence of a membrane potential ($\Delta\Psi$) and generally requires ATP hydrolysis by mhsp70 on the matrix side for unidirectional translocation. The TIM23 complex acts independently of the TOM complex although the two can be reversibly asssociated while a precuror is in transit.[85] During transient association, the super TOM-TIM23 complex is approximately 600 kDa.[86] All components of the TIM23 translocase are essential for viability in *S. cerevisiae*. The TIM23 complex of the inner membrane thus is a complicated machine with broad similarities to the *Sec* machinery of bacteria and the eukaryotic endoplasmic reticulum (ER).

In contrast to the outer membrane, the inner membrane is necessarily ion impermeable. The TIM channels must therefore be highly regulated during opening to prevent ion leakage and to accommodate a peptide chain in transit. The TIM23 channel of the inner membrane is comprised of two related proteins, Tim17p and Tim23p. The size of this channel is approximately 22 Å as shown by studies of mitochondrial precursor proteins tagged with different sized particles.[87] Both Tim17p and Tim23p are essential for viability in yeast. While Tim17p functions only in channel formation, Tim23p is a multifunctional protein, similar to Tom22p. Tim17p and Tim23p have four putative membrane spanning domains, and Tim23p contains a negatively-charged domain in the intermembrane space that recognizes precursors taking the general import route. Tim23p has been proposed to form a dimer in the presence of a membrane potential such that the import channel is assembled.[88] Binding of the Tim23p intermembrane space domain to the precursor then triggers dimer dissociation, allowing the precursor to pass through the import channel. Another intriguing observation is that the amino-terminal domain of Tim23p inserts into the outer membrane and tethers both inner and outer membranes.[89] However, specific binding to the TOM complex has not been identified so the relevance to protein import is not clear.

Initiation of translocation across the inner membrane depends on the membrane potential $\Delta\Psi$, which is negative on the matrix side. The positively-charged presequence of precursor proteins passes across the inner membrane because of the electrophoretic effect of the membrane potential.[90] For the completion of translocation, the matrix-sided components, Tim44p, mHsp70, and mGrpE function as the ATP-dependent translocation motor.[51] Tim44p is stably associated with the inner membrane but is mainly exposed at the matrix side. mHsp70 has three domains: an amino-terminal ATPase domain, a central peptide-binding domain, and a shorter carboxy-terminal segment.[91,92] The interaction with Tim44p is dependent on the mhsp70 ATPase domain and is stabilized by the other two mHsp70 domains.[93] After the initial $\Delta\Psi$-driven translocation of the amino-terminal targeting sequence, mHsp70 is required for the translocation of the remainder of the precursor across the inner membrane.[94,95] The cochaperone mGrpE is a matrix protein homologous to the nucleotide exchange factor GrpE of bacteria.[51,96] mGrpE interacts with mHsp70 bound to a precursor and promotes the reaction cycle of mHsp70, thereby allowing nucleotide release.[97]

After translocation into the matrix, the imported proteins fold into their active conformations. The diverse nature of the imported proteins is reflected by the array of folding mediators, including mHsp70, the Hsp60-Hsp10 system, and the peptidyl-prolyl cis/trans isomerases (PPIases). Different precursors have different requirements for assistance in protein folding.[55] Mitochondrial Hsp70 cooperates with cochaperone Mdj1, the homolog of bacterial DnaJ, to mediate folding in the matrix.[51,97] The Hsp60-Hsp10 system is homologous to the prokaryotic GroEL-GroES complex. Hsp60 promotes productive folding of proteins by enclosing them in a central cavity that is covered by Hsp10.[98] The mode of action of Hsp60 is based on detailed analysis of the bacterial system.[99] Interestingly, Hsp60 deficiency was observed in fibroblasts from a patient with mitochondrial encephalomyopathy,[100] and it was proposed to be the primary cause of mitochondrial dysfunction, however, no gene defect has been identified.[101] PPIases catalyze the cis/trans isomerization of peptide bonds preceding a prolyl residue.[102] This isomerization is slow in the absence of PPIases and is a rate-limiting step in protein folding. The mitochondrial PPIase can bind to the immunosuppressive drug cyclosporin A and is hence termed cyclophilin 20 (corresponding to its apparent molecular weight).[103,104]

Additional proteins in this TIM machinery have been identified, but their specific role in protein import has not been determined. Tim11p was identified because of its intimate association with the Tim23p channel.[105] A cytochrome b_2 arrested translocation intermediate and a cross-linker with a short spacer arm cross-link Tim11p with very high specificity. Further studies revealed Tim11p as the γ-subunit of ATP synthase and imply it acts as an ATPase assembly factor.[106] Studies by Endo and colleagues, based on the presence of site-specific crosslinks with a mitochondrial precursor with a classical targeting sequence, have identified other proteins that also might play a role in import.[107] Of these, a 50 kDa protein is identified as a potential new import component.[107]

The TIM22 Import Pathway

Many inner membrane proteins lack a cleavable targeting sequence, carrying instead their targeting and sorting information within the "mature" part of the polypeptide chain. This category of proteins includes at least 34 members of the yeast mitochondrial carrier family,[108] which span the inner membrane six times, as well as the TIM components. The mechanism by which inner membrane proteins cross the hydrophilic intermembrane space and insert correctly into the inner membrane has been recently elucidated along with a new protein import pathway (designated TIM22) that acts specifically on these proteins (Fig. 4).[56-58,109-111] Components in this pathway are located both in the mitochondrial intermembrane space and inner membrane.

A family of small proteins in the mitochondrial intermembrane space mediates import of inner membrane proteins across the intermembrane space.[56,57,109-111] Five proteins, Tim8p, Tim9p, Tim10p, Tim12p, and Tim13p have been identified in the yeast intermembrane space. Similar complements are also found in other metazoans. The amino acid sequences of the small Tim proteins are 25% identical and 50% similar to each other. They also share a "twin CX₃C" motif, in which two cysteine residues are separated by three amino acids and each cysteine

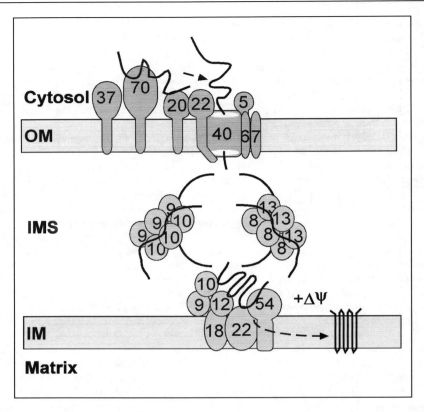

Figure 4. Import of membrane proteins into the mitochondrial inner membrane. As the precursor protein emerges from the TOM complex (consisting of Tom5, 6, 7, 20, 22, 37, 40 and 70 proteins), it binds to the Tim9p-Tim10p or Tim8p-Tim13p complexes of the intermembrane space (IMS). The bound precursor is then usually delivered to an insertion complex composed of Tim9p, Tim10p, Tim12p, Tim18p, Tim22p and Tim54p that catalyzes the membrane potential ($\Delta\Psi$)-dependent insertion of the precursor into the inner membrane. OM, outer membrane; IM, inner membrane. See text for additional details and relevant references.

block is separated from the other by 11-16 amino acids.[110] This motif is reminiscent of a canonical zinc finger, but with a longer spacer. Recombinant Tim10p and Tim12p fusion proteins bind zinc, suggesting that the small Tim proteins bind zinc in vivo and that zinc binding is required for their function.

Tim10p and Tim12p were the first two components of the intermembrane space shown to mediate protein import.[56,57] Fractionation of yeast mitochondria demonstrates that most of Tim10p is located in the soluble intermembrane space while Tim12p is peripherally bound to the outer surface of the inner membrane. Both proteins could be cross-linked chemically to a partially imported AAC precursor, indicating that they interact directly with the imported protein. However, the different intramitochondrial locations of Tim10p and Tim12p reflect their different functions in the import pathway. Inactivation or depletion of Tim12p does not interfere with import of AAC into the intermembrane space, but prevents insertion of AAC into the inner membrane. In contrast, inactivation or depletion of Tim10p blocks import of AAC, P_iC and Tim22p across the outer membrane. Thus, Tim10p functions before Tim12p, probably by binding the incoming precursor as it emerges from the TOM complex.

Through genetic and biochemical approaches Tim9p was shown to functionally associate with Tim10p.[109,111] Tim9p is primarily localized to the mitochondrial intermembrane space with Tim10p in a soluble 70 kDa complex;[109,111] the remainder is present in the 300 kDa insertion complex. The other two yeast proteins related to Tim10p and Tim12p, Tim8p and Tim13p,[110] are found in the intermembrane space as a distinct 70 kDa complex that can be separated from the Tim9p-Tim10p complex by ion exchange chromatography.[110] Deletion of Tim8p or Tim13p, alone or in combination, has no notable effect on cell growth and does not significantly affect import of AAC or P_iC into isolated mitochondria. Studies with a broader spectrum of precursor proteins in yeast strains lacking Tim8p or Tim13p reveal that Tim8p-Tim13p complex mediates import of Tim23p into mitochondria.[112-114] Thus the Tim8p-Tim13p complex most likely works in parallel with the Tim9p-Tim10p complex by mediating the import of a subset of integral inner membrane proteins.

The specific route taken by substrates to reach the inner membrane is still uncertain. One possibility is that the small Tim complexes act as chaperone-like molecules to guide the precursors across the aqueous intermembrane space, yielding a soluble intermediate in which the precursor is bound to the 70 kDa complexes in the intermembrane space. This model is supported by import studies in yeast strains containing temperaturesensitive *tim10* and *tim12* mutations, and by the fact that an AAC translocation intermediate bound to Tim10p in intact mitochondria is protected from added protease.[57,109] It predicts a transient complex in which Tim9p-Tim10p or Tim8p-Tim13p is bound directly to the precursor. Equally plausible is a model in which the 70 kDa complexes form a link between the TOM and the TIM complexes. In this model, the precursor is not released into the intermembrane space, but binds to the small Tim proteins as it emerges from the TOM complex. Further transfer to the Tim22p-Tim54p complex could then occur without release into the intermembrane space. This model is supported by the recent finding that an AAC translocation intermediate is partially degraded by added protease.[115] It predicts a transient complex in which TOM and the small Tim proteins bind the precursor.

Tim22p, an essential inner membrane protein, was the first component of the inner membrane complex identified, based on homology to Tim17p and Tim23p.[116] Surprisingly, depletion of Tim22p did not affect the general import pathway but inhibited the insertion of inner membrane proteins, particularly those of the carrier family. A second component, Tim54p, was identified through a two hybrid interaction with the mitochondrial outer membrane protein Mmm1p.[58] Subsequent analysis revealed that Tim54p is an integral inner membrane protein and partners with Tim22p. Inactivation of Tim54p in a temperaturesensitive *tim54* mutant inhibits import of AAC into isolated mitochondria.[58] Tim18p was recently identified through its genetic interactions with a temperaturesensitive *tim54* mutant[117] and through coimmunoprecipitation with Tim54p.[118] Tim18 is an integral inner membrane protein that is 40% identical to Sdh4p, the membrane anchor of succinate dehydrogenase.[119] Tim18p, Tim22p, and Tim54p with the tiny Tim proteins of the intermembrane space form a 300 kDa complex. While a direct role in protein import has not been established, Tim18p may regulate assembly of the 300 kDa complex as depletion of Tim18p yields a functional complex of 250 kDa.[117,118]

Novel Type of Mitochondrial Disease Marked by Defective Protein Import

Humans contain at least six homologs of the small Tim proteins found in the yeast mitochondrial intermembrane space. One of these homologs is termed deafness-dystonia peptide (DDP1) because its loss results in the severe X-linked Mohr-Tranebjaerg syndrome, characterized by deafness, dystonia, muscle weakness, dementia and blindness.[120,121] DDP1 is most similar to yeast Tim8p and, when expressed in monkey or yeast cells, is localized to mitochondria.[110] Mohr-Tranebjaerg syndrome is thus almost certainly a new type of mitochondrial disease caused by a defective protein import system of mitochondria. Loss of DDP1 function probably lowers the abundance of some inner membrane proteins that are critical for the function, development or maintenance of the sensorineural system in mammals. The findings in yeast suggest that DDP1functions as a complex with related partner proteins, perhaps including hTim13.

Mitochondrial Protein Export

Recent studies of protein export pathways for mitochondrially-coded proteins have revealed new membrane components. While the topology of mitochondrial export resembles that of bacterial secretion, yeast lacks a detectable homolog to the bacterial *Sec* translocase.[122] However, at least two pathways have been identified for protein export from the matrix to the inner membrane (Fig. 1). Oxa1p is a nuclear-coded inner membrane protein that mediates export of amino- and carboxy-tails of the mitochondrially-coded precursor protein cytochrome c oxidase subunit II (Cox2p) and also plays a role in ATP synthase formation.[123,124] Oxa1p interacts directly with nascent mitochondrially synthesized polypeptides.[124] However, its precise role in membrane insertion is not clear as *oxa1* mutants are suppressed by mutations in the nuclear gene coding for the cytochrome c_1 subunit of the *bc1* complex,[123] thus suggesting the conserved Oxa1p function can be bypassed in the membrane insertion process. Interestingly, Oxa1p has homologs in bacteria, YidC,[125] and chloroplasts, termed ALB3 in *Arabidopsis thaliana*.[126] YidC is essential for bacterial viability and mediates the membrane insertion of Sec-independent proteins,[125] while ALB3 is an essential protein mediating integration of the light harvesting chlorophyll-binding protein into thylakoid membranes.[126] Recently, a second protein Mba1p with overlapping functions has been identified that functions independently of Oxa1p. Mba1p also mediates the export of mitochondrial translation products and nuclear-coded proteins that are conservatively sorted.[127]

Additional factors are also required for the export of the carboxy-terminus of Cox2p. Pnt1p was first identified in an elegant genetic screen to identify yeast mutants defective for the export of mitochondrially-coded proteins.[128] Pnt1p is an integral inner membrane protein facing into the mitochondria matrix. However, its precise role in export has not been determined because deletion of *PNT1* in *S. cerevisiae* does not impair Cox2p processing.[128] Two additional proteins Cox18p and Mss1p were identified that interact genetically and associate with Pnt1p to facilitate export of the Cox2p carboxy-terminus.[129]

The Protein Surveillance System of the Mitochondrion

Mitochondrial biogenesis and maintenance depend on a complex proteolytic system. Components include the processing peptidases in the matrix and intermembrane space and the ATP-dependent proteases in the inner membrane and matrix. In contrast to the protein import components, the proteolytic system is highly conserved, including homology with prokaryotic proteases. In yeast, the proteolytic system operates predominantly during starvation conditions for the nonselective degradation of mitochondrial proteins, but also is important for assembly of protein complexes and for presequence cleavage.[130,131] Mitochondrial peptidases are divided into three groups: processing peptidases, oligopeptidases, and ATP-dependent proteases.

Processing peptidases are present in the mitochondrial matrix and intermembrane space for the cleavage of the presequence of nascent polypeptides. The mitochondrial processing peptidase (MPP) is located in the matrix and is responsible for the first processing step removal of the presequence.[132] This heterodimeric Zn^{2+}-metallopeptidase consists of two subunits, α- and β-MPP, and is essential for viability in yeast.[132] The α-MPP subunit recognizes and binds to the presequence followed by cleavage via the β-MPP subunit.[133] Maturation of some matrix and intermembrane space proteins depends on a second processing step. A subset of matrix proteins undergoes an additional processing step by the mitochondrial intermediate peptidase

(MIP).[134] After MPP cleavage, MIP cleaves amino-terminal octapeptides from some matrix proteins, including iron-utilizing proteins and components of the electron transport chain, the tricarboxylic acid cycle and the mitochondrial genetic machinery.[135,136] The physiological relevance of MIP processing remains to be elucidated. The intermembrane space contains the inner membrane protease (IMP),[137] which is homologous to eubacterial and eukaryotic signal peptidases.[138] IMP is composed of two related subunits with nonoverlapping substrate specificities; both subunits are integral membrane proteins and expose their catalytic sites to the intermembrane space.[139] After processing in the matrix by MPP, IMP cleaves off the remainder of the bipartite signal sequence from proteins such as cytochrome b_2 and cytochrome c_1.

In contrast to the specific proteolytic events mediated by the above described processing peptidases, ATP-dependent proteases mediate the complete turnover of mitochondrial proteins. These proteases are located in the matrix and the inner membrane and have evolved from prokaryotic ancestors.[131,140] Interestingly, these proteases have two functions, they degrade nonassembled and misfolded polypeptides and act as chaperones to mediate the assembly of protein complexes that are crucial for mitochondrial function.[131,140] The matrix proteases are the Lon/Pim1 protease and the Clp-like proteases. Substrates of Lon include nonassembled polypeptides, subunits of the F_1F_0-ATP synthase, and ribosomal proteins.[141,142] Yeast mitochondria lacking the Lon protease accumulate inclusion bodies that most likely contain aggregated proteins and accumulate extensive mutations in mitochondrial DNA. The Lon protease has been shown to bind single-stranded DNA in a site-specific manner suggesting that Lon might play a direct role in mitochondrial DNA metabolism.[143] A role for the Lon protein in cell stress pathways has been shown recently because Lon expression was enhanced by hypoxia or ER stress, and in vivo by brain ischemia. These observations suggest that changes in nuclear gene expression triggered by ER stress have the potential to alter mitochondrial processes such as the assembly and/or degradation of inner membrane complexes. The Clp proteases have been identified in mammalian mitochondria but are absent in lower eukaryotes, including yeast.[144] The Clp proteases form hetero-oligomeric complexes with the ATPase and proteolytic subunits; and these complexes can unfold misfolded polypeptides allowing either refolding by other chaperone systems, or if associated with the proteolytic subunit, their degradation.[145]

The inner membrane is rich in proteins and has its own quality control system that consists of two ATP-dependent proteases, termed AAA proteases (for ATPases associated with a variety of cellular activities).[146-148] AAA proteases expose their catalytic sites to opposite membrane surfaces, specifically the intermembrane space or matrix side for the i- and m-AAA proteases, respectively. In both the i- and m-AAA proteases, the proteolytic domain is present at the carboxy-terminus while the amino-terminus anchors the protease to the membrane. Mutant yeast strains lacking the i-AAA protease lose respiratory competence at elevated temperature and accumulate mitochondria with a punctate, nonreticulated morphology.[149-151] Turnover of mitochondria by the vacuole is increased resulting in an increased rate of mitochondrial DNA escape.[149] The only identified substrate of the i-AAA is a subunit of cytochrome oxidase, though others likely exist.[149] In yeast, the m-AAA protease is composed of two subunits, Yta10p (Afg3p) and Yta12p (Rca1p).[152,153] Substrates consist of nonassembled subunits of the respiratory complexes and of the F_1F_0-ATP synthase.[154,155] The m-AAA protease is, therefore, essential for the maintenance of oxidative phosphorylation. Two orthologs of yeast m-AAA protease subunits have been identified in humans.[156] Mutation in one, paraplegin, causes an autosomal recessive form of hereditary spastic paraplegia.[156] Deficiencies in oxidative phosphorylation were observed in these cells, similar to defects observed in yeast.

What is the fate of the degraded mitochondrial proteins? Proteolysis of nonassembled mitochondrially-coded proteins by AAA proteases results in the formation of a heterogeneous array of peptides and free amino acids within the mitochondria.[157] The degraded products are exported from the mitochondrial matrix by a mitochondrial ABC (ATP-binding cassette) transporter, Mdl1p, to the intermembrane space.[158] Mdl1p is similar to the transporter associated with antigen presentation in higher eukaryotic cells, which transports peptides into the lumen of the endoplasmic reticulum.[159] The degraded products then exit to the cytosol by passive diffusion, via porin or possibly the TOM complex. The physiological role of peptide export is not known. Peptides derived from mitochondrially coded membrane proteins have been detected at the cell surface of mammalian cells, where they are presented by class I MHC molecules. It has been postulated that the mitochondrially coded minor histocompatability antigens are generated by AAA proteases in the mitochondria and then released to the cytosol, from where they enter the conventional class I antigen presentation pathway.[160] Alternatively, the exported peptides may be involved in signaling pathways between the mitochondrion and the nucleus.[161]

Metal Ion Transport

One of the most recent topics to unfold in the studies of mitochondrial function and maintenance is that of the pathways for metal ion trafficking, particularly for copper and iron. Studies in mammalian systems as well as *S. cerevisiae* have been important for identifying components of this trafficking machinery. Moreover, defects in metal ion trafficking have been linked to a broad spectrum of human diseases. The mitochondrion is the key site for the assembly of iron-sulfur (Fe/S) clusters, and copper is an essential component of cytochrome oxidase (Fig. 5).

Copper is required in mitochondrial respiration because it is a component of cytochrome oxidase.[162] The mechanism by which copper ions are inserted into the enzyme, however, is not known, though two proteins involved in copper utilization have been identified among the collection of assembly factors. These are Cox17p, a soluble protein that acts as a metallochaperone,[163] and Sco1p, a mitochondrial inner membrane protein that mediates insertion of copper into cytochrome oxidase.[164] The observed genetic interaction between the *SCO1* and *COX17* genes in *S. cerevisiae* suggests that the two proteins function in a common pathway.[164] Cox17p is a small protein with six cysteines that are highly conserved among eukaryotes.[165] Yeast Cox17p localizes to the cytosol and intermembrane space and, thus, most likely shuttles copper to the mitochondria.[163] At the inner membrane, Sco1p, which faces the intermembrane space, mediates the transfer the copper from Cox17p to Cox2p.[164] The molecular basis for the transfer is not known but two mechanisms have been hypothesized. Because Sco1p shares similarity with Cox2p, including two conserved copper-binding cysteinyl ligands, Sco1p may transfer copper directly.[164,166] Alternatively, Sco1p is homologous to disulfide reductases and may reduce the cysteine residues (copper ligands) as a prerequisite for copper binding.[167] Mutations in Sco1p have been identified in a patient presenting hepatic failure and encephalopathy as a result of a cytochrome oxidase deficiency.[168] Humans and yeast also contain *SCO2* that is homologous to *SCO1*, though its specific role in cytochrome oxidase assembly is not known.[162] However, mutations in *SCO2* have been identified in patients presenting early fatal encephalomyopathy associated with cytochrome oxidase deficiencies, with the most severe occurring in highly aerobic tissues such as muscle and heart.[169] Sco2p thus seems to play a role in cytochrome oxidase assembly.

Recently, a role for copper has been shown in the mitochondrial intermembrane space because the Cu,Zn-superoxide dismutase (Sod1p) and its copper chaperone CCS (Lys7p in *S. cerevisiae*) localize to the intermembrane space in addition to the cytosol.[170] Sod1p and Sod2p (the mitochondrial Mn-superoxide dismutase in the matrix) protect the cell from reactive oxygen species by catalyzing the disproportionation of superoxide to hydrogen peroxide and water. Defects in Sod1p have been linked to amyotrophic lateral sclerosis (ALS), a fatal, adult-onset neurodegenerative disease.[171,172] Various mitochondrial pathologies have been associated with

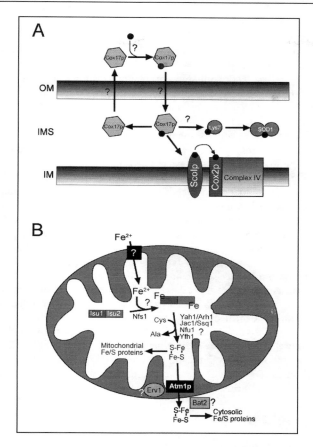

Figure 5. Hypothetical models for metal ion transport in the mitochondrion of S. cerevisiae. A) Cox17p translocates Cu^{2+} from the cytosol to the mitochondrial inner membrane. Sco1p transfers Cu^{2+} to cytochrome oxidase subunit 2 of respiratory complex IV. Lys7p (the CCS copper chaperone) transfers Cu^{2+} to an intermembrane space pool of Cu,Zn-superoxide dismutase (Sod1p). B) Fe/S cluster assembly pathway of the mitochondrion. Fe^{2+} is transported into the mitochondrion via an unidentified transporter and transferred via Nfs1p to Isu1p/Isu2p. Sulfur is donated from cysteine to yield alanine. The proteins Yah1p, Arh1, Jac1, Ssq1, Nfu1, and frataxin (Yfh1 in *S. cerevisiae*) mediate assembly of the Fe/S cluster. The assembled cluster is then incorporated into mitochondrial Fe/S proteins or exported via Atm1p. Erv1p and Bat2p assist in assembly of the Fe/S cluster into cytosolic proteins.

ALS including damage to mitochondrial DNA, defects in respiratory chain enzymes, and abnormal mitochondrial morphology.[173] ALS thus may involve an interplay between oxidative damage and mitochondrial dysfunction.[174]

Proteins with Fe/S cluster cofactors are ubiquitous in both eukaryotic and prokaryotic organisms. They play central roles in various cellular processes that include redox reactions, metabolic catalysis, and the sensing of iron and ambient oxygen levels. In the past few years, the factors involved in Fe/S protein cluster assembly have been identified and the molecular pathway of Fe/S cluster biogenesis has started to unfold. Much of the early work started from the link between Friedreich's ataxia, a neurodegenerative disease characterized by progressive gait and limb ataxia and cardiomyopathy, and a defect in iron metabolism in the mitochondria.[175]

The responsible gene was named frataxin and the protein was localized to the mitochondria.[176] Electron micrograph studies show that iron accumulates in patient's mitochondria.[177] The function of frataxin in iron metabolism is under much debate but its hypothesized role is in storage or transport of iron or assembly of Fe/S proteins.[178,179]

Fe/S protein biogenesis is the only biosynthetic process for which the mitochondrion is essential for life of the yeast cell,[180] indicating the evolutionary importance of this pathway. In prokaryotes, the proteins are encoded by the *isc* (iron-sulfur cluster assembly) operon[181] and the *nif* gene cluster of nitrogen-fixing bacteria, where they participate in the formation of the Fe/S cofactors of nitrogenase.[182] Pioneering investigations in bacteria have provided an outline of this pathway in higher organisms. In eukaryotes, the mitochondrion contains a complex apparatus termed the ISC (iron–sulfur cluster) assembly machinery consisting of at least ten proteins.[7,180] The ISC assembly machinery contains proteins with diverse functions. Nfs1p, a cysteine desulfurase, was the first component identified and is essential for viability in yeast.[183] Nfs1p is the functional ortholog of the bacterial cysteine desulfurases NifS and IscS, which produce elemental sulfur from cysteine for incorporation into Fe/S proteins.[181] Two factors that play an integral role in assembly of the Fe/S cluster are the matrix Isu1p and Isu2p proteins.[184,185] Deletion of both *ISU1* and *ISU2* is lethal, and the Isu proteins play a role in generating the Fe/S cluster, potentially by binding to the iron substrate. Nfu1p also interacts genetically with Isu1p, but its precise role in Fe/S cluster assembly is not known.

After the initial synthesis of the intermediate Fe/S cluster, additional steps are needed to release, remodel, and transfer the Fe/S cluster to the apoprotein. Only some of the key players in this process have been identified. The ferredoxin Yah1p and its reductase Arh1p mediate reduction that is required for Fe/S cluster assembly by an electron transport chain.[186-188] And Fe/S cluster assembly also involves the chaperones Jac1p and Ssq1p,[189-191] which are homologs of the heat-shock proteins Hsp40p/DnaJ and Hsp70p/DnaK, respectively. Jac1p is essential in yeast but deletion of Ssq1p yields a cold-sensitive phenotype.[189] The site of action of these chaperones has not been identified but a genetic interaction between Ssq1p and Nfu1p has been reported.

In eukaryotes, Fe/S proteins are located predominantly in the mitochondrion. However, examples of cytosolic proteins are known and include glutamate synthase, isopropyl malate dehydrogenase, the mammalian iron regulatory protein 1, and the RNase inhibitor, Rli1p. In addition to the mitochondrial ISC machinery, two components that specifically mediate biogenesis of the extra-mitochondrial Fe/S proteins have been identified. These are the inner membrane ABC transporter Atm1p[192,193] and the sulfhydryl oxidase Erv1p in the intermembrane space.[194] The specific export mechanism is not known, but Atm1p most likely transports an Fe/S cluster intermediate[195] and Erv1p acts downstream to maintain the assembly competence of the cluster into the apoprotein or to mediate disulfide bond formation.[196] In the cytosol, Bat2p, originally identified as a branched-chain amino acid transaminase, also seems to play a role in Fe/S protein biogenesis.[197] Loss of Bat2p resulted in a defect in de novo assembly of Fe/S proteins.

Atm1 is highly conserved and the homologs in man (hABC7) and plants (Sta1 in *Arabidopsis thaliana*) replace the function of the yeast mitochondrial ABC transporter. Mutations in hABC7 result in an increase in mitochondrial iron levels and are linked to the iron storage disease X-linked sideroblastic anemia and ataxia (XLSA/A).[198] Patients with XLSA/A display two to three fold lower activity in the biogenesis of cytosolic Fe/S proteins.[199] Defects in the plant ABC transporter Sta1 result in dwarfism and chlorosis, though interestingly no significant increase in mitochondrial iron levels is apparent in mutant cells.[200] The *A. thaliana* genome, however, contains two additional gene, STA2 and STA3, that are most likely functionally redundant with STA1. A homolog of Erv1p, termed hepatopoetin (HPO)/augmenter of liver regeneration,[201] also is a novel human hepatotrophic factor. Recently, HPO was shown to act as a putative mitogen for hepatoma cell lines via HPO-specific receptors on the cell surface.[201] Because the biogenesis of Fe/S proteins is complicated, future studies should lead to the identification of new components and subsequent elucidation of the biosynthetic pathway.

Perspectives

Over the last ten years, a better understanding of the link between mitochondrial dysfunction and disease has and continues to develop. In addition, the molecular mechanisms of mitochondrial biogenesis and maintenance including protein import and export, ion trafficking, and mitochondrial dynamics are being dissected. Defects in mitochondrial biogenesis, ion homeostasis, and energy production have been shown to cause a wide array of human diseases. Examples include apoptosis or programmed cell death, Friedreich's ataxia, deafness/dystonia syndrome, ALS, paraplegia, and myopathies and neuropathies. As genomes are sequenced and polymorphisms are identified, the role of the mitochondrion in diverse cellular circuits will be deciphered.

References

1. Altman R. Die Elementarorganismen und Ihre Beziehungen zur den Zellen. Liepzig: Veit; 1890.
2. Tzagoloff A. Mitochondria. New York: Plenum Press, 1982.
3. Tyler D. The mitochondrion in health and disease. New York: VCH Publishers, 1992.
4. Lehninger AL. The mitochondrion. New York: Benjamin, 1964.
5. Baker KP, Schatz G. Mitochondrial proteins essential for viability mediate protein import into yeast mitochondria. Nature 1991; 349:205-208.
6. Mühlenhoff U, Lill R. Biogenesis of iron-sulfur proteins in eukaryotes: A novel task of mitochondria that is inherited from bacteria. Biochim Biophys Acta 2000; 1459:370-382.
7. Craig EA, Voisine C, Schilke B. Mitochondrial iron metabolism in the yeast Saccharomyces cerevisiae. Biol Chem 1999; 380:1167-1173.
8. Koshkin V, Greenberg ML. Oxidative phosphorylation in cardiolipin-lacking yeast mitochondria. Biochem J 2000; 347:687-691.
9. Shaw JM, Nunnari J. Mitochondrial dynamics and division in budding yeast. Trends Cell Biol 2002; 12:178-184.
10. Berger KH, Yaffe MP. Mitochondrial DNA inheritance in Saccharomyces cerevisiae. Trends Microbiol 2000; 8:508-513.
11. Jensen RE, Hobbs AE, Cerveny KL et al. Yeast mitochondrial dynamics: Fusion, division, segregation, and shape. Microsc Res Tech 2000; 51:573-583.
12. Hales KG, Fuller MT. Developmentally regulated mitochondrial fusion mediated by a conserved, novel, predicted GTPase. Cell 1997; 90:121-129.
13. Hermann GJ, Thatcher JW, Mills JP et al. Mitochondrial fusion in yeast requires the transmembrane GTPase Fzo1p. J Cell Biol 1998; 143:359-373.
14. Sesaki H, Jensen RE. UGO1 encodes an outer membrane protein required for mitochondrial fusion. J Cell Biol 2001; 152:1123-1134.
15. Labrousse AM, Zappaterra MD, Rube DA et al. C. elegans dynamin-related protein DRP-1 controls severing of the mitochondrial outer membrane. Mol Cell 1999; 4:815-826.
16. Bleazard W, McCaffery JM, King EJ et al. The dynamin-related GTPase Dnm1 regulates mitochondrial fission in yeast. Nat Cell Biol 1999; 1:298-304.
17. Hinshaw JE. Dynamin and its role in membrane fission. Annu Rev Cell Dev Biol 2000; 16:483-519.
18. Jones BA, Fangman WL. Mitochondrial DNA maintenance in yeast requires a protein containing a region related to the GTP-binding domain of dynamin. Genes Dev 1992; 6:380-389.
19. Pelloquin L, Belenguer P, Menon Y et al. Identification of a fission yeast dynamin-related protein involved in mitochondrial DNA maintenance. Biochem Biophys Res Commun 1998; 251:720-726.
20. Shepard KA, Yaffe MP. The yeast dynamin-like protein, Mgm1p, functions on the mitochondrial outer membrane to mediate mitochondrial inheritance. J Cell Biol 1999; 144:711-720.

21. Wong ED, Wagner JA, Gorsich SW et al. The dynamin-related GTPase, Mgm1p, is an intermembrane space protein required for maintenance of fusion competent mitochondria. J Cell Biol 2000; 151:341-352.

22. Tieu Q, Nunnari J. Mdv1p is a WD repeat protein that interacts with the dynamin-related GTPase, Dnm1p, to trigger mitochondrial division. J Cell Biol 2000; 151:353-366.

23. Mozdy AD, McCaffery JM, Shaw JM. Dnm1p GTPase-mediated mitochondrial fission is a multi-step process requiring the novel integral membrane component Fis1p. J Cell Biol 2000; 151:367-380.

24. Fekkes P, Shepard KA, Yaffe MP. Gag3p, an outer membrane protein required for fission of mitochondrial tubules. J Cell Biol 2000; 151:333-340.

25. Cerveny KL, McCaffery JM, Jensen RE. Division of mitochondria requires a novel DMN1-interacting protein, Net2p. Mol Biol Cell 2001; 12:309-321.

26. Smirnova E, Griparic L, Shurland DL et al. Dynamin-related protein Drp1 is required for mitochondrial division in mammalian cells. Mol Biol Cell 2001; 12:2245-2256.

27. Boldogh IR, Yang HC, Pon LA. Mitochondrial inheritance in budding yeast. Traffic 2001; 2:368-374.

28. Hollenbeck PJ. The pattern and mechanism of mitochondrial transport in axons. Front Biosci 1996; 1:d91-d102.

29. Pereira AJ, Dalby B, Stewart RJ et al. Mitochondrial association of a plus end-directed microtubule motor expressed during mitosis in Drosophila. J Cell Biol 1997; 136:1081-1090.

30. Nangaku M, Sato-Yoshitake R, Okada Y et al. KIF1B, a novel microtubule plus end-directed monomeric motor protein for transport of mitochondria. Cell 1994; 79:1209-1220.

31. Simon VR, Karmon SL, Pon LA. Mitochondrial inheritance: Cell cycle and actin cable dependence of polarized mitochondrial movements in Saccharomyces cerevisiae. Cell Motil Cytoskeleton 1997; 37:199-210.

32. Boldogh IR, Yang HC, Nowakowski WD et al. Arp2/3 complex and actin dynamics are required for actin-based mitochondrial motility in yeast. Proc Natl Acad Sci USA 2001; 98:3162-3167.

33. Simon VR, Swayne TC, Pon LA. Actin-dependent mitochondrial motility in mitotic yeast and cell-free systems: Identification of a motor activity on the mitochondrial surface. J Cell Biol 1995; 130:345-354.

34. Hermann GJ, King EJ, Shaw JM. The yeast gene, MDM20, is necessary for mitochondrial inheritance and organization of the actin cytoskeleton. J Cell Biol 1997; 137:141-153.

35. Fisk HA, Yaffe MP. Mutational analysis of Mdm1p function in nuclear and mitochondrial inheritance. J Cell Biol 1997; 138:485-494.

36. Boldogh I, Vojtov N, Karmon S et al. Interaction between mitochondria and the actin cytoskeleton in budding yeast requires two integral mitochondrial outer membrane proteins, Mmm1p and Mdm10p. J Cell Biol 1998; 141:1371-1381.

37. Sogo LF, Yaffe MP. Regulation of mitochondrial morphology and inheritance by Mdm10p, a protein of the mitochondrial outer membrane. J Cell Biol 1994; 126:1361-1373.

38. Berger KH, Sogo LF, Yaffe MP. Mdm12p, a component required for mitochondrial inheritance that is conserved between budding and fission yeast. J Cell Biol 1997; 136:545-553.

39. Roeder AD, Hermann GJ, Keegan BR et al. Mitochondrial inheritance is delayed in Saccharomyces cerevisiae cells lacking the serine/threonine phosphatase PTC1. Mol Biol Cell 1998; 9:917-930.

40. Fisk HA, Yaffe MP. A role for ubiquitination in mitochondrial inheritance in Saccharomyces cerevisiae. J Cell Biol 1999; 145:1199-1208.

41. Zoladek T, Tobiasz A, Vaduva G et al. MDP1, a Saccharomyces cerevisiae gene involved in mitochondrial/cytoplasmic protein distribution, is identical to the ubiquitin-protein ligase gene RSP5. Genetics 1997; 145:595-603.

42. MacAlpine DM, Perlman PS, Butow RA. The numbers of individual mitochondrial DNA molecules and mitochondrial DNA nucleoids in yeast are coregulated by the general amino acid control pathway. EMBO J 2000; 19:767-775.

43. Hobbs AE, Srinivasan M, McCaffery JM et al. Mmm1p, a mitochondrial outer membrane protein, is connected to mitochondrial DNA (mtDNA) nucleoids and required for mtDNA stability. J Cell Biol 2001; 152:401-410.

44. Gray MW, Burger G, Lang BF. Mitochondrial Evolution. Science 1999; 283:1476-1481.

45. Pfanner N, Douglas MG, Endo T et al. Uniform nomenclature for the protein transport machinery of the mitochondrial membranes. Trends Biochem Sci 1996; 21:51-52.

46. Pfanner N. Protein sorting: Recognizing mitochondrial presequences. Curr Biol 2000; 10(11):R412-415.
47. Neupert W. Protein import into mitochondria. Annu Rev Biochem, 1997; 66:863-917.
48. Schatz G, Dobberstein B. Common principles of protein translocation across membranes. Science 1996; 271:1519-1526.
49. Ryan KR, Jensen RE. Mas6p can be cross-linked to an arrested precursor and interacts with other proteins during mitochondrial protein import. J Biol Chem 1993; 268:23743-23746.
50. Martin J, Mahlke K, Pfanner N. Role of an energized inner membrane in mitochondrial protein import: ΔΨ• drives the movement of presequences. J Biol Chem 1991; 266:18051-18057.
51. Kang PJ, Ostermann J, Shilling J et al. Requirement for hsp70 in the mitochondrial matrix for translocation and folding of precursor proteins. Nature 1990; 348:137-143.
52. Horst M, Oppliger W, Feifel B et al. The mitochondrial protein import motor: Dissociation of mitochondrial hsp70 from its membrane anchor requires ATP binding rather than ATP hydrolysis. Protein Sci 1996; 5:759-767.
53. Voos W, von Ahsen O, Muller H et al. Differential requirement for the mitochondrial Hsp70-Tim44 complex in unfolding and translocation of preproteins. EMBO J 1996; 15:2668-2677.
54. Hawlitschek G, Schneider H, Schmidt B et al. Mitochondrial protein import: Identification of processing peptidase and of PEP, a processing enhancing protein. Cell 1988; 53:795-806.
55. Rospert S, Looser R, Dubaquie Y et al. Hsp60-independent protein folding in the matrix of yeast mitochondria. EMBO J 1996; 15:764-774.
56. Sirrenberg C, Endres M, Folsch H et al. Carrier protein import into mitochondria mediated by the intermembrane proteins Tim10/Mrs11 and Tim12/Mrs5. Nature 1998; 391:912-915.
57. Koehler CM, Jarosch E, Tokatlidis K et al. Import of mitochondrial carriers mediated by essential proteins of the intermembrane space. Science 1998; 279:369-373.
58. Kerscher O, Holder J, Srinivasan M et al. The Tim54p-Tim22p complex mediates insertion of proteins into the mitochondrial inner membrane. J Cell Biol 1997; 139:1663-1675.
59. Dekker PJ, Muller H, Rassow J et al. Characterization of the preprotein translocase of the outer mitochondrial membrane by blue native electrophoresis. Biol Chem 1996; 377:535-538.
60. Ahting U, Thun C, Hegerl R et al. The TOM core complex: The general protein import pore of the outer membrane of mitochondria. J Cell Biol 1999; 147:959-968.
61. van Wilpe S, Ryan MT, Brix J et al. Tom22 is a multifunctional organizer of the mitochondrial preprotein translocase. Nature 1999; 401:485-489.
62. Künkele KP, Heins S, Dembowski M et al. The preprotein translocation channel of the outer membrane of mitochondria. Cell 1998; 93:1009-1019.
63. Ramage L, Junne T, Hahne K et al. Functional cooperation of mitochondrial protein import receptors in yeast. EMBO J 1993; 12:4115-4123.
64. Brix J, Rudiger S, Bukau B et al. Distribution of binding sequences for the mitochondrial import receptors Tom20, Tom22, and Tom70 in a presequence-carrying preprotein and a noncleavable preprotein. J Biol Chem 1999; 274:16522-16530.
65. Abe Y, Shodai T, Muto T et al. Structural basis of presequence recognition by the mitochondrial presequence receptor Tom20. Cell 2000; 100:551-560.
66. Hines V, Brandt A, Griffiths G et al. Protein import into yeast mitochondria is accelerated by the outer membrane protein MAS70. EMBO J 1990; 9:3191-3200.
67. Wiedemann N, Pfanner N, Ryan MT. The three modules of ADP/ATP carrier cooperate in receptor recruitment and translocation into mitochondria. EMBO J 2001; 20:951-960.
68. Brix J, Ziegler GA, Dietmeier K et al. The mitochondrial import receptor Tom70: Identification of a 25 kDa core domain with a specific binding site for preproteins. J Mol Biol 2000; 303:479-488.
69. Bömer U, Pfanner N, Dietmeier K. Identification of a third yeast mitochondrial Tom protein with tetratrico peptide repeats. FEBS Lett 1996; 382:153-158.
70. Schlossmann J, Lill R, Neupert W et al. Tom71, a novel homologue of the mitochondrial preprotein receptor Tom70. J Biol Chem 1996; 271:17890-17895.
71. Lithgow T, Junne T, Suda K et al. The mitochondrial outer membrane protein Mas22p is essential for protein import and viability of yeast. Proc Natl Acad Sci USA 1994; 91:11973-11977.
72. Ryan MT, Muller H, Pfanner N. Functional Staging of ADP/ATP Carrier Translocation across the Outer Mitochondrial Membrane. J Biol Chem 1999; 274:20619-20627.

73. Gratzer S, Lithgow T, Bauer RE et al. Mas37p, a novel receptor subunit for protein import into mitochondria. J Cell Biol 1995; 129:25-34.
74. Armstrong LC, Komiya T, Bergman BE et al. Metaxin is a component of a preprotein import complex in the outer membrane of the mammalian mitochondrion. J Biol Chem 1997; 272:6510-6518.
75. Abdul KM, Terada K, Yano M et al. Functional analysis of human metaxin in mitochondrial protein import in cultured cells and its relationship with the Tom complex. Biochem Biophys Res Comm 2000; 276:1028-1034.
76. Armstrong LC, Saenz AJ, Bornstein P. Metaxin 1 interacts with metaxin 2, a novel related protein associated with the mammalian mitochondrial outer membrane. J Cell Biochem 1999; 74:11-22.
77. Hill K, Model K, Ryan MT et al. Tom40 forms the hydrophilic channel of the mitochondrial import pore for preproteins. Nature 1998; 395:516-521.
78. Künkele KP, Juin P, Pompa C et al. The isolated complex of the translocase of the outer membrane of mitochondria. Characterization of the cation-selective and voltage- gated preprotein-conducting pore. J Biol Chem 1998; 273:31032-31039.
79. Kurz M, Martin H, Rassow J et al. Biogenesis of Tim proteins of the mitochondrial carrier import pathway: Differential targeting mechanisms and crossing over with the main import pathway. Mol Biol Cell 1999; 10:2461-2474.
80. Dekker PJ, Ryan MT, Brix J et al. Preprotein translocase of the outer mitochondrial membrane: Molecular dissection and assembly of the general import pore complex. Mol Cell Biol 1998; 18:6515-6524.
81. Krimmer T, Rapaport D, Ryan MT et al. Biogenesis of porin of the outer mitochondrial membrane involves an import pathway via receptors and the general import pore of the TOM complex. J Cell Biol 2001; 2001:289-300.
82. Schatz G. Just follow the acid chain. Nature 1997; 388:121-122.
83. Komiya T, Rospert S, Koehler C et al. Interaction of mitochondrial targeting signals with acidic receptor domains along the protein import pathway: Evidence for the 'acid chain' hypothesis. EMBO J 1998; 17:3886-3898.
84. Brix J, Dietmeier K, Pfanner N. Differential recognition of preproteins by the purified cytsolic domains of the mitochondrial import receptors Tom20, Tom22, and Tom70. J Biol Chem 1997; 272:20730-20735.
85. Horst M, Hilfiker-Rothenfluh S, Oppliger W et al. Dynamic interaction of the protein translocation systems in the inner and outer membranes of yeast mitochondria. EMBO J 1995; 14:2293-2297.
86. Dekker PJ, Martin F, Maarse AC et al. The Tim core complex defines the number of mitochondrial translocation contact sites and can hold arrested preproteins in the absence of matrix Hsp70-Tim44. EMBO J 1997; 16:5408-5419.
87. Schwartz MP, Matouschek A. The dimensions of the protein import channel in the outer and inner mitochondrial membranes. Proc Natl Acad Sci USA 1999; 98:13086-13090.
88. Bauer MF, Sirrenberg C, Neupert W et al. Role of Tim23 as voltage sensor and presequence receptor in protein import into mitochondria. Cell 1996; 87:33-41.
89. Donzeau M, Kaldi K, Adam A et al. Tim23 links the inner and outer mitochondrial membranes. Cell 2000; 101:401-412.
90. Geissler A, Krimmer T, Bomer U et al. Membrane potential-driven protein import into mitochondria. The sorting sequence of cytochrome b_2 modulates the deltaΨ-dependence of translocation of the matrix-targeting sequence. Mol Biol Cell 2000; 11:3977-3991.
91. Hartl FU. Molecular chaperones in cellular protein folding. Nature 1996; 381:571-579.
92. Bukau B, Horwich AL. The Hsp70 and Hsp60 chaperone machines. Cell 1998; 92:351-366.
93. Krimmer T, Rassow J, Kunau WH et al. The mitochondrial protein import motor: The ATPase domain of matrix Hsp70 is crucial for binding to Tim44, while the peptide binding domain and the carboxy-terminal segment play a stimulatory role. Mol Cell Biol 2000; 20:5879-5887.
94. Gambill BD, Voos W, Kang PJ et al. A dual role for mitochondrial heat shock protein 70 in membrane translocation of preproteins. J Cell Biol 1993; 123:109-117.
95. Kronidou NG, Oppliger W, Bolliger L et al. Dynamic interaction between Isp45 and mitochondrial hsp70 in the protein import system of the yeast mitochondrial inner membrane. Proc Natl Acad Sci USA 1994; 91:12818-12822.

96. Bolliger L, Deloche O, Glick BS et al. A mitochondrial homolog of bacterial GrpE interacts with mitochondrial hsp70 and is essential for viability. EMBO J 1994; 13:1998-2006.

97. Voos W, Gambill BD, Laloraya S et al. Mitochondrial GrpE is present in a complex with hsp70 and preproteins in transit across membranes. Mol Cell Biol 1994; 14:6627-6634.

98. Ostermann J, Horwich AL, Neupert W et al. Protein folding in mitochondria requires complex formation with hsp60 and ATP hydrolysis. Nature 1989; 341:125-130.

99. Fenton WA, Weissman JS, Horwich AL. Putting a lid on protein folding: Structure and function of the cochaperonin, GroES. Chem Biol 1996; 3:157-161.

100. Briones P, Vilaseca MA, Ribes A et al. A new case of multiple mitochondrial enzyme deficiencies with decreased amount of heat shock protein 60. J Inherit Metab Dis 1997; 20:569-577.

101. Huckriede A, Heikema A, Wilschut J et al. Transient expression of a mitochondrial precursor protein. A new approach to study mitochondrial protein import in cells of higher eukaryotes. Eur J Biochem 1996; 237:288-294.

102. Schmid FX. Prolyl isomerases: Enzymatic catalysis of slow protein-folding reactions. Annu Rev Biophys Biomol Struct 1993; 22:123-143.

103. Rassow J, Mohrs K, Koidl S et al. Cyclophilin 20 is involved in mitochondrial protein folding in cooperation with molecular chaperones Hsp70 and Hsp60. Mol Cell Biol 1995; 15:2654-2662.

104. Matouschek A, Rospert S, Schmid K et al. Cyclophilin catalyzes protein folding in yeast mitochondria. Proc Natl Acad Sci USA 1995; 92:6319-6323.

105. Tokatlidis K, Junne T, Moes S et al. Translocation arrest of an intramitochondrial sorting signal next to Tim11 at the inner-membrane import site. Nature 1996; 384:585-588.

106. Arnold I, Pfeiffer K, Neupert W et al. Yeast mitochondrial F1F0-ATP synthase exists as a dimer: Identification of three dimer-specific subunits. EMBO J 1998; 17:7170-7178.

107. Kanamori T, Nishikawa S, Shin I et al. Probing the environment along the protein import pathways in yeast mitochondria by site-specific photocrosslinking. Proc Natl Acad Sci USA 1997; 94:485-490.

108. Palmieri F, Bisaccia F, Capobianco L et al. Mitochondrial metabolite transporters. Biochim Biophys Acta 1996; 1275:127-132.

109. Koehler CM, Merchant S, Oppliger W et al. Tim9p, an essential partner subunit of Tim10p for the import of mitochondrial carrier proteins. EMBO J 1998; 17:6477-6486.

110. Koehler CM, Leuenberger D, Merchant S et al. Human deafness dystonia syndrome is a mitochondrial disease. Proc Natl Acad Sci USA 1999; 96:2141-2146.

111. Adam A, Endres M, Sirrenberg C et al. Tim9, a new component of the TIM22.54 translocase in mitochondria. EMBO J 1999; 18:313-319.

112. Paschen SA, Rothbauer U, Kaldi K et al. The role of the TIM8-13 complex in the import of Tim23 into mitochondria. EMBO J 2000; 19:6392-6400.

113. Davis AJ, Sepuri NB, Holder J et al. Two intermembrane space TIM complexes interact with different domains of Tim23p during its import into mitochondria. J Cell Biol 2000; 150:1271-1282.

114. Leuenberger D, Bally NA, Schatz G et al. Different import pathways through the mitochondrial intermembrane space for inner membrane proteins. EMBO J 1999; 17:4816-4822.

115. Endres M, Neupert W, Brunner M. Transport of the ADP/ATP carrier of mitochondria from the TOM complex to the TIM22.54 complex. EMBO J 1999; 18:3214-3221.

116. Sirrenberg C, Bauer MF, Guiard B et al. Import of carrier proteins into the mitochondrial inner membrane mediated by Tim22. Nature 1996; 384:582-585.

117. Kerscher O, Sepuri NB, Jensen RE. Tim18p is a new component of the Tim54p-Tim22p translocon in the mitochondrial inner membrane. Mol Biol Cell 2000; 11:103-116.

118. Koehler CM, Murphy MP, Bally N et al. Tim18p, a novel subunit of the inner membrane complex that mediates protein import into the yeast mitochondrial inner membrane. Mol Cell Biol 2000; 20:1187-1193.

119. Oyedotun KS, Lemire BD. The carboxyl terminus of the Saccharomyces cerevisiae succinate dehydrogenase membrane subunit, SDH4p, is necessary for ubiquinone reduction and enzyme stability. J Biol Chem 1997; 272:31382-31388.

120. Tranebjaerg L, Schwartz C, Eriksen H et al. A new X linked recessive deafness syndrome with blindness, dystonia, fractures, and mental deficiency is linked to Xq22. J Med Genet 1995; 32:257-263.

121. Jin H, May M, Tranebjaerg L et al. A novel X-linked gene, DDP, shows mutations in families with deafness (DFN-1), dystonia, mental deficiency and blindness. Nat Genet 1996; 14:177-180.

122. Glick BS, Von Heijne G. Saccharomyces cerevisiae mitochondria lack a bacterial-type sec machinery. Protein Sci 1996; 5:2651-2652.

123. Hamel P, Lemaire C, Bonnefoy N et al. Mutations in the membrane anchor of yeast cytochrome c1 compensate for the absence of Oxa1p and generate carbonate-extractable forms of cytochrome c1. Genetics 1998; 150:601-611.

124. Hell K, Herrmann J, Pratje E et al. Oxa1p mediates the export of the N- and C-termini of pCoxII from the mitochondrial matrix to the intermembrane space. FEBS Lett 1997; 418:367-370.

125. Samuelson JC, Chen M, Jiang F et al. YidC mediates membrane protein insertion in bacteria. Nature 2000; 406:637-641.

126. Sundberg E, Slagter JG, Fridborg I et al. ALBINO3, an Arabidopsis nuclear gene essential for chloroplast differentiation, encodes a chloroplast protein that shows homology to proteins present in bacterial membranes and yeast mitochondria. Plant Cell 1997; 9:717-730.

127. Preuss M, Leonhard K, Hell K et al. Mba1, a Novel Component of the Mitochondrial Protein Export Machinery of the Yeast Saccharomyces cerevisiae. J Cell Biol 2001; 153:1085-1096.

128. He S, Fox TD. Mutations affecting a yeast mitochondrial inner membrane protein, pnt1p, block export of a mitochondrially synthesized fusion protein from the matrix. Mol Cell Biol 1999; 19:6598-6607.

129. Saracco SA, Fox TD. Cox18p Is Required for Export of the Mitochondrially Encoded Saccharomyces cerevisiae Cox2p C-Tail and Interacts with Pnt1p and Mss2p in the Inner Membrane. Mol Biol Cell 2002; 13:1122-1131.

130. Rep M, Grivell LA. The role of protein degradation in mitochondrial function and biogenesis. Curr Genet 1996; 30:367-380.

131. Langer T, Neupert W. Regulated protein degradation in mitochondria. Experientia 1996; 52:1069-1076.

132. Geli V, Yang MJ, Suda K et al. The MAS-encoded processing protease of yeast mitochondria. Overproduction and characterization of its two nonidentical subunits. J Biol Chem 1990; 265:19216-19222.

133. Luciano P, Geli V. The mitchondrial processing peptidase: Function and specificity. Experientia 1996; 52:1077-1082.

134. Isaya G, Kalousek F, Fenton WA et al. Cleavage of precursors by the mitochondrial processing peptidase requires a compatible mature protein or an intermediate octapeptide. J Cell Biol 1991; 113:65-76.

135. Kalousek F, Isaya G, Rosenberg LE. Rat liver mitochondrial intermediate peptidase (MIP): Purification and initial characterization. EMBO J 1992; 11:2803-2809.

136. Isaya G, Miklos D, Rollins RA. MIP1, a new yeast gene homologous to the rat mitochondrial intermediate peptidase gene, is required for oxidative metabolism in Saccharomyces cerevisiae. Mol Cell Biol 1994; 14:5603-5616.

137. Schneider A, Behrens M, Scherer P et al. Inner membrane protease I, an enzyme mediating intramitochondrial protein sorting in yeast. EMBO J 1991; 10:247-254.

138. Dalbey RE, Lively MO, Bron S et al. The chemistry and enzymology of the type I signal peptidase. Protein Sci 1997; 6:1129-1138.

139. Nunnari J, Fox TD, Walter P. A mitochondrial protease with two catalytic subunits of nonoverlapping specificities. Science 1993; 262:1997-2004.

140. Suzuki CK, Rep M, Maarten van Dijl J et al. ATP-dependent proteases that also chaperone protein biogenesis. Trends Biochem Sci 1997; 22:118-123.

141. Suzuki CK, Suda K, Wang N et al. Requirement for the yeast gene LON in intramitochondrial proteolysis and maintenance of respiration. Science 1994; 264:891.

142. Wagner I, Arlt H, van Dyck L et al. Molecular chaperones cooperate with PIM1 protease in the degradation of misfolded proteins in mitochondria. EMBO J 1994; 13:5135-5145.

143. Fu GK, Markovitz DM. The human Lon protease binds to mitochondrial promoters in a single-stranded, site-specific, strand-specific manner. Biochemistry 1998; 37:1905-1909.

144. Bross P, Andresen BS, Knudsen I et al. Human ClpP protease: cDNA sequence, tissue-specific expression and chromosomal assignment of the gene. FEBS Lett 1995; 377:249-252.

145. Gottesman S, Maurizi MR, Wickner S. Regulatory subunits of energy-dependent proteases. Cell 1997; 91:435-438.

146. Patel S, Latterich M. The AAA team: Related ATPases with diverse functions. Trends Cell Biol 1998; 8:65-71.

147. Beyer A. Sequence analysis of the AAA protein family. Protein Sci 1997; 6:2043-2058.

148. Leonhard K, Herrmann JM, Stuart RA et al. AAA proteases with catalytic sites on opposite membrane surfaces comprise a proteolytic system for the ATP-dependent degradation of inner membrane proteins in mitochondria. EMBO J 1996; 15:4218-4229.

149. Weber ER, Hanekamp T, Thorsness PE. Biochemical and functional analysis of the YME1 gene product, an ATP and zinc-dependent mitochondrial protease from S. cerevisiae. Mol Biol Cell 1996; 7:307-317.

150. Thorseness PE, White KH, Fox TD. Inactivation of YME1, a member of the ftsH-SEC18-PAS1-CDC48 family of putative ATPase-encoding genes, causes increased escape of DNA from mitochondria in Saccharomyces cerevisiae. Mol Cell Biol 1993; 13:54118-55426.

151. Campbell CL, Tanaka N, White KH et al. Mitochondrial morphological and functional defects in yeast caused by yme1 are suppressed by mutation of a 26S protease subunit homologue. Mol Biol Cell 1994; 5:899-905.

152. Guelin E, Rep M, Grivell LA. Sequence of the AFG3 gene encoding a new member of the FstH/Yme1/Tma subfamily of the AAA-protein family. Yeast 1994; 10:1389-1394.

153. Tauer R, Mannhaupt G, Schnall R et al. Yta10p, a member of a novel ATPase family in yeast, is essential for mitochondrial function. FEBS Lett. 1994; 353:197-200.

154. h'Arlt H, Tauer R, Feldmann H et al. The YTA10-12 complex, an AAA protease with chaperone-like activity in the inner membrane of mitochondria. Cell 1996; 85:875-885.

155. Guelin E, Rep M, Grivell LA. Afg3p, a mitochondrial ATP-dependent metalloprotease, is involved in the degradation of mitochondrially-encoded Cox1, Cox3, Cob, Su6, Su8, and Su9 subunits of the inner membrane complexes III, IV and V. FEBS Lett 1996; 381:42-46.

156. Casari G, De Fusco M, Ciarmatori S et al. Spastic paraplegia and OXPHOS impairment caused by mutations in paraplegin, a nuclear-encoded mitochondrial metalloprotease. Cell 1998; 93:973-983.

157. Desautels M, Goldberg AL. Liver mitochondria contain an ATP-dependent, vanadate-sensitive pathway for the degradation of proteins. Proc Natl Acad Sci USA 1982; 79:1869-1873.

158. Young L, Leonhard K, Tatsuta T et al. Role of the ABC transporter Mdl1 in peptide export from mitochondria. Science 2001; 291:2135-2138.

159. Elliott T, Young L, Leonhard K et al. Transporter associated with antigen processing between mitochondria and their cellular environment. Adv Immunol 1997; 65:47-109.

160. Lindahl KF, Byers DE, Dabhi VM et al. H2-M3, a full-service class Ib histocompatibility antigen. Annu Rev Immunol 1997; 15:851-879.

161. Hallstrom TC, Moye-Rowley WS. Multiple signals from dysfunctional mitochondria activate the pleiotropic drug resistance pathway in Saccharomyces cerevisiae. J Biol Chem 2000; 275:37347-37356.

162. Barrientos A, Barros MH, Valnot I et al. Cytochrome oxidase in health and disease. Gene 2002; 286:53-63.

163. Glerum DM, Shtanko A, Tzagoloff A. Characterization of COX17, a yeast gene involved in copper metabolism and assembly of cytochrome oxidase. J Biol Chem 1996; 271:14504-14509.

164. Glerum DM, Shtanko A, Tzagoloff A. SCO1 and SCO2 act as high copy suppressors of a mitochondrial copper recruitment defect in Saccharomyces cerevisiae. J Biol Chem 1996; 271:20531-20535.

165. Beers J, Glerum DM, Tzagoloff A. Purification, characterization, and localization of yeast Cox17p, a mitochondrial copper shuttle. J Biol Chem 1997; 272:33191-33196.

166. Nittis T, George GN, Winge DR. Yeast Sco1, a protein essential for cytochrome c oxidase function is a Cu(I)-binding protein. J Biol Chem 2001; 276:42520-42526.

167. Chinenov YV. Cytochrome c oxidase assembly factors with a thioredoxin fold are conserved among prokaryotes and eukaryotes. J Mol Med 2000; 78:239-242.

168. Valnot I, Osmond S, Gigarel N et al. Mutations of the SCO1 gene in mitochondrial cytochrome c oxidase deficiency with neonatal-onset hepatic failure and encephalopathy. Am J Hum Gene 2000; 67:1104-1109.

169. Papadopoulou LC, Sue CM, Davidson MM et al. Fatal infantile cardioencephalomyopathy with COX deficiency and mutations in SCO2, a COX assembly gene. Nat Genet 1999; 23:333-337.

170. Sturtz LA, Diekert K, Jensen LT et al. A fraction of yeast Cu,Zn-superoxide dismutase and Its metallochaperone, CCS, localize to the intermembrane space of mitochondria. A physiological role for SOD1 in guarding against mitochondrial oxidative damage. J Biol Chem 2001; 276:38084-38089.

171. Deng HX, Hentati A, Tainer JA et al. Amyotrophic lateral sclerosis and structural defects in Cu,Zn superoxide dismutase. Science 1993; 261:1047-1051.

172. Gurney ME, Pu H, Chiu AY et al. Motor neuron degeneration in mice that express a human Cu,Zn superoxide dismutase mutation. Science 1994; 264:1772-1775.

173. Vielhaber S, Kunz D, Winkler K et al. Mitochondrial DNA abnormalities in skeletal muscle of patients with sporadic amyotrophic lateral sclerosis. Brain 2000; 123:1339-1348.

174. Klivenyi P, Ferrante RJ, Matthews RT et al. Neuroprotective effects of creatine in a transgenic animal model of amyotrophic lateral sclerosis. Nat Med 1999; 5:347-350.

175. Campuzano V, Montermini L, Molto MD et al. Friedreich's ataxia: Autosomal recessive disease caused by an intronic GAA triplet repeat expansion. Science 1996; 271:1423-1427.

176. Campuzano V, Montermini L, Lutz Y et al. Frataxin is reduced in Friedreich ataxia patients and is associated with mitochondrial membranes. Hum Mol Genet 1997; 6:1771-1780.

177. Rotig A, de Lonlay P, Chretien D et al. Aconitase and mitochondrial iron-sulphur protein deficiency in Friedreich ataxia. Nat Genet 1997; 17:215-217.

178. Cavadini P, O'Neill HA, Benada O et al. Assembly and iron-binding properties of human frataxin, the protein deficient in Friedreich ataxia. Hum Mol Genet 2002; 11:217-227.

179. Chen OS, Kaplan J. YFH1-mediated iron homeostasis is independent of mitochondrial respiration. FEBS Lett 2001; 509:131-134.

180. Mühlenhoff U, Lill R. Biogenesis of iron-sulfur proteins in eukaryotes: a novel task of mitochondria that is inherited from bacteria. Biochim Biophys Acta 2000; 1459:370-382.

181. Zheng L, Cash VL, Flint DH et al. Assembly of iron-sulfur clusters. Identification of an iscSUA-hscBA-fdx gene cluster from Azotobacter vinelandii. J Biol Chem 1998; 273:13264-13272.

182. Peters JW, Fisher K, Dean DR. Nitrogenase structure and function: A biochemical-genetic perspective. Annu Rev Microbiol 1995; 49:335-366.

183. Strain J, Lorenz CR, Bode J et al. Suppressors of superoxide dismutase (SOD1) deficiency in Saccharomyces cerevisiae. Identification of proteins predicted to mediate iron-sulfur cluster assembly. J Biol Chem 1998; 273:31138-31144.

184. Schilke B, Voisine C, Beinert H et al. Evidence for a conserved system for iron metabolism in the mitochondria of Saccharomyces cerevisiae. Proc Natl Acad Sci USA 1999; 96:10206-10211.

185. Garland SA, Hoff K, Vickery LE et al. Saccharomyces cerevisiae ISU1 and ISU2: Members of a well-conserved gene family for iron-sulfur cluster assembly. J Mol Biol 1999; 294:897-907.

186. Barros MH, Nobrega FG. YAH1 of Saccharomyces cerevisiae: A new essential gene that codes for a protein homologous to human adrenodoxin. Gene 1999; 233:197-203.

187. Lange H, Kaut A, Kispal G et al. A mitochondrial ferredoxin is essential for biogenesis of cellular iron-sulfur proteins. Proc Natl Acad Sci USA 2000; 97:1050-1055.

188. Manzella L, Barros MH, Nobrega FG. ARH1 of Saccharomyces cerevisiae: A new essential gene that codes for a protein homologous to the human adrenodoxin reductase. Yeast 1998; 14:839-846.

189. Voisine C, Cheng YC, Ohlson M et al. Jac1, a mitochondrial J-type chaperone, is involved in the biogenesis of Fe/S clusters in Saccharomyces cerevisiae. Proc Natl Acad Sci USA 2001; 98:1483-1488.

190. Lutz T, Westermann B, Neupert W et al. The mitochondrial proteins Ssq1 and Jac1 are required for the assembly of iron sulfur clusters in mitochondria. J Mol Biol 2001; 307:815-825.

191. Voisine C, Schilke B, Ohlson M et al. Role of the mitochondrial Hsp70s, Ssc1 and Ssq1, in the maturation of Yfh1. Mol Cell Biol 2000; 20:3677-3684.

192. Leighton J, Schatz G. An ABC transporter in the mitochondrial inner membrane is required for normal growth of yeast. EMBO J 1995; 14:188-195.

193. Kispal G, Csere P, Guiard B et al. The ABC transporter Atm1p is required for mitochondrial iron homeostasis. FEBS Lett 1997; 418:346-350.

194. Lee J, Hofhaus G, Lisowsky T. Erv1p from Saccharomyces cerevisiae is a FAD-linked sulfhydryl oxidase. FEBS Lett 2000; 477:62-66.

195. Kispal G, Csere P, Prohl C et al. The mitochondrial proteins Atm1p and Nfs1p are essential for biogenesis of cytosolic Fe/S proteins. EMBO J 1999; 18:3981-3989.

196. Lange H, Lisowsky T, Gerber J et al. An essential function of the mitochondrial sulfhydryl oxidase Erv1p/ALR in the maturation of cytosolic Fe/S proteins. EMBO Rep 2001; 2:715-720.
197. Kispal G, Steiner H, Court DA et al. Mitochondrial and cytosolic branched-chain amino acid transaminases from yeast, homologs of the myc oncogene-regulated Eca39 protein. J Biol Chem 1996; 271:24458-24464.
198. Allikmets R, Raskind WH, Hutchinson A et al. Mutation of a putative mitochondrial iron transporter gene (ABC7) in X-linked sideroblastic anemia and ataxia (XLSA/A). Hum Mol Genet 1999; 8:743-749.
199. Bekri S, Kispal G, Lange H et al. Human ABC7 transporter: Gene structure and mutation causing X-linked sideroblastic anemia with ataxia with disruption of cytosolic iron-sulfur protein maturation. Blood 2000; 96:3256-3264.
200. Kushnir S, Babiychuk E, Storozhenko S et al. A Mutation of the Mitochondrial ABC Transporter Sta1 Leads to Dwarfism and Chlorosis in the Arabidopsis Mutant starik. Plant Cell 2001; 13:89-100.
201. Li Y, Xing G, Wang Q et al. Hepatopoietin acts as an autocrine growth factor in hepatoma cells. DNA Cell Biol 2001; 20:791-795.

CHAPTER 9

The Biogenesis and Cell Biology of Peroxisomes in Human Health and Disease

Stanley R. Terlecky and Paul A. Walton

Abstract

Recent results have demonstrated that the molecular mechanisms of peroxisomal membrane biogenesis and the post-translational import of proteins into the organelle do not follow those paradigms established for other subcellular organelles. As such, we have much to learn about the peroxisome, and the human diseases that occur as a result of its malfunction. In this review, we describe how peroxisomes arise through these seemingly non-conventional processes, specifically focusing on how the organelle membrane assembles its constituent proteins, and how appropriate enzymes are imported. Particular emphasis is placed on identifying the role of specific peroxins at each step in the biosynthetic mechanism.

Introduction

Peroxisomes are single-membrane bound organelles found in almost all eukaryotic cells (Fig. 1). The study of peroxisomes began in the 1950s with the electron microscopic discovery by Rhodin that mouse kidney cells contain small structures with diameters between 0.1-1.0 μm surrounded by a single lipid bilayer membrane, which were named microbodies.[1] The enzymatic characterization of peroxisomes was first carried out by de Duve and Baudhuin who, in 1966, demonstrated that microbodies contained enzymes involved in the production and degradation of hydrogen peroxide.[2] Therefore, these structures were renamed peroxisomes.

Peroxisomes contain some 50 enzymes involved in such metabolic processes as plasmalogen, sterol and bile acid synthesis, as well as very-long-chain fatty acid β-oxidation and nitrogenous waste processing among many others.[3-5] Peroxisomal constituents and functions of this biochemically diverse organelle appear to depend upon cell type and metabolic conditions. Mammalian cells typically contains hundreds of peroxisomes, though their abundance can be increased in response to extracellular stimuli such as high fat diets,[6] thyroid hormones[7] and diabetes.[8] Other peroxisome proliferation agents include hypolipidemic drugs such as fibrates,[9] plasticizers and chlorinated hydrocarbons.[10]

Classically defined as containing both hydrogen peroxide-producing oxidases and catalase, peroxisomes are thought to provide an isolated environment in which toxic hydrogen peroxide can be eliminated before it can cause oxidative damage to other cellular components.[11,12] The absence of DNA in peroxisomes requires that all peroxisomal proteins be encoded by the nuclear genome. Thus, peroxisomal proteins are synthesized on free polysomes and then imported from the cytosol directly to the organelle lumen.[13] Related organellar structures were

The Biogenesis of Cellular Organelles, edited by Chris Mullins. ©2005 Eurekah.com and Kluwer Academic/Plenum Publishers.

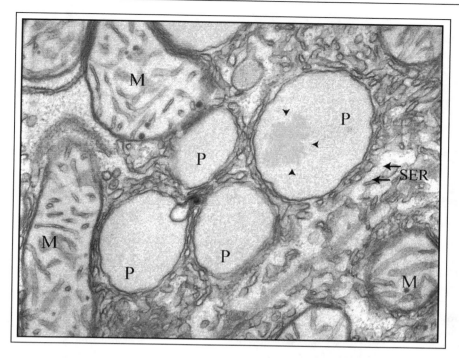

Figure 1. Electron micrograph of rat liver. Ultrastructure of rat liver peroxisomes (P), mitochondria (M), and smooth ER (SER). The peroxisomal core composed of crystalline urate oxidase is indicated by arrowheads. (Image kindly provided by Dr. Eveline Baumgart-Vogt, Justus-Liebig-Universitaet Giessen, Giessen, Germany)

also discovered and named depending on their specialized biochemical functions and in the organisms in which they were found. In plants, these organelles were involved in the glyoxylate pathway and therefore were named glyoxysomes.[14] In trypanosomes, they were named glycosomes because they were involved in the glycolytic pathway.[15]

Our knowledge of the function of peroxisomes in human cell metabolism has been obtained primarily by the study of patients with peroxisomal dysfunctions.[16,17] Indeed, peroxisomes have been shown to be required for normal human development.[18,19] A class of autosomal recessive diseases known as peroxisomopathies (including Zellweger syndrome, rhizomelic chondrodysplasia punctata, infantile Refsum's disease and X-linked adrenoleukodystrophy) is characterized by severe neurological, hepatic and renal defects. The most severe of these diseases, Zellweger syndrome, is marked by disorders of peroxisomal membrane biogenesis and protein import, and results in death within the first few months or years after birth.[16,20] Levels of mRNA for peroxisomal proteins are normal in cells from these patients, but the enzyme activities are reduced or undetectable.[21-23] Activities that remain (e.g., catalase) are non-sedimentable by centrifugation, indicating that they are found in the cytosol.

Peroxisome biogenesis disorders exist as 12 distinct complementation groups as characterized by cell fusion studies.[19] The genes responsible for many of these human pathologies have been recently identified (Table 1).[19,24]

In some forms of Zellweger syndrome typical peroxisomes are absent, although peroxisomal "ghosts" can be detected.[25,26] These structures are two to four times larger and less dense than normal peroxisomes, but do possess normal amounts of some peroxisomal membrane

Table 1. Complementation groups and respective genes linked to human peroxisome disorders

Complementation Group	Affected Gene
1	*PEX1*
2	*PEX5*
3	*PEX12*
4	*PEX6*
7	*PEX10*
8	*unknown*
9	*PEX16**
10	*PEX2*
11	*PEX7*
12	*PEX3**
13	*PEX13*
14	*PEX19**

* Genes implicated in the second form of Zellweger syndrone, in which peroxisomes are undetectable (see text for details). Table adapted from refs. 19 and 24.

proteins.[27,28] Evidence suggests these peroxisomal ghosts are capable of proliferation and sorted normally to daughter cells during mitosis. In the second form of Zellweger syndrome (marked by asterisks in Table 1) peroxisomes are undetectable. The molecules responsible for these complementation groups (Pex3p,* Pex16p and Pex19p—discussed further below) appear to be involved in the earliest stages of peroxisomal biogenesis (i.e., membrane assembly) rather than the later stages of matrix protein import. Thus, peroxisomopathies are a very heterogeneous group of diseases displaying a marked variation in the assembly of peroxisomal membranes, and the synthesis, import and processing of peroxisomal proteins.[16]

Biogenesis of Peroxisomal Membranes

Although much is understood about the biochemical functions of peroxisomes, details regarding the early steps in biogenesis of this organelle are not resolved and various models have been postulated.

Originally, Novikoff and Shin proposed that peroxisomes formed by budding from the endoplasmic reticulum (ER), based upon electron microscopic images that appeared to show interconnections between the organelles.[29] Subsequent investigations did not provide support for this hypothesis, and an analysis of the proteins and lipids of the peroxisome showed them to be quite different from the endoplasmic reticulum.[30] The source of the lipids and the mechanisms by which they are trafficked to the peroxisome membrane remain interesting and largely un-addressed problems.

It is now widely believed that new peroxisomes, required in times of cellular growth, are formed from pre-existing peroxisomes,[13] although recent evidence indicates that this may not be universally so.[31,32] It is presently unknown whether the proliferation of the peroxisomes in mammalian cells occurs by budding and fission of pre-existing peroxisomes alone, or in

---

* A "Pexp" designation indicates a protein which acts at a particular point in the formation of peroxisomes. These molecules are called peroxins; to date, 32 have been identified. Their respective numbers refer to the order in which they were discovered.

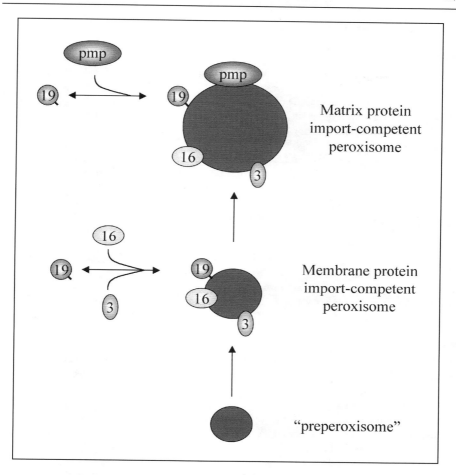

Figure 2. Model for early steps of peroxin-mediated organelle assembly. In this view, the peroxins Pex3p, Pex16p, and Pex19p (designated 3, 16 and 19, respectively) play a role in the earliest stages of peroxisome biogenesis. Their collective action results in the stepwise maturation of organelles poised first to assemble peroxisomal membrane proteins (pmp), and, subsequently, to import matrix proteins. The existence of a "preperoxisome" is considered in the text.

combination with other mechanisms. Serial electron microscopic sections of regenerating rat liver have shown the formation of a peroxisomal reticulum at early times, and the subsequent return of single peroxisomes.[33-35] Using molecular genetic screens in yeast, cell lines from human Zellweger syndrome patients and Chinese hamster ovary cell mutants, a number of genes have been identified that appear to be involved specifically in the initial steps of peroxisome biogenesis (Fig. 2). These are the molecules that contribute to those complementation groups that show an absence of detectable peroxisomes. As discussed here, their role in peroxisome biogenesis occurs early, involving the formation of vesicles that will ultimately contain peroxisomal enzymes.

Early Acting Peroxins

Pex3p

The absence of peroxisomal ghosts in fibroblast cells taken from CG12 patients with Zellweger syndrome indicates that Pex3p is involved in the biogenesis of the organelle membrane. Pex3p itself is an integral membrane protein of approximately 42 kDa; it is targeted to the peroxisomal membrane by an amino-terminal sequence of approximately 37 amino acids.[36] This peroxisomal membrane targeting signal (mPTS) is sufficient to direct GFP to the organelle membrane.[37] Interestingly, this hybrid mPTS-GFP is also targeted to vesicles in Δ*PEX3* cells,[38] which implies that this molecule is able to insert into a preperoxisomal membrane lacking other peroxisomal proteins. Although the exact function of Pex3p is not clear, an emerging model is that it serves as a peroxisomal membrane assembly "initiator". That is, it is the first peroxin associated with the nascent organelle and, once in place, other peroxins and peroxisomal membrane proteins are able to assemble. Consistent with this model is the finding that cells devoid of Pex3p degrade or mistarget a number of peroxisomal proteins, including the critical docking peroxin, Pex14p (see below).[39]

One clue as to how Pex3p facilitates the downstream assembly of peroxisomal membrane proteins may be the fact that the molecule's carboxy-terminus, which is exposed to the cytosol, interacts with a second early acting peroxin, Pex19p.[37,40] This critically important peroxin has been described, among other ways, as an "assembly factor for peroxisomal membrane proteins".[24]

Pex19p

Pex19p is a 33 kDa hydrophilic protein found predominately in the cytosol, but with a small amount also associated with the peroxisomal membrane.[41-43] The molecule contains a carboxy-terminal farnesyl group,[44] although it is unclear whether this lipid modification is required for the peroxin's function.[41-43] Pex19p associates with many peroxisomal membrane proteins, including the aforementioned Pex3p and the third early acting peroxin, Pex16p.[41-43] For most of the interactions examined, Pex19p's association with peroxisomal membrane proteins occurs at regions distinct from those responsible for targeting the proteins to the organelle (i.e., the mPTSs).[42] Therefore, the molecule does not appear to be acting as a general mPTS "import receptor" for peroxisomal membrane proteins per se. Indeed, it is even unclear precisely where in the cell Pex19p and peroxisomal membrane proteins interact (i.e., in the cytosol or on the organelle membrane). Irrespective, the importance of this peroxin cannot be overemphasized; it is now generally accepted that Pex19p plays an important role in facilitating the import and/or assembly of a wide variety of peroxisomal membrane proteins.[41-43] Among these are membrane proteins, to be discussed below, which are involved in the import of peroxisomal matrix proteins. Perhaps not surprisingly, in cells from CG14 Zellweger syndrome patients, the absence of Pex19p results in the degradation of many peroxisomal membrane proteins, which presumably fail to find their proper subcellular location.[41]

The suggestion that Pex19p acts downstream of Pex3p is supported by the observation that—using sophisticated detection methods in one yeast species—Pex3p-positive membrane "structures" (preperoxisomes?) are seen in Δ*PEX19* cells.[45] Whether or not similar structures exist in higher eukaryotes awaits further examination.

Pex16p

In contrast to other peroxins which exhibit a broad species distribution, Pex16p is found only in mammalian cells, and in one species of yeast. This 39 kDa protein is anchored in the peroxisomal membrane by two transmembrane domains.[46] The function of Pex16p is unknown,

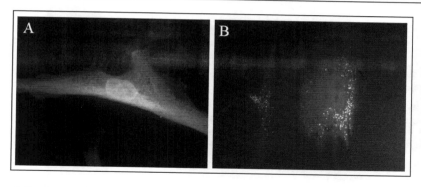

Figure 3. Restoration of peroxisomal membrane biogenesis and matrix protein import in a human cell. Subcellular localization of GFP coupled to a PTS1-peptide in a peroxisome-deficient (ΔPEX16) human fibroblast (A), and 48 hr after a (ΔPEX16) cell was complemented by microinjection of plasmids containing PEX16 (B). Expression of PEX16 resulted in the de novo biogenesis of peroxisomes—including membrane lipid and protein assembly and matrix protein import.

but its involvement in peroxisomal biogenesis is implicated by the lack of demonstrable peroxisomes in ΔPEX16 cells. However, following the expression of this gene (for example, after needle microinjection of PEX16 DNA in Fig. 3) peroxisomal membranes can be seen to form de novo and import peroxisomal matrix proteins.

The "Preperoxisome": A Precursor Organelle to the Peroxisome?

The reformation of peroxisomes that occurs following the expression of PEX3, PEX19 or PEX16 in CG12, CG14 and CG9 cells, respectively, appears to violate the tenet that organelles cannot be created de novo. That this restoration occurs implies that there exists a structure in apparently peroxisome-deficient cells, which occupies a position upstream in the biogenesis pathway to those vesicles identified as peroxisomes. This hypothetical structure has been called the "preperoxisome". The origin of the preperoxisome is unknown, but there is evidence for, and against, the hypothesis that it is derived from the endoplasmic reticulum.

In addition to evidence obtained in lower eukaryotes reviewed in refs. 32,33, experimental results that support the role of the ER in the assembly of mammalian peroxisomes has come from the studies of Pex11pα in rat liver and CHO cells.[47] Pex11pα is found associated with the peroxisome membrane via two putative transmembrane spanning domains and contains a cytoplasmic-facing dilysine motif at the carboxy-terminus.[47] Interestingly, the presence of such motifs have been shown to be involved in binding COPI coatomer subunits to generate vesicles for the retrograde retrieval of ER resident proteins from the "ER-Golgi-intermediate compartment" back to the endoplasmic reticulum.[48] Studies undertaken with purified rat liver peroxisomes revealed that Pex11pα indeed associated with ADP-ribosylation factor 1 (ARF) and coatomer subunits in a GTP-γS-dependent manner.[47] (Note: Small GTP-binding proteins have been previously identified as associated with peroxisomal membranes.[49]) This association of Pex11pα and elements of the retrograde secretory pathway implies that the ER may be connected in some manner to the biogenesis of peroxisomes. It is certainly an interesting hypothesis, but there have been concerns raised which make the link form Pex11pα to the ARF/COP1 coatomer components tenuous. For example Abe et al[50] report that mutating the dilysine motif, moving it away from the carboxy-terminus, or deleting it altogether has no effect on the localization or functioning of Pex11pα. And, perhaps consistent with this is the fact that the dilysine motif is not conserved through evolution; for example, it is not found in any yeast or trypanosome Pex11p molecules.

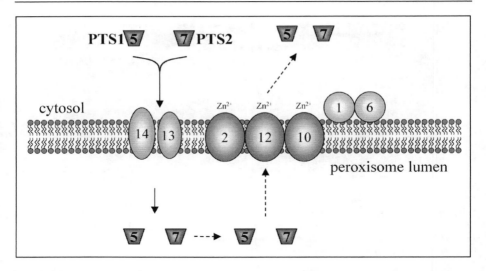

Figure 4. Model for later steps of peroxin-mediated matrix protein import. Identified in this scheme are the peroxins (designated by their respective numbers) which play a role in the import of matrix proteins and/ or the trafficking of PTS-receptors.

Arguing against an ER connection, Gould and coworkers have demonstrated quite convincingly that mammalian peroxisomal proteins do not require transit through this organelle in order to be associated with the peroxisomes.[41,51] For example, treatment of cells with brefeldin A had no effect on the reformation of peroxisomes following expression of Pex3p or Pex16p, nor did it effect the subcellular localization of these proteins in normal cells. Likewise, incubation of cells at 15°C, a temperature which blocks vesicle-mediated transport, did not affect the subcellular localization of expressed peroxisomal membrane proteins.[41] Lastly, inhibition of COPII-mediated vesiculation from the endoplasmic reticulum by expression of a dominant negative version of SAR1, had no effect on Pex3p localization or Pex3p-mediated peroxisomal restoration.[51]

Taken together, while the origin and components of the preperoxisome remain a mystery, there exists strong evidence that in mammalian cells, known peroxisomal proteins probably do not travel through the endoplasmic reticulum as part of there normal trafficking pathway.

Molecular Mechanisms of Peroxisomal Protein Import

Peroxisomal protein import is signal-mediated. With only a select few exceptions, enzymes destined for the peroxisome matrix contain a remarkably simple carboxy-terminal targeting signal which is recognized post-translationally by the cycling receptor, Pex5p (Fig. 4).[52,53] In most cases, this signal, called peroxisomal targeting signal 1 (PTS1), is related to the tripeptide, serine-lysine-leucine.[54] There are, however, peroxisomal proteins which contain a PTS1 seemingly unrelated to the "consensus". The critical antioxidant enzyme, catalase, is such an example; it contains a necessary and sufficient carboxy-terminal PTS which interacts with Pex5p, but consists of the four amino acids, lysine-alanine-asparagine-leucine.[55] Although not yet well analyzed, it is reasonable to assume that distinct PTS1s interact with Pex5p to varying extents, and that this will contribute to differences in the overall import efficiency of one enzyme versus another.

Of the few non-PTS1-containing peroxisomal enzymes, some contain a loose consensus sequence of nine amino acids, near the amino terminus.[56,57] Called PTS2, this determinant is recognized by a second soluble receptor, Pex7p, which mediates its import.[52] Peroxisomal enzymes devoid of a PTS1 and PTS2 exist, at least in lower eukaryotes;[38] how they are recognized and trafficked to the organelle is unclear.

Pex5p's direct binding to PTS1 is mediated by tetratricopeptide repeats (TPR) contained within the receptor protein.[52] Once complexed, the receptor and ligand move to the peroxisome membrane and engage downstream components of the import apparatus. Pex7p appears to function analogously, binding its PTS2-containing ligand in the cytosol, and delivering same to the peroxisome membrane.[52] The situation is slightly more complex in human and other mammalian cells, where Pex5p exists in a long and a short form—reflecting the presence or absence of a 37 amino acid insert.[58-60] This sequence, which lies outside the TPR regions, mediates Pex7p's binding to Pex5p, an interaction required for PTS2 protein import.[61,62] Thus, in these organisms there appears to exist a dynamic interplay between the two matrix protein import pathways.

The pathways intersect again at the peroxisome membrane, with both import receptors docking with Pex14p.[63-65] This membrane bound peroxin occupies a pivotal point in the import mechanism. Ligand-complexed receptors not only assemble at the membrane via Pex14p, but presumably also initiate the downstream interactions culminating in translocation across the membrane bilayer. For PTS1-Pex5p, the downstream components include Pex13p[66] and the RING-family peroxins, Pex10p and Pex12p.[67,68] Other peroxins which appear to act after docking to mediate import include Pex1p,[38,69] Pex2p[61,70] and Pex6p.[38,69] Unfortunately, the precise manner by which these proteins function remains largely ill-defined. Also unclear is the extent to which these molecules, either alone or in combination with other proteins, contribute to the peroxisomal translocon.

In a mechanism akin to the cycling of nuclear import receptors, Pex5p not only ferries its substrate to the peroxisome, but actually enters the organelle as part of its functional cycle.[71] Having released its cargo the receptor recycles back to the cytosol presumably to initiate another round of import. This mechanism requires that the peroxisomal protein import apparatus accommodate fully folded oligomeric proteins, a feature already well described in a number of previous studies.

Indeed, documented substrates for peroxisomal protein import include PTS-containing dimers and trimers, and a variety of stably-folded proteins.[52] Peroxisomal enzymes will even deliver, in piggy-back fashion, pre-bound antibody molecules to the organelle lumen.[72] Remarkably, this machinery will also accommodate PTS-coated gold spheres[73] This is perhaps the best illustration that import occurs without major perturbations of (protein) conformation. Most of the information regarding the import-competence of various substrates has been gleaned from in vitro assays in which the import process is reconstituted. Several powerful assays have been developed with each adding to a biochemical understanding of peroxisomal protein translocation.

These assays include: (i) microinjecting substrates into the cytosol of cells and looking, by immunofluorescence microscopy, for time-dependent redistribution to peroxisomes,[74] as well as (ii) isolating peroxisomes, adding the substrate, and gauging import by protease protection,[75] and (iii) adding substrates to bacterial cytolysin-treated or mechanically disrupted cells, and monitoring import by immunofluorescence microscopy or ELISA, respectively.[76,77,70] Collectively, these approaches have revealed that peroxisomal protein import is a signal, temperature and time-dependent event. Substrates associate with the peroxisome membrane in an ATP-independent manner, but require the energy of ATP-hydrolysis for translocation. Import is saturable, and perhaps not surprisingly, requires direct action of the peroxins, Pex5p, Pex14p (and Pex2p). Zinc stimulates import perhaps via functioning of the zinc-binding peroxins, Pex2p, Pex10p and Pex12p. Whole cytosol is stimulatory, with the molecular chaperones Hsc70 and Hsp40 among the responsible factors. Goals for future studies include trying to understand where and how these Hsps act, as well as to determine what factors are present in cytosol which promote import to levels beyond those thus far achieved with purified components. A final point; although most of the results included here were obtained using PTS1 substrates, recent reconstitution and characterization of PTS2 protein import in vitro suggests that most of the biochemical properties are conserved between pathways.[72]

Conclusions and the Future of Peroxisome Cell Biology

An understanding of peroxisome biogenesis at the molecular level has begun to emerge. Peroxins involved in all facets of the organelle's biosynthesis have been identified and, in many cases, characterized. How these molecules interact with one another as well as with other components of the biogenesis machinery is reasonably well understood. Yet questions remain; what proteins specifically constitute the peroxisomal membrane and matrix protein import machineries, and how is their assembly/disassembly and activity controlled. Also, are these stable complexes or dynamic ones which come together (and apart) in a regulated manner?

Peroxisome cell biology is not simply of interest to basic scientists. As discussed above, there is compelling medical relevance to advancing these studies in humans. In the next few years, the molecular basis of many peroxisomal disorders will be clarified and with such advances will come a call for therapeutic intervention. Can strategies and pharmaceuticals be developed which ameliorate or altogether eliminate peroxisomal disease? There will likely be a push for gene therapy. However, it remains to be determined if such cutting edge technology be applied to restoring peroxisome function and assuring patient health. Continued progress in the development of animal models expressing not only complete gene-knockouts, but also tissue specific and inducible ones will be extremely important in these efforts to develop novel therapeutic strategies.

Finally, new areas for peroxisome research will be revealed. For example, what is the exact role of the organelle in important processes including human development or aging? At this point, there is only limited information available. It will be a combination of old and new foci, established perspectives and new insights, and traditional approaches coupled with new technologies that will sustain interest in the cell biology of peroxisomes for many years to come.

Acknowledgements

The authors gratefully acknowledge Prof. Dr. Eveline Baumgart-Vogt (Justus-Liebig-Universitat Giessen) for providing Figure 1, Julie Legakis (Wayne State University School of Medicine) for producing Figures 2 and 4, and Holly Edwards for editorial assistance. S.R.T. is supported by NIH grant DK56299; P.A.W. is supported by a CIHR operating grant.

References

1. Rhodin J. Correlation of ultrastructure organization and function in normal and experimentally treated proximal convoluted tubule cells of the mouse kidney. Doctoral thesis, Karolinska Institute, Stockholm 1954.
2. de Duve C, Baudhuin P. Peroxisomes (microbodies and related particles). Physiol Rev 1966; 46:323-357.
3. Reddy JK, Mannaerts GP. Peroxisomal lipid metabolism. Ann Rev Nutr 1994; 14:343-370.
4. Krisans SK. Cell compartmentalization of cholesterol biosynthesis. In: Reddy JK, Suga T, Mannaerts GP et al, eds. Peroxisomes: Biology and role in toxicology and disease. New York: New York Academy of Sciences, 1996:142-164.
5. Mannaerts GP, Van Veldhoven PP, Casteels M. Peroxisomal lipid degradation via β- and α-oxidation in mammals. Cell Biochem Biophys 1999; 31:321-335.
6. Ishii H, Fukumori N, Horie S et al. Effects of fat content in the diet on hepatic peroxisomes of the rat. Biochem Biophys Acta 1980; 617:1-11.

7. Fringes B, Reith A. Time course of peroxisome biogenesis during adaptation to mild hyperthyroidism in rat liver: A morphometric, stereologic study by electron microscope. Lab Invest 1982; 47:19-26.

8. Horie S, Ishii H, Sugar T. Changes in peroxisomal fatty acid oxidation in the diabetic rat liver. J Biochem 1981; 90:1691-1696.

9. Reddy JK, Azarnoff DL, Hignite CE. Hypolipidaemic hepatic peroxisome proliferators from a novel class of chemical carcinogens. Nature 1980; 283:397-398.

10. Bremer J, Osmundsen H, Christiansen RZ et al. Methods Enzymol 1981; 72:516-517.

11. Lazarow PB, de Duve C. The synthesis and turnover of rat liver peroxisomes: Intracellular pathway of catalase synthesis. J Cell Biol 1973; 59:507-524.

12. Singh I. Mammalian peroxisomes: Metabolism of oxygen and reactive oxygen species. In: Reddy JK, Suga T, Mannaerts GP et al, eds. Peroxisomes: Biology and role in toxicology and disease. New York: New York Academy of Sciences, 1996:612-627.

13. Lazarow PB, Fujiki Y. Biogenesis of Peroxisomes. Ann Rev Cell Biol 1985; 1:489-530.

14. Breidenbach RW, Beevers H. Association of the glyoxylate cycle enzymes in a novel subcellular particle from castor bean endosperm. Biochem Biophys Res Commun 1967; 27:462-469.

15. Opperdoes FR, Borst P. Localisation of nine glycolytic enzymes in a microbody-like organelle in Trypanosoam brucei: The glycosome. FEBS Lett 1977; 80:360-364.

16. Moser HW, Begin A, Cornblath D. Peroxisomal disorders. Biochem Cell Biol 1991; 69:463-474.

17. Motley AM, Hettema EH, Distel B et al. Differential protein import deficiencies in human peroxisome assembly disorders. J Cell Biol 1994; 125:755-767.

18. Goldfisher S, Collins J, Rapin I et al. Peroxisome abnormalities in metabolic diseases. J Pediatr 1986; 108:25-32.

19. Gould SJ, Valle D. Peroxisome biogenesis disorders: Genetics and cell biology. Trends Genet 2000; 16:340-345.

20. Zellweger H. Peroxisomes and peroxisomal disorders. Alab J Med Sci 1988; 25:54-58.

21. Lazarow PB, Black V, Shio H et al. Zellweger syndrome: Biochemical and morphological studies on two patients treated with clofibrate. Ped Res 1985; 19:1356-1364.

22. Suzuki Y, Shimozawa N, Orii T et al. Molecular analysis of peroxisomal beta-oxidation enzymes in infants with Zellweger syndrome and Zellweger-like syndrome: Further heterogeneity of the peroxisomal disorder. Clin Chem Acta 1988; 172:65-76.

23. Wanders PA, Kos M, Roest B et al. Activity of peroxisomal enzymes and intracellular distribution of catalase in Zellweger syndrome. Biochem Biophys Res Commun 1984; 123:1054-1061.

24. Subramani S, Koller A, Snyder WB. Import of peroxisomal matrix and membrane proteins. Ann Rev Biochem 2000; 69:399-418.

25. Santos MJ, Imanaka T, Shio H et al. Peroxisomal membrane ghosts in Zellweger syndrome – aberrant organelle assembly. Science 1988; 239:1536-1538.

26. Santos MJ, Imanaka T, Shio H et al. Peroxisomal integral membrane proteins in control and Zellweger fibroblasts. J Biol Chem 1988; 263:10502-10509.

27. Lazarow PB, Fujiki Y, Small GM et al. Presence of the peroxisomal 22-kDa integral membrane protein in the liver of a person lacking recognizable peroxisomes (Zellweger syndrome). Proc Nat Acad Sci USA 1986; 83:9193-9196.

28. Small GM, Santos MJ, Imanaka T et al. Peroxisomal integral membrane proteins are present in livers of patients with Zellweger syndrome, infantile Refsum's disease and X-linked adrenoleukodystrophy. J Inher Metab Dis 1988; 11:358-371.

29. Novikoff AB, Shin WY. The endoplasmic reticulum in the Golgi zone and its relation to microbodies, Golgi apparatus and autophagic vacuoles in rat liver cells. J Microscopy 1964; 3:187-206.

30. Fujiki Y, Fowler S, Shio H et al. Polypeptide and phospholipid composition of the membrane of rat liver peroxisomes: Comparison with endoplasmic reticulum. J Cell Biol 1982; 93:103-110.

31. Kunau WH, Erdmann R. Peroxisome biogenesis: Back to the endoplasmic reticulum. Curr Biol 1998; 8:R299-R302.

32. Titorenko VI, Rachubinski RA. Dynamics of peroxisome assembly and function. Trends Cell Biol 2001; 11:22-29.

33. Wendel FP, Berger EP. On the quantitative stereomorphology of microbodies in rat hepatocytes. J Ultrastruct Res 1975; 51:153-165.

34. Yamamoto K, Fahimi HD. Three-dimensional reconstruction of a peroxisomal reticulum in regeneration rat liver: Evidence of interconnections between heterogenous segments. J Cell Biol 1987; 105:713-722.
35. Yakota S, Himeno M, Kato K. Formation of autophagosomes during degradation of excess peroxisomes induced by di-(2-ethylhexyl)-phthalate treatment. III. Fusion of early autophagosomes with lysosomal compartments. Eur J Cell Biol 1995; 66:15-24.
36. Baerends RJS, Rasmussen SW, Hillbrands RE et al. The Hansenula polymorpha PER9 gene encodes a peroxisomal membrane protein essential for peroxisomal assembly and integrity. J Biol Chem 1996; 271:8887-8894.
37. Ghaedi K, Tamura S, Okumoto K et al. The peroxin Pex3p initiates membrane assembly in peroxisome biogenesis. Mol Biol Cell 2000; 11:2085-2102.
38. Purdue PE, Lazarow PB. Peroxisome biogenesis. Ann Rev Cell Dev Biol 2001; 17:701-752.
39. Muntau AC, Mayerhofer PU, Paton BC et al. Defective peroxisome membrane synthesis due to mutations in human PEX3 causes Zellweger syndrome, complementation group G. Am J Hum Genet 2000; 67:967-975.
40. Soukupova M, Sprenger C, Gorgas K et al. Identification and characterization of the human peroxin PEX3. Eur J Cell Biol 1999; 78:357-374.
41. Sacksteder KA, Jones JM, South ST et al. PEX19 binds multiple peroxisomal membrane proteins, is predominantly cytoplasmic, and is required for peroxisome membrane synthesis. J Cell Biol 2000; 148:931-44.
42. Fransen M, Wylin T, Brees C et al. Human Pex19p binds peroxisomal integral membrane proteins at regions distinct from their sorting sequences. Mol Cell Biol 2001; 21:4413-4424.
43. Snyder WB, Koller A, Choy AJ et al. The peroxin Pex19p interacts with multiple, integral membrane proteins at the peroxisomal membrane. J Cell Biol 2000; 149:1171-1177.
44. James GL, Goldstein JL, Pathak RK et al. PxF, a prenylated protein of peroxisomes. J Biol Chem 1994; 269:14182-14190.
45. Snyder WB, Faber KN, Wenzel TJ et al. Pex19 interacts with Pex3p and Pex10p and is essential for peroxisome biogenesis in Pichia pastoris. Mol Cell Biol 1999; 10:1745-1761.
46. South ST, Gould SJ. Peroxisome synthesis in the absence of preexisting peroxisomes. J Cell Biol 1999; 144:255-266.
47. Passreiter M, Lay D, Frank R et al. Peroxisomal biogenesis: Involvement of ARF and coatomer. J Cell Biol 1998; 141:373-383.
48. Letourneur F, Gaynor EC, Hennecke S et al. Coatomer is essential in retrieval of di-lysine-tagged proteins to the endoplasmic reticulum. Cell 1994; 79:1199-1207.
49. Verheyden K, Fransen M, Van Veldhoven BB et al. Presence of small GTP-binding proteins in the peroxisomal membrane. Biochem Biophys Acta 1992; 1109:48-54.
50. Abe I, Okumoto K, Tamura S et al. Clofibrate-inducible, 28-kDa peroxisomal membrane protein is encoded by Pex11. FEBS Lett 1998; 431:468-472.
51. South ST, Sacksteder KA, Li XL et al. Inhibitors of COPI and COPII do not block PEX3-mediated peroxisome synthesis. J Cell Biol 2000; 149:1345-1359.
52. Subramani S. Components involved in peroxisome import, biogenesis, proliferation, turnover, and movement. Physiol Rev 1998; 78:171-188
53. Elgersma Y, Tabak HF. Proteins involved in peroxisome biogenesis and functioning. Biochem Biophys Acta 1996; 1286:269-283.
54. Gould SJ, Keller GA, Hosken N et al. A conserved tripeptide sends proteins to peroxisomes. J Cell Biol 1989; 108:1657-1664.
55. Purdue PE, Lazarow PB. Targeting of human catalase to peroxisomes is dependent upon a novel COOH-terminal peroxisomal targeting sequence. J Cell Biol 1996; 134:849-862.
56. Osumi T, Tsukamoto T, Hata S et al. Amino-terminal presequence of the precursor of peroxisomal 3-ketoacyl-CoA thiolase is a cleavable signal peptide for peroxisomal targeting. Biochem Biophys Res Comm 1991; 181:947-954.
57. Swinkels BW, Gould SJ, Bodnar AG et al. A novel, cleavable peroxisome targeting signal at the amino-terminus of the rat 3-ketoacyl-CoA thiolase. EMBO J 1991; 10:3255-3262.
58. Braverman N, Dodt G, Gould SJ et al. An isoform of Pex5p, the human PTS1 receptor, is required for the import of PTS2 proteins into the peroxisome. Human Mol Genet 1998; 7:1195-1205.
59. Otera H, Tateishi K, Okumoto K et al. Peroxisome targeting signal type 1 (PTS1) receptor is involved in import of both PTS1 and PTS2: Studies with PEX5-defective CHO cell mutants. Mol Cell Biol 1998; 18:388-399.

60. Dodt G, Braverman N, Wong CS et al. Mutations in the PTS1 receptor gene, PXR 1, define complementation group 2 of the peroxisome biogenesis disorders. Nat Genet 1995; 9:115-125.
61. Otera H, Harano T, Honsho M et al. The mammalian peroxin, Pex5pL, the longer isoform of the mobile peroxisome targeting signal (PTS) type 1 transporter, translocates the Pex7p-PTS2 protein complex into peroxisomes via its initial docking site, Pex14p. J Biol Chem 2000; 275:21703-21714.
62. Matsumura T, Otera H, Fujiki Y. Disruption of the interaction of the longer isoform of Pex5p, Pex5pL, with Pex7p abolished peroxisome targeting signal type 2 protein import in mammals. J Biol Chem 2000; 275:21715-21721.
63. Shimizu N, Itoh R, Hirono Y et al. The peroxin Pex14p: CDNA cloning by functional complementation on a Chinese hamster ovary cell mutant, characterization, and functional analysis. J Biol Chem 1999; 274:12593-12604.
64. Albertini M, Rehling P, Erdmann R et al. Pex14p a peroxisomal membrane protein binding both receptors of the two PTS-dependent import pathways. Cell 1997; 89:83-92.
65. Fransen M, Terlecky SR, Subramani S. Identification of a human PTS1 receptor docking protein directly required for peroxisomal protein import. Proc Natl Acad Sci USA 1998; 95:8087-8092.
66. Urquhart AJ, Kennedy D, Gould SJ et al. Interaction of Pex5p, the type 1 peroxisome targeting signal receptor, with the peroxisomal membrane proteins Pex14p and Pex13p. J Biol Chem 2000; 275:4127-4136.
67. Chang CC, Warren DS, Sacksteder KA et al. PEX12 interacts with PEX5 and PEX10 and acts downstream of receptor docking in peroxisomal matrix protein import. J Cell Biol 1999; 147:761-774.
68. Dodt G, Gould SJ. Multiple PEX genes are required for proper subcellular distribution and stability of Pex5p, the PTS1 receptor: Evidence that PTS1 protein import is mediated by a cycling receptor. J Cell Biol 1996; 135:1763-1774.
69. Gould SJ, Collins CS. Peroxisomal-protein import: Is it really that complex? Nat Rev Mol Cell Biol 2002; 3:382-389.
70. Terlecky SR, Legakis JE, Hueni SE et al. Quantitative analysis of peroxisomal protein import in vitro. Exp Cell Res 2001; 263:98-106.
71. Dammai V, Subramani S. The Human peroxisomal targeting signal receptor, Pex5p, is translocated into the peroxisomal matrix and recycled to the cytosol. Cell 2001; 105:187-196.
72. Legakis JE, Terlecky SR. PTS2 protein import into mammalian peroxisomes. Traffic 2001; 2:252-260.
73. Walton PA, Hill PE, Subramani S. Import of stably folded proteins into peroxisomes. Mol Biol Cell 1995; 6:675-683.
74. Walton PA, Gould SJ, Feramisco JR et al. Transport of microinjected proteins into peroxisomes of mammalian cells: Inability of Zellweger cell lines to import proteins with the SKL tripeptide peroxisomal targeting signal. Mol Cell Biol 1992; 12:531-541.
75. Lazarow P, Thieringer R, Cohen G et al. Small G. Protein import into peroxisomes in vitro. Meth Cell Biol 1991; 34:303-326.
76. Wendland M, Subramani S. Cytosol-dependent peroxisomal protein import in a permeabilized cell system. J Cell Biol 1993; 120:675-685.
77. Rapp S, Soto U, Just WW. Import of firefly luciferase into peroxisomes of permeabilized Chinese hamster ovary cells: A model system to study peroxisomal protein import in vitro. Exp Cell Res 1993; 205:59-65.

INDEX

E

Early endosome antigen 1 (EEA1) 49, 50, 56, 57

Endocytosis 4, 9, 20, 23, 26, 27, 32, 35, 36, 49, 52, 53, 57, 111-113, 117, 141

Endoplasmic reticulum (ER) 2, 4, 5, 7-10, 12, 13, 19, 20, 29-32, 45-48, 50, 63-86, 96-105, 113, 128-130, 132, 146, 151, 152, 165, 166, 169, 170

Endosomal carrier vesicle (ECV) 30

Endosome 2, 4, 7, 11, 20, 22, 26, 28, 30, 31, 35, 45-50, 54-57, 78, 111-118

Erv1p 153, 154

F

Fibrillar center (FC) 132

Fibrillarin 132, 133

Fluorescence loss in photobleaching (FLIP) 73, 74, 79

Fluorescence recovery after photobleaching (FRAP) 69, 72-74, 79, 80

Friedreich's ataxia 153, 155

Fusion 5-9, 11-13, 22, 23, 32, 36, 46-48, 50-52, 55-57, 66, 71-75, 77-79, 82, 99, 101-103, 111-113, 115-118, 129-133, 138-141, 148, 152, 165

Fusion machinery 5, 8, 74, 99, 140

G

G protein 5, 53, 67, 105, 116

Golgi 2-5, 7, 8, 10-13, 18, 20, 23, 24, 26, 29-33, 35, 38-50, 53-55, 64-68, 72, 74, 77, 79, 89-105, 112-116, 132, 169

Golgi-localized, γ-ear-containing, ARF-binding protein (GGA) 7, 33-36, 49, 50, 53-55, 101, 114

Granular components (GCs) 132

GTPase-activating protein (GAP) 22, 31, 32, 34, 49

Guanine nucleotide exchange factor (GEF) 21, 31, 32, 49, 51, 53, 54

H

Hepatopoetin (HPO) 154, 155

Hermansky-Pudlak syndrome (HPS) 28

Hsp70 65, 144, 146, 147

I

Importin b 130-132

Inositol 1,4,5-triphosphate (IP3) receptor 68

Ion transport 138, 152, 153

ISU1 154

K

Kinesin 8, 53, 69, 70, 76-78, 118, 141

L

Lamin 66, 68, 130-132

Late endosome 11, 20, 30, 35, 47, 49, 54, 111-117

Lipid synthesis 66-68, 83, 84

Lysosome 2-5, 7, 11, 13, 20, 22, 26, 28, 30, 45-47, 49, 54, 101, 111-119

M

Mannose 6-phosphate receptor (M6PR) 7, 26, 28, 33, 54, 111, 114-116

Matrix 5, 10, 13, 50, 56, 69, 72, 97, 128, 142-144, 146, 147, 150-152, 154, 166-172

mdm1 142

Membrane 1-13, 19-36, 45-57, 63-86, 96-105, 111-117, 127-130, 132, 138-154, 164-172

Membrane proliferation 82-84

Membrane traffic 1, 5-8, 11, 13, 49, 96, 103, 117

Microtubule associated protein (MAP) 69, 142

Date Due